THERAPEUTICS IN
NEUROLOGY

THERAPEUTICS IN NEUROLOGY

DONALD B. CALNE

BSc, DM, MRCP
Consultant Neurologist
Royal Postgraduate Medical School
Hammersmith Hospital, London

BLACKWELL SCIENTIFIC PUBLICATIONS

OXFORD LONDON EDINBURGH MELBOURNE

© 1975 Blackwell Scientific Publications
Osney Mead, Oxford
85 Marylebone High Street, London W1M 3DE
9 Forrest Road, Edinburgh
P.O. Box 9, North Balwyn, Victoria, Australia

ISBN 0 632 00621 8

First published 1975

Distributed in the United States of America by
J. B. Lippincott Company, Philadelphia
and in Canada by
J. B. Lippincott Company of Canada Ltd, Toronto

Printed in Great Britain by
Billing & Sons Limited, Guildford and London

TO ALL THOSE PATIENTS
WHO HAVE TAKEN PART IN
STUDIES ON NEW DRUGS
FOR THE TREATMENT OF
NEUROLOGICAL DISEASES

CONTENTS

Treatment for consequences of neurological disease

PREFACE

This book is concerned with the use of drugs in treating diseases of the nervous system. It is intended primarily for physicians involved in the management of neurological disorders. Emphasis is placed upon the practical aspects of therapeutics, but the mechanisms of drug action are also considered in an attempt to bridge the gap between the clinician and the pharmacologist.

Many accuse neurologists of having an obsession with diagnosis and the documentation of obscure clinicopathological correlations. This is an unfair criticism. The commonest neurological disturbances, migraine and epilepsy, have been treated effectively for many years. It is unfortunately true that there are many diseases which do not respond well to therapy, but this problem is not confined to neurology —the same applies to a number of much commoner disorders encountered in general medical practice such as atheroma and chronic bronchitis.

Accidental observation is a recurrent theme in the history of treating diseases of the nervous system, so therapy is often based upon nothing more than a chance finding. A logically structured approach to treatment is, therefore, not always possible. It is difficult, for example, to give an adequate account of the neuropharmacology of corticosteroids when the mechanism of their most important action in neurology—reduction of cerebral oedema—is not understood. Nevertheless, the techniques developed to study the actions of drugs in general medicine have been applied to neurological therapeutics and in consequence a reasonably coherent new body of knowledge has emerged—clinical neuropharmacology.

In this book both the rational and the pragmatic aspects of treatment are considered. First, the importance of human pharmacological studies are outlined, citing examples bearing upon the management of neurological patients. Some basic neuropharmacological developments are then briefly reviewed, stressing the action of drugs which modify synaptic transmission. There follows a discussion of treating the causes and the consequences of neurological diseases—it is not always possible to place therapy firmly into one or other of these categories, so some compromises are inevitable.

The scope of this book is limited to pharmacotherapy; surgery, radiotherapy, physiotherapy, psychotherapy and occupational therapy are not discussed. The references are intended to provide access to sources of more detailed information, priority being given to those which are recent. To avoid repetition, drugs which are used in different clinical contexts are fully considered once only, with cross references when they recur. Where numerous drugs are employed for a group of related conditions, a general review of treatment precedes the more detailed appraisal of individual therapeutic agents. The generic names of drugs are employed throughout, doses being appropriate for an adult weighing 70 kg. Psychiatric, cardiovascular and endocrinological aspects of neuropharmacology are only considered in outline. Attention is concentrated on common neurological diseases, widely used drugs, and adverse reactions which are frequently encountered; in this way it is hoped that the salient points in treating diseases of the nervous system are kept in perspective.

London, April 1974   DONALD B. CALNE

ACKNOWLEDGEMENTS

I am indebted to Miss E.Allbutt, Mrs C.Chmaj and Mrs F.Lewin for typing the manuscript. I wish to thank my colleagues at Hammersmith Hospital for their comments; in particular Dr A.Breckenridge, Dr L.E.Claveria, Dr J.Darrell, Professor V.Dubowitz, Dr. R. Eastman, Dr. T.Eisler, Dr. F.Fogelman, Professor R.Fraser, Dr C.George, Dr D.Gompertz, Dr O.Holmes, Dr G.Hughes, Dr P.Lewis and Dr C.Pallis. I am also grateful for the help that I received from Dr H.Davson, Dr L.Iversen, Professor J.Marshall Dr G.H.Ree and Dr P.K.Thomas. Miss F.Cuthill and Mr R.Meakin kindly prepared the illustrations in collaboration with the photographic department of the Royal Postgraduate Medical School. Miss E.M. Read and her library staff provided invaluable assistance with the references. Mr J.Robson combined patience with efficiency in supervising publication. Finally, I wish to thank my wife and children for their tolerance of my distraction while writing this book.

CLINICAL NEUROPHARMACOLOGY

CHAPTER 1
CLINICAL PHARMACOLOGY
IN NEUROLOGY

The first treatment to have any impact in neurology was the use of bromides in epilepsy. These drugs were introduced by Locock in 1857 because they had a reputation for reducing libido, and masturbation—'the convulsive habit'—was at the time thought to be a common cause of fits. This background of error and confusion is typical of the setting from which many therapeutic advances have arisen, but in recent years interest in clinical pharmacology has generated a more rational approach to developing new drugs and improving upon the results obtained with old ones. In this Chapter aspects of clinical pharmacology which are relevant to neurology will be considered in the following stages: (1) Old drugs and new drugs; (2) Efficacy; (3) Toxicity; (4) Pharmacodynamics; (5) Pharmacokinetics; (6) Pharmacogenetics; (7) Drug interactions; (8) Plasma concentrations.

OLD DRUGS AND NEW DRUGS

The value of a drug depends on the balance between its therapeutic and toxic effects. For treatment which has been in use over many years, an adequate appraisal will have emerged from an accumulation of widespread experience; for example the efficacy and safety of phenobarbitone in the management of epilepsy were established long before the advent of the 'double-blind' 'cross-over' trial or recognition of the importance of anticonvulsant plasma concentra-

3

tions. However, it is still possible for substantial progress to be made by employing the methods of clinical pharmacology to re-examine old drugs. Pursuing the same example of phenobarbitone, this approach has revealed binding to plasma proteins, induction of inactivating enzymes, substrate competition with other drugs, pharmacogenetic variation in the rate of metabolism, and acceleration of excretion by alkaline diuresis—all of which have important implications in the treatment of epileptic patients. Furthermore, these findings have led to new therapeutic uses for drugs; for example, the administration of phenobarbitone (to increase the activity of enzymes that conjugate bilirubin) in certain types of jaundice.

Clinical pharmacology has an even greater bearing on the problems of introducing new drugs (Dollery and Davies 1970; Melmon and Morelli 1972; Laurence 1973; Turner and Richens 1973). The World Health Organisation report on this subject* comments that 'the administration of biologically active substances to human beings must always be accompanied by some element of risk that cannot be avoided by the most careful and exhaustive scientific study of the drug before it is introduced'. To ensure that this risk is justified, a number of minimal requirements are currently being delineated. A new drug normally goes through the following stages of development:

1   Pharmacological activity is established in animals.
2   Acute toxicity is investigated in several animal species and chronic toxicity (including teratogenic studies) is studied in at least two.
3   Purity and stability of the drug are demonstrated.
4   First administration is undertaken in man. Single doses are given to a limited number of normal volunteers. Initially a very small fraction of the predicted effective dose is given, with biochemical or isotopic monitoring of absorption, protein binding, metabolism and excretion of the drug.
5   Evidence is presented to government bodies controlling the introduction of new drugs. If independent prediction of efficacy and safety is favourable, further investigation is approved.
6   Small groups of patients are treated for short periods to find

* *World Health Organisation Technical Report Series*, No. 403.

suitable dose regimens for repeated administration and to enable a comparison to be made between the effects of the drug in health and disease.

7 Formal clinical trials are conducted to determine details of efficacy and toxicity. Women of childbearing age, children and psychiatric patients unable to give informed consent are excluded from early studies unless the new drug is specifically intended for them.

8 The drug is released generally, with continued surveillance for adverse reactions, which may only become apparent after widespread experience.

Taken together the precautions which have been discussed are as much as can be done to set a sensible course between unreasonable opposition to all innovation and irresponsible pursuit of every novelty.

EFFICACY

The decision on whether a drug is therapeutically active or not may be difficult, particularly when dealing with diseases which undergo spontaneous fluctuations. The evaluation of drug action in such cases becomes a major undertaking. The tool for this problem depends on the circumstances, but the essential component is comparison (Harris and Fitzgerald 1970). If economy of time and effort is important, for example where it is ethically desirable to know as quickly as possible whether a new drug is preferable to previous therapy, sequential analysis of the results of two forms of treatment is appropriate (Armitage 1960). As an alternative to sequential analysis, treatment can be evaluated in different patients who are randomly allocated into separate groups, the new drug being compared with conventional ones or an intentionally inactive (placebo) product. In diseases which run a sufficiently prolonged course, the precision of assessment can be increased by a comparative analysis of the effects of different therapy in the same patient; this technique eliminates variation between patients. To prevent bias being introduced by suggestibility of either patient or assessor it is desirable to keep both unaware of changes in treatment by adopting a double-blind design. For both practical and ethical reasons, patients taking part in a within-patient comparison should be told, before they submit to investigation, that their therapy may be altered without warning at some stage of the study. The order of *test* and *control* regimens is randomised to avoid difficulties of interpretation arising from drugs or their metabolites persisting in the tissues after administration has been stopped and to reduce the chance of observations being influenced by a spontaneous trend to improve or deteriorate. If possible, the maximum tolerated dosage is given, otherwise it is difficult to interpret negative results. However, the use of maximum tolerated dosage creates further problems, such as decoding consequent upon adverse reactions. Furthermore it may become impossible to randomise the order of treatment because an initial build up of placebo to a toxic level of intake is hardly feasible!

The measurement of drug actions is often difficult. Objective techniques are ideal but these must be simple; when they become elaborate, they usually yield results which are not reproducible. For example, there are so many variables involved in measuring limb rigidity with a torque meter that more meaningful observations can be obtained by simple clinical methods. An arbitrary scoring protocol, based on the history and examination, can provide more reliable information than that derived from complex studies which introduce distortions because of the alarm and anxiety which they generate in the patient.

Having acquired quantitative observations, these must be submitted to statistical analysis to determine the confidence with which conclusions can be drawn.

In summary, studies designed to evaluate treatment should incorporate (1) a comparison of regimens administered in randomised order to the same patient if possible—otherwise, random allocation of patients to groups receiving different therapy, (2) blind technique, (3) adequate dosage, (4) satisfactory methods of measuring efficacy, (5) statistical analysis of the results. Such complex designs pose many administrative problems and are not always practicable; nevertheless they represent the most satisfactory approach available for breaking away from the traditional rustic testimonial of clinical impression.

TOXICITY

By the time late adverse reactions develop, patients are often taking many different medications at the same time, so it may be impossible to decide which, out of a number of drugs, is responsible for a toxic effect. This problem is exemplified by the difficulty in establishing the relative contribution of different anticonvulsants to the folate deficiency and osteomalacia occasionally encountered in patients on prolonged antiepileptic therapy. The dangers of an uncritical approach are exemplified by 'the scientist who, having become intoxicated on successive occasions from drinking scotch and soda, bourbon and soda and rye and soda, concluded that soda was inebriating' (Gilman 1964).

Experience in the management of adverse reactions to drugs is becoming more important (Wade 1970) because fixed dose regimens for all patients are frequently inappropriate, even when based upon body weight. Individual variation in response is such that optimum therapeutic results commonly depend upon titration of dosage to maximum tolerated levels.

Toxicity due to known pharmacological actions of the drug

Predictable adverse reactions consequent upon the known pharmacology of a drug generally become documented over initial clinical studies. These effects are usually dose dependent and reversible.

Teratogenicity

It is seldom possible to exclude human teratogenicity until a drug has been widely used for a considerable time. Reports of congenital abnormalities induced by phenobarbitone and phenytoin have only recently been accumulating, although these drugs have been prescribed extensively for many years (Spiedal and Meadow 1972; Loughnan *et al* 1973).

Hypersensitivity

Hypersensitivity reactions comprise fever, skin eruptions, bronchospasm and anaphylactic shock, which are thought to represent an immunological response to sensitisation consequent upon previous exposure to the drug.

Idiosyncrasy

Idiosyncrasy is a term employed for those rare reactions to a drug which are unrelated to known pharmacological effects, teratogenicity or previous exposure—and for which no explanation is currently available. Drugs tend to produce relatively specific types of idiosyncratic response, such as the retroperitoneal fibrosis of methysergide.

PHARMACODYNAMICS

The pharmacodynamics of a drug—its biological actions—may be therapeutic, toxic, or irrelevant to the health of the patient. It is desirable to document biological effects in man as precisely as possible in order to formulate an adequate appraisal of the actions and interactions of drugs. Pharmacodynamic processes can be measured by changes in biochemistry (for example the fall in serum copper in Wilson's disease achieved with penicillamine); physiology (for example the improvement in neuromuscular conduction in myasthenia gravis following administration of acetylcholinesterase inhibitors); or morphology (for example the atrophy of type II muscle fibres in myopathy induced by corticosteroids).

Measurement of drug actions usually reveals a relationship with dosage such that above a certain threshold (D_{min} in Fig. 1), the intensity of the effect is related to the logarithm of the dose up to a maximum response (E_{max} in Fig. 1). Over the dotted portion of the dose-response curve in Fig. 1, $E = m \log D + c$ (where m is the slope and c is a constant).

In clinical pharmacology it is always desirable to investigate drug effects at several dosages (i.e. determine the dose-response relationship) in order to avoid drawing incorrect conclusions from observations unwittingly made below D_{min} or above E_{max}.

When one drug interferes with the action of another by competitive inhibition, the dose response curve is shifted to the right, but remains parallel. It may thus be possible to establish the mechanism of drug interaction by simply investigating dose-response relationships.

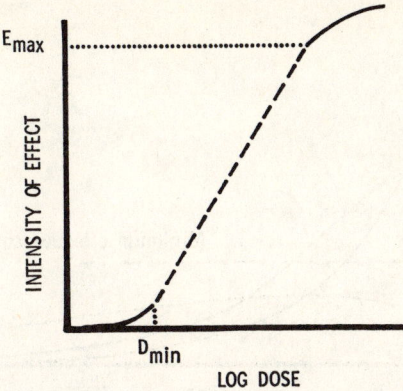

Fig. 1. Relationship between the dose of a drug and the intensity of its effect. Below a threshold dose (D_{min}) the effect is very limited. The response then rises to a maximum (E_{max}) as the dose is increased. Further augmentation of the dose has little effect (after Barr (1968) *Amer. J. Pharm. Educ.* **32,** 958).

PHARMACOKINETICS

Rational use of drugs is based upon knowledge of their pharmacokinetics—absorption, distribution, metabolism and excretion. It is important to know, for example, that neostigmine is rapidly inactivated in the gastrointestinal tract, so a parenteral dose of only 1 mg corresponds to some 30 mg taken orally. Many of the pharmacokinetic details which are discussed in subsequent Chapters derive from Goodman and Gilman (1970) or Martindale (1973) who provide a comprehensive and authoritative source of information on this subject.

Absorption

For most drugs, absorption is directly related to lipid solubility and inversely related to the extent of ionisation. The degree of ionisation varies with pH. As the pH differs considerably from one region of the gastrointestinal tract to another, knowledge of the pKa of a drug (that pH at which a substance is 50% ionised) allows prediction of the site of maximum absorption.

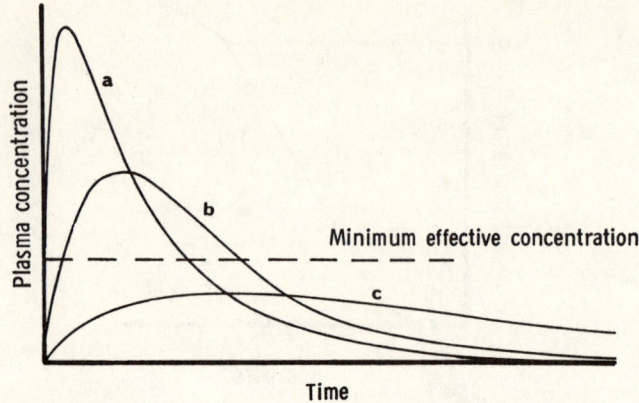

Fig. 2. The temporal profile of the plasma concentrations of drugs which are absorbed (a) very rapidly; (b) at a moderate rate; (c) very slowly. Although the quantity of drug absorbed is the same in each case, very slow absorption may preclude any therapeutic action (after Rowland (1972) in: *Clinical Pharmacology*, Ed. Melmon and Morelli, Macmillan, New York).

If the action of a drug depends upon its plasma concentration, rapid absorption leads to a response which is often transient, while slower absorption results in a delayed but more sustained action. Drugs which are very slowly absorbed may never reach therapeutic concentrations although the same quantity (area under the curve in Fig. 2) eventually enters the plasma.

Distribution

When considering distribution, it is useful to bear in mind the proportions of the major body constituents, which are illustrated in Fig. 3.

Following absorption, many drugs become loosely bound to plasma proteins. While the formation of drug-protein complexes exposes the patient to the hazards of certain interactions with other drugs (see on), protein binding can be helpful by providing a relatively stable pool from which free pharmacologically active agent is only slowly released. This prolongs the period of therapeutic action and allows the intervals between dosage to be extended.

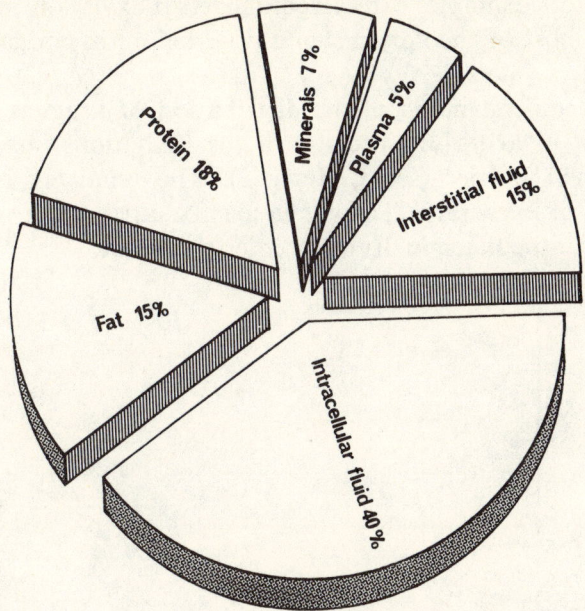

Fig. 3. Diagrammatic summary of the proportions of major body constituents (by weight).

To establish the dynamic relationships between the concentrations of a drug in different parts of the body, the concept of single and multiple compartment models has been introduced. Out of this has grown the notion of apparent volumes of distribution. If, for example, the body is considered as a single compartment and it is envisaged that the drug is evenly distributed at a concentration equal to that in the plasma, then $Q = C \times V$ where Q is the quantity of drug in the body, C is the concentration of drug in the plasma and V is the apparent volume of distribution. There is no real compartment that fulfills this relationship. V is merely a ratio with the dimensions of volume.

Drugs enter the various compartments over a distributive phase and then establish an equilibrium with concentration gradients which depend on permeability between compartments and the rate of disappearance of the drug from each. Peripheral metabolism can reduce the amount of drug available to enter the central nervous system—for example extracerebral decarboxylation of levodopa removes most of the administered dose before it can gain access to the brain.

Some understanding of the distribution of drugs is particularly important in neurology because of the limitations imposed by the blood–brain barrier (see Chapter 2). The relatively high current incidence of intracranial leukaemia may be attributable to the failure of many antileukaemic drugs to enter the brain.

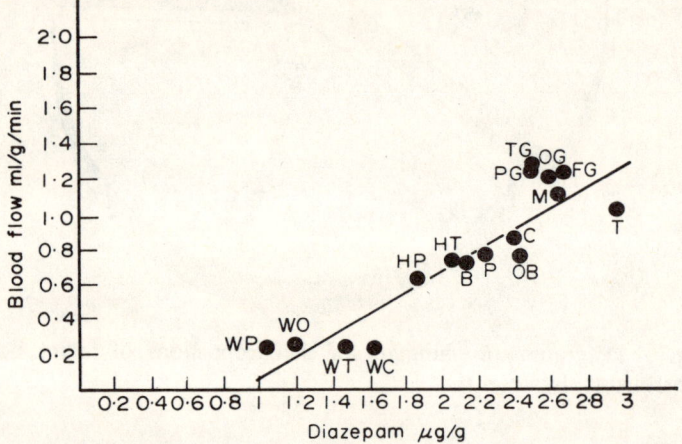

Fig. 4. Relationship between vascularity and drug distribution in different regions of the cat's brain. The localised blood flow in various areas (ml/g/min) is plotted against the focal concentration of diazepam (μg/g) one minute after intravenous injection. FG = frontal grey; OG = occipital grey; TG = temporal grey; PG = parietal grey; M = mesencephalon; T = thalamus; C = cerebellum grey; OB = optic bulb; P = pons; B = bulb; HT = hypothalamus; HP = hippocampus; WC = cerebellar white; WT = temporal white; WO = occipital white; WP = parietal white (after Morselli *et al* (1973) in *The Benzodiazepines* Ed. Garattini, Mussini and Randall, Raven Press, New York.)

Having crossed the blood–brain barrier, drugs are not distributed uniformly throughout the central nervous system; vascularity determines the initial pattern (Fig. 4). Subsequent partitioning depends upon such factors as lipid solubility, tissue binding and rates of metabolism. The relative concentrations in grey and white matter can undergo substantial changes with time (Fig. 5).

CORTEX 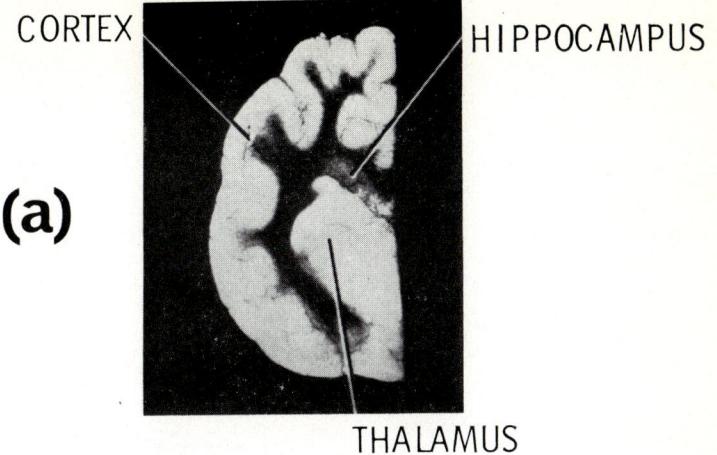 HIPPOCAMPUS

(a)

THALAMUS

CORTEX 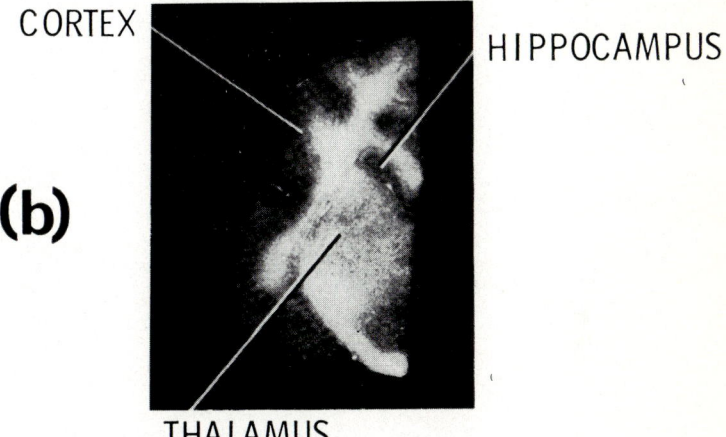 HIPPOCAMPUS

(b)

THALAMUS

Fig. 5. Alteration in the relative distribution of drug between grey and white matter. Autoradiograms of the cat's cerebral hemisphere; light areas having high concentrations. (a) 1 minute and (b) 1 hour after intravenous injection of diazepam (Morselli *et al* 1973 in: *The Benzodiazepines*, Ed. Garattini, Mussini and Randall, Raven Press, New York).

facing p. 12

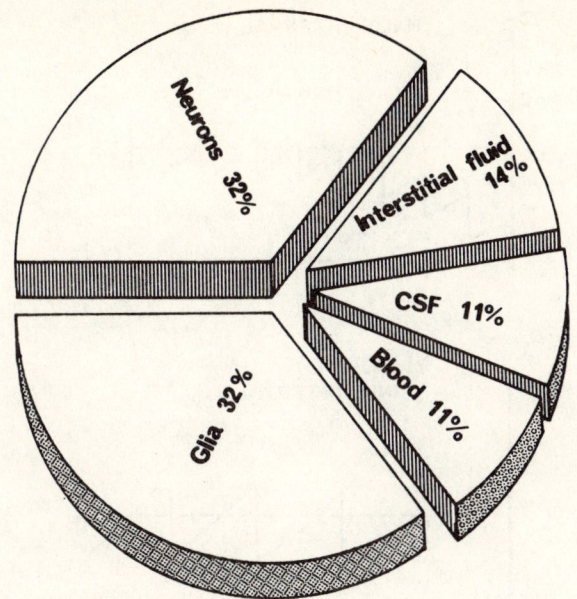

Fig. 6. Diagrammatic summary of the proportions of various intra-cranial components (by volume).

The intracranial contents (Fig. 6) comprise the neurons (450 ml), the glia (450 ml), the interstitial fluid (200 ml) and the cerebrospinal fluid (150 ml). The rate of exchange of materials can be extremely rapid; the normal cerebral blood flow is 750 ml/min (15–20% of the cardiac output). Some 90% of the blood in the brain is replaced in 5 seconds.

Metabolism

Metabolism generally renders ingested toxic materials, including drugs, less active pharmacologically and more water soluble—hence easier to excrete. One common method of increasing water solubility is conjugation to form, in particular, sulphates and glucuronides. Paracetamol, for example, is conjugated in the liver. Since there are only a limited number of metabolic transformations available for drugs, many share the same enzyme systems; enzymes of the hepatic endoplasmic reticulum (microsomal fraction) are

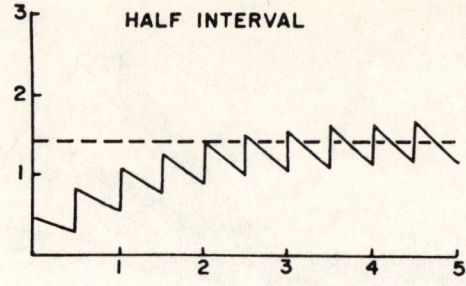

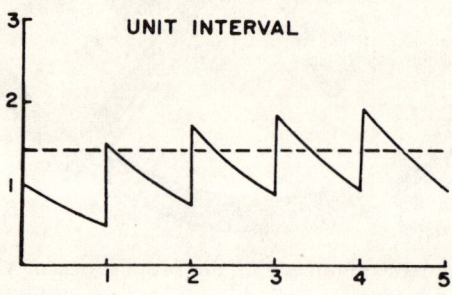

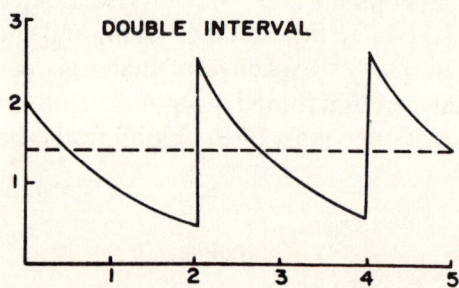

Fig. 7. Plasma concentrations on starting treatment with the same daily dose, administered at different intervals. (a) The interval is half the plasma *half-life*. (b) The interval is one plasma *half-life*. (c) The interval is twice the plasma *half-life*. Absorption is assumed to be immediate. Concentrations are plotted on the ordinate and time on the abscissa. The dotted line represents the mean steady state concentrations (after Fingl 1972, in: *Antiepileptic Drugs*, Ed. Woodbury, Penry and Schmidt, Raven Press, New York, 1972).

important in these biochemical changes. Prediction and interpretation of the interactions of drugs can often be based upon knowledge of their metabolism.

In addition to the inactivation of drugs, hepatic metabolism can produce therapeutic agents, such as phenobarbitone from primidone.

Impairment of liver function may make it necessary to adjust drug dosage according to the role of hepatic metabolism. Considering the importance of the liver in drug metabolism, it is surprising that hepatic disease does not have a greater impact on treatment.

Excretion

Knowledge of the mechanism of excretion of a drug may be important when treating a patient with kidney disease; in renal failure a normal dose of nitrofurantoin leads to excessive plasma concentrations with a consequent risk of producing peripheral neuropathy.

The plasma half-life and steady state levels

Absorption, distribution, metabolism and excretion together determine the rate at which the concentration of a drug rises and falls in the plasma. The plasma half-life of a drug (time taken for the concentration to fall by 50%) is a useful guide to how frequently doses should be given in order to maintain reasonably constant blood levels and how long it will take to achieve these concentrations (Fig. 7). On starting treatment at constant dosage a period of 5 half-lives is required to reach a steady state. The plasma half-life also gives some indication of the duration for which toxic effects are likely to persist after administration is stopped, though precise prediction is not possible because plasma concentration may not reflect pharmacological activity.

The steady state concentration of a drug is directly related to the half-life and the fraction of the dose absorbed. It is inversely related to the apparent volume of distribution and the interval between doses. To reach steady state levels rapidly, it is self evident that high initial dosage is required (Fig. 8).

The salient factors which interact to determine the tissue concentrations of a drug are summarised in Fig. 9.

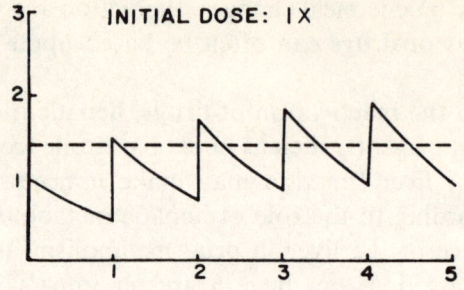

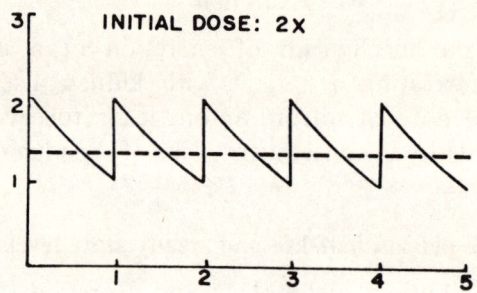

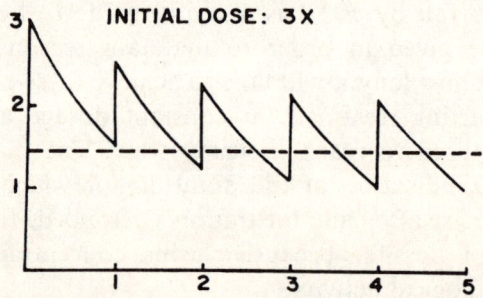

Fig. 8. Plasma concentrations following different initial doses. (a) The first dose is the same as the subsequent doses. (b) The first dose is twice the subsequent doses. (c) The first dose is thrice the subsequent doses. Absorption is assumed to be immediate. Concentrations are plotted on the ordinate and time on the abscissa. The dotted line represents the mean steady state concentrations (after Fingl 1972 in: *Antiepeleptic Drugs,* Ed. Woodbury, Penry and Schmidt, Raven Press, New York, 1972).

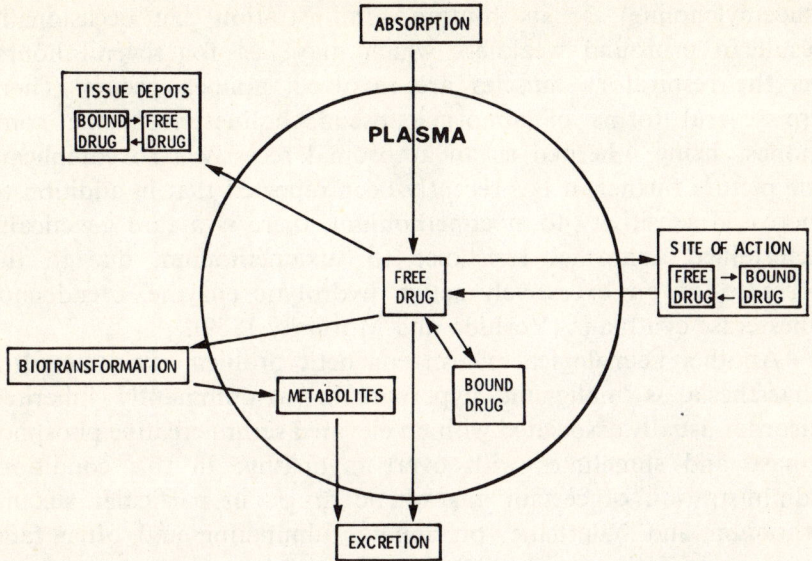

Fig. 9. Diagrammatic summary of the major factors which determine the tissue concentration of a drug.

PHARMACOGENETICS

Individuals react to the same drug in different ways (Evans 1969; Paterson 1972; Smith and Rawlins 1973). This is mainly due to genetically determined variation in pharmacokinetics, for example the extent to which drugs become bound to plasma proteins (Alexanderson and Borga 1972). Similarly there are marked hereditary differences in the rate of metabolism of drugs—most people are capable of metabolising up to 700 mg/day of phenytoin but certain subjects progressively accumulate unmetabolised drug when taking a routine dose of 300 mg/day (Kutt 1971). These slow metabolisers, who are often grouped in families, develop prominent toxicity on normal doses. Conversely, other patients metabolise phenytoin very rapidly, so an unusually high dosage is required to achieve therapeutic effects.

Abnormal pseudocholinesterase may cause acute drug induced paralysis. Approximately 1 in 2,500 of the population inherit an anomalous enzyme which does not hydrolyse suxamethonium (succinylcholine), so its routine administration can occasionally result in profound weakness which may last for several hours. As the respiratory muscles are involved, apnoea occurs. There are several forms of abnormal pseudocholinesterase, the commonest being inherited as an autosomal recessive. To complicate the picture further, it has recently been reported that in addition to increased sensitivity to suxamethonium, there is a rare genetically determined abnormal resistance to suxamethonium due to the presence of an excessively active hydrolytic enzyme, pseudocholinesterase cynthiana (Yoshida and Motulsky 1969).

Another neurological pharmacogenetic problem encountered in anaesthesia is malignant hyperpyrexia—a dominantly inherited disorder usually associated with an elevated serum creatine phosphokinase and sometimes with overt myopathy. In this condition, administration of certain anaesthetic drugs, in particular suxamethonium and halothane, precipitate fulminating and often fatal hyperpyrexia (Ellis *et al* 1972).

Isoniazid is inactivated by acetylation. As a final example of the importance of pharmacogenetic variation, patients treated with isoniazid fall into two approximately equal groups—fast and slow acetylators. The slow acetylators incur a greater risk of developing isoniazid toxicity, in particular peripheral neuropathy. The interactions between isoniazid and anticonvulsants are virtually confined to slow acetylators.

DRUG INTERACTIONS

Each year more drugs are being administered to an increasing number of patients, so the adverse consequences of drug interactions present a problem which is growing in both size and complexity (Dollery *et al* 1972):

Before administration

Interactions can occur before drugs even reach the patient. Precipitation occurs if phenytoin for injection is mixed with other drugs such as phenobarbitone, penicillins, tetracycline, chloramphenicol, aminophylline or promethazine.

In the gastrointestinal tract

Absorption of one drug may be modified by another. Anticholinergic drugs employed in the treatment of Parkinsonism delay gastro-intestinal transit times, reducing the rate of absorption of other orally administered agents. Similarly drugs which modify gastro-intestinal pH or gut flora can interfere with absorption.

Displacement from plasma protein complexes

There is considerable variation in the affinity of different drugs for binding with plasma proteins. For example, phenylbutazone competes with warfarin; administration of phenylbutazone to a patient already receiving warfarin can therefore precipitate haem-orrhage by displacing anticoagulant from plasma protein complexes. This type of interaction is transient because homeostatic mechanisms tend to restore stable drug levels.

Substrate competition

Reference has already been made to the limited number of metabolic pathways available to a very large number of drugs. Where two drugs share the same inactivating enzyme system, they may interact by substrate competition to result in an increase in the plasma concentration of both. Sulthiame competes with phenytoin for metabolic pathways; administration of sulthiame to a patient already receiving phenytoin may, by competitive inhibition of metabolism, lead to a 100% increase in the plasma concentration of phenytoin and so precipitate an acute toxic reaction.

Enzyme induction

Some drugs induce increased activity of the microsomal hepatic enzymes concerned with their inactivation. Many barbiturates are potent enzyme inducers in man; administration of phenobarbitone to a patient already receiving, for example, phenytoin may sub-stantially reduce the plasma concentration of the latter. Other drugs have been shown to induce hepatic microsomal enzymes in

animals, but it has not been firmly established that they have the
same action in man. A further complicating factor is the considerable
variation in the extent of enzyme induction that occurs in different
individuals (Breckenridge *et al* 1973).

The same drugs that induce inactivating enzymes may also
display substrate competition. The outcome of such drug interactions
is therefore difficult to predict in terms of plasma concentrations,
therapeutic effect and toxicity.

Blockade of transport systems

The adrenergic neuron blocking drugs—bretylium, bethanidine,
guanethidine and debrisoquine—act at presynaptic endings where
they are concentrated by an active uptake system. The antidepressants amitriptyline and imipramine block this active transport
mechanism; administration of a tricyclic antidepressant to a patient
receiving an adrenergic neuron blocking drug can therefore result
in a rise in blood pressure (Mitchell *et al* 1967; Simpson and Hodge
1967).

Interference at the site of pharmacological action

Drugs may interfere with each other at their ultimate site of action.
A bactericidal agent, which exerts maximum effect on dividing cells,
will be rendered less active by concomitant administration of a
bacteriostatic drug which stops cells multiplying. It has been shown,
for example, that penicillins and tetracyclines are antagonistic rather
than synergistic in pneumonococcal meningitis.

Advantageous interactions

Drugs are sometimes deliberately given together in order to increase
efficacy or decrease toxicity. High doses of anticholinesterase drugs
may cause undesirable parasympathetic reactions in myasthenic
patients, such as colic and excessive salivation, which can be corrected
by giving a muscarinic blocking agent. Adverse effects of levodopa
resulting from peripheral decarboxylation to catecholamines can
be reduced by administration of an extracerebral decarboxylase
inhibitor.

PLASMA CONCENTRATIONS

Some of the practical problems which have been discussed can be resolved by analysing the concentration of drugs in the plasma (Davies and Prichard 1973). In this way crucial information determining the adjustment of dosage may be obtained in certain drug interactions; in genetically determined variations of pharmacokinetics; and in the management of patients with diseases affecting absorption, metabolism or excretion of drugs. However, it is possible to place too much emphasis on blood levels, because these may not correlate well with therapeutic activity or toxicity. In neurology in particular, plasma concentrations may be misleading owing to the limitations imposed by the blood–brain barrier. Other factors which complicate the interpretation of blood levels are the formation of active metabolites, binding to plasma proteins, and attachment to cell components.

There is one common situation where estimations of plasma concentrations of a drug may be invaluable. Epileptic patients are frequently encountered who have seizures which are controlled by administering anticonvulsants in hospital, but who deteriorate dramatically following discharge to the outpatient clinic. A comparison of plasma levels of anticonvulsants in the ward and the clinic can provide irrefutable evidence that the patient is not taking his drugs at home in their prescribed dosage. This simple point is often impossible to establish by merely questioning the patient.

CHAPTER 2
THE BLOOD–BRAIN BARRIER

Almost a century ago Erlich observed that following intravenous injection of a number of dyes, one tissue failed to become stained—the central nervous system. Thus arose the concept of a blood–brain barrier, due to limited permeability of the intracranial and spinal vascular beds. The blood–brain barrier is of considerable importance in determining the extent of penetration and hence the neuropharmacological action of many drugs.

Capillary permeability is not uniform throughout the neural parenchyma. In certain regions substances readily penetrate from plasma to the neural extracellular space—for example at the area postrema, the median eminence and the pineal. Increased permeability at these sites may be biologically important. The area postrema is close to the emetic centre and chemoreceptor trigger zone, so the concentration of toxic materials in the plasma can be monitored and reduced by vomiting if necessary. The median eminence and pineal control the output of hormones—sampling of plasma can take place for negative feedback control to maintain homeostasis.

The blood–brain barrier is not the only factor determining the distribution of drugs to the central nervous system. Regions of high vascularity, such as grey matter, allow more rapid entry and exit of materials than areas of relatively low blood flow, such as white matter. Subsequent distribution depends upon the affinity of tissue components for the drug and upon local differences in the rate of metabolism. To illustrate the varied patterns of distribution after crossing the blood–brain barrier; chlorpromazine, butyrophenones, imipramine and amitriptyline tend to accumulate in the hippocampus and caudate nucleus whereas diazepam, phenytoin and barbiturates collect in cerebral and cerebellar cortex, thalamus and midbrain (Morselli *et al* 1973).

It is useful to employ the terms *blood–CSF barrier* when referring to transport of material into the cerebrospinal fluid, and *blood–brain barrier* when considering the passage of substances into the neural parenchyma. This Chapter discusses these barriers in the following stages: (1) Anatomy; (2) The interstitial space; (3) The CSF; (4) Transport of drugs; (5) Significance of the blood–brain barrier in therapeutics.

ANATOMY

Transport of materials between the blood and the extracellular fluid of the central nervous system occurs at three specialised sites—the parenchymal capillary, the choroidal capillary and the arachnoid villus.

Parenchymal capillaries

The capillary walls of the brain and spinal cord parenchyma have three unusual morphological features: (1) the endothelial cells possess exceptionally tight intercellular junctions; (2) they contain few cytoplasmic vesicles; (3) they are surrounded by processes from neighbouring glia—astrocytic feet. The tight junctions appear to impose some limitation on permeability (Reese and Karnovsky 1967). It is not known whether the other structural findings are relevant.

·Choroidal capillaries

Capillary endothelium of the choroid plexus is morphologically unlike that of the brain parenchyma, possessing none of the special elements mentioned above. Choroidal capillaries are essentially similar to extracranial capillaries, but they are covered by a layer of epithelial cells which have the same tight junctions that are found in brain capillaries. It is probable that the tight junctions of the choroidal epithelium restrict the passage of solutes in the same way as the tight junctions of the parenchymal capillaries (Davson 1972).

Arachnoid villi

While the parenchymal and choroidal capillaries are primarily concerned with controlling the entry of material to the central nervous system, the arachnoid villi are drainage channels. They consist of small evaginations of arachnoid membrane into the dural venous sinuses. The precise anatomy of the endothelial lining of the villus is controversial. Some workers have reported microscopically visible channels which can open up, according to pressure gradients between subarachnoid space and venous sinus, to provide valve-like, collapsible microtubular communications for the transit of particles up to the size of erythrocytes (Courtice and Simmonds 1951; Welch and Friedman 1960). Others claim that the endothelium has no pores, particles being transported by phagocytosis (Shabo and Maxwell 1968 a and b).

THE INTERSTITIAL SPACE

The various major compartments of the central nervous system are illustrated in Fig. 10. Before reaching neurons, drugs crossing the blood–brain barrier must enter the interstitial space. Physiological studies with labelled material indicate that this occupies some 10–15% of the brain parenchyma (Davson 1967; 1970). The recent dispute by electron microscopists over the existence of an extracellular space has now been resolved; controversial early reports were the result of fixation artefacts consequent upon rapid absorption of interstitial fluid. When precautions were taken to freeze and fix the brain rapidly, the presence of an extracellular space was confirmed (Van Harreveld *et al* 1965).

The brain and spinal cord have no lymphatic system, so drainage occurs through the pericellular regions surrounding neurons and glia to reach the cerebrospinal fluid, ultimate discharge into the bloodstream occurring via the arachnoid villi.

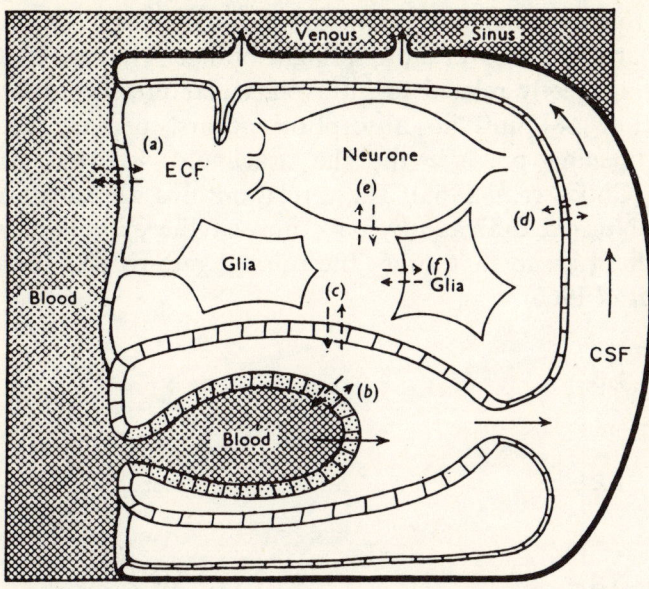

Fig. 10. Diagrammatic summary of the intracranial compartments. Continuous arrows indicate major directions of fluid flow. Interrupted arrows indicate where diffusion of water and solutes may occur (a) across the blood–brain barrier (capillary to interstitial fluid); (b) across the epithelium of the choroid plexus; (c) across the ependyma; (d) across the pial membrane; (e) across the cell membranes of neurons; (f) across the cell membranes of glia. The thick outline represents the arachnoid-dural membranes (Davson and Bradbury 1965, *Symp. Soc. Exp. Biol.* **19**, 349).

THE CEREBROSPINAL FLUID

Cerebrospinal fluid is secreted at the choroid plexuses; the contribution, if any, of the parenchymal brain capillaries is controversial (Davson 1972). The rate of formation of CSF in man is 0.35–04. ml/minute (500–800 ml/day). As its volume is about 150 ml, the CSF is renewed about 6 times a day (Rubin *et al* 1966; Cutler *et al* 1968).

A threefold increase in the rate of formation is required to raise the CSF pressure to 200 mm CSF (Bercaw and Greer 1970). The

rate of formation is not influenced by short term alterations in
ventricular pressure over a physiological range. The rate of drainage
of CSF is directly related to intraventricular pressure over 68–250
mm. Below 68 mm, no absorption occurs, perhaps because a
critical opening pressure for the arachnoid villi has not been
reached (Cutler *et al* 1968). These relationships are summarised in
Fig. 11. Normal drainage by bulk flow at the arachnoid villi can
remove fluid at up to 4 times the normal rate of CSF production
(Rubin *et al* 1966).

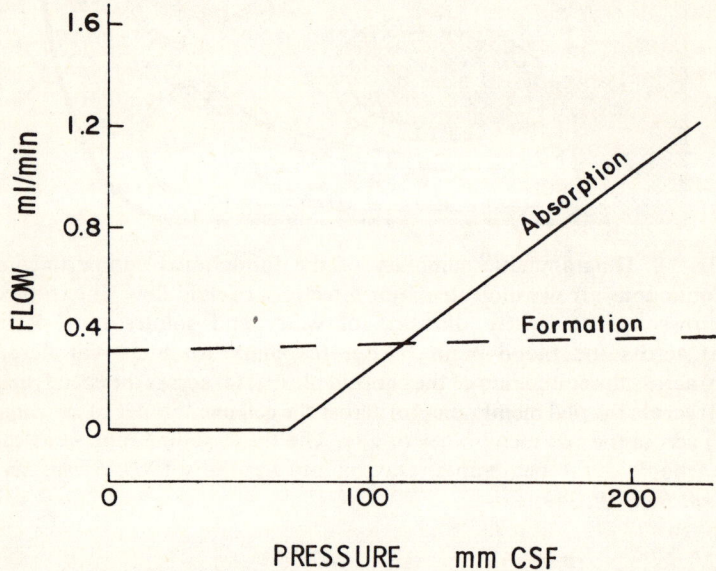

Fig. 11. Relationship between the flow and pressure of human CSF.
(From Cutler *et al* 1968, *Brain*, **91**, 707.)

It has been suggested that if the drainage of CSF is blocked by
pathological occlusion of pathways proximal to the arachnoid villi,
the chronically increased hydrocephalic pressure may force CSF
back through brain parenchyma to reach the subarachnoid space
and villi. If the arachnoid villi are themselves blocked, it is likely
that subsidiary drainage channels develop, for example around the
subarachnoid space of cranial and spinal nerves (Davson 1970).

TRANSPORT OF DRUGS

From a pharmacokinetic viewpoint, the interstitial fluid of the central nervous system and the CSF resemble the intracellular space—free access to all these compartments is generally limited to drugs which readily cross membranes (Rall 1971). Substances enter by diffusion, filtration or active transport at the parenchymal and choroidal capillaries.

Removal of drugs is mainly achieved by the bulk flow of CSF back into the bloodstream at the arachnoidal villi. The rate of CSF flow is therefore a critical factor in determining the elimination of drugs from the central nervous system. Certain drugs are also actively transported out of the CSF at the choroid plexuses and some are inactivated by metabolism in the brain.

Examples of drugs which enter the brain very readily are caffeine, ethanol and imipramine. Access is poor for aminoglycosides, ascorbic acid, aspirin, azathioprine, cephalosporins, chloroquine, guanethidine, methotrexate, morphine, neostigmine, penicillins, pimozide and polyenes. Barbiturates, hydantoins and levodopa occupy intermediate positions (Oldendorf 1971). It is notable that in many cases the site of the therapeutic action of drugs is not related to the facility of passage across the blood–brain barrier—some agents employed for their central action, such as morphine, enter the brain with difficulty while others which are used for their peripheral effects, such as procaine, readily penetrate.

The factors determining the permeability of drugs are lipid solubility (a direct relationship) and the extent of ionisation (an inverse relationship). In these respects the blood–brain barrier resembles the gastrointestinal tract, though drugs readily absorbed from the gut do not necessarily gain easy access to the brain; ionisation depends on pH—the stomach and jejunal contents have respectively lower and higher values than the brain capillary (pH 7.4).

1 *Relatively ionised (polar) drugs.* The rate of entry of highly polar drugs depends upon the proportion of material unionised at pH 7.4.
2 *Relatively unionised (non-polar) drugs.* These enter the brain at a rate which correlates with their lipid solubility (lipid/water partition

coefficient at pH 7.4) rather than their degree of ionisation (Brodie *et al* 1960).

A number of substances which would enter the brain very slowly according to the above criteria appear to have specialised carrier systems to transport them (Bradbury and Davson 1964; Oldendorf 1973 a and b); sugars, aminoacids and short chain fatty acids are examples. It is possible that certain drugs may employ some of these carrier systems.

Substances which cross the blood–brain barrier very slowly may attain higher concentrations in the parenchyma than the CSF, because a steady state concentration gradient is established in the interstitial fluid by the continuous drainage of CSF (Davson *et al* 1961).

Protein binding is another factor influencing the transport of drugs into the central nervous system. Passage is related to the free rather than the total concentration of drug in the plasma because the fraction bound to protein is held back. Drugs which are taken up into lipid or protein components of the brain parenchyma may accumulate.

As already mentioned, partitioning of drugs between the blood and brain will depend on the pH. A reduction in plasma pH leads to a fall in the plasma concentration of phenobarbitone and an increase in the brain level. Conversely a rise in plasma pH results in augmentation of the plasma concentration of phenobarbitone and a decrease in the brain level (Waddell and Butler 1957).

SIGNIFICANCE OF THE BLOOD–BRAIN BARRIER IN THERAPEUTICS

The existence of a blood–brain barrier may be useful. For example quaternary ammonium anticholinesterase drugs such as neostigmine and pyridostigmine can be given to patients with myasthenia gravis in very high dosage without increasing the concentration of acetylcholine in the brain. This is only possible because the quaternary ammonium compounds are highly polar and therefore fail to gain significant access to the brain.

Similarly, the blood–brain barrier is exploited in treating

Parkinsonian patients with carbidopa in order to reduce certain unwanted effects of levodopa. Carbidopa inhibits decarboxylation of levodopa (pharmacologically inert) to dopamine (pharmacologically active) but the hydrazine moiety of carbidopa precludes transport across the blood–brain barrier so that dopamine can still be formed in the striatum where it is needed. In addition to conferring protection from adverse reactions due to the peripheral formation of catecholamines, carbidopa reduces nausea, probably by inhibiting formation of dopamine in a region of the central nervous system where the brain capillaries are exceptionally permeable so that no effective barrier exists—the area postrema.

Unfortunately, the blood–brain barrier creates more therapeutic problems than it solves. For example, modern antileukaemic therapy is proving very effective in prolonging life, but a progressively increasing incidence of neurological complications are being encountered because many antileukaemic drugs do not readily cross the blood–brain barrier. The brain is emerging as a privileged area for the growth of leukaemic deposits. Attempts have been undertaken to overcome this by lumbar intrathecal injection of methotrexate or intraventricular infusion via an Ommaya reservoir. While these approaches may reduce the prevalence of intracranial leukaemia, they introduce new difficulties because high localised concentrations of methotrexate are neurotoxic. There have been several reports of paraplegia and encephalopathy (Back 1969; Bagshaw *et al* 1969; Rosner *et al* 1970; Kay *et al* 1972).

The blood–brain and blood–CSF barriers also pose therapeutic problems in the treatment of infections of the central nervous system. As already mentioned, aminoglycosides (e.g. streptomycin, gentamicin), cephalosporins (e.g. cephaloridine, cephalothin), penicillins (e.g. ampicillin, benzylpenicillin) and the polyenes (e.g. amphotericin B) only gain limited access to the normal brain and CSF (Goodman and Gilman 1970). Inflammation increases the permeability of the parenchymal and choroidal capillaries so that drugs are able to penetrate the nervous system during the acute phases of infection (Lithander 1966; Belsey and Tardo 1967). However, as recovery occurs inflammation recedes and the blood–brain and blood–CSF barriers become re-established so that therapy is less effective and there is a risk of low grade chronic infection persisting. Antimicrobial agents which do not readily cross the blood–brain and blood–CSF barriers may even contribute to the development of meningitis when administered for infection outside the central nervous system. In this context cephalothin in particular, has been implicated (Mangi *et al* 1973). As in the case of antileukaemic treatment, selective therapy to peripheral tissues leads to vulnerability of the central nervous system.

Efforts to find drugs which modify the barriers are unlikely to be therapeutically rewarding because such agents would almost certainly be cell poisons whose actions could not be confined to the membranes of the central nervous system (Schanker 1966). Moreover, disturbance of the highly complex homeostasis imposed by the elaborate permeability barriers around the brain and spinal cord could be deleterious. It would therefore be preferable to concentrate on developing therapeutic agents with properties appropriate for their desired distribution. To facilitate entry to the brain, minimum ionisation and maximum lipid solubility are the salient requirements; the converse obtains for drugs intended to have a selectively peripheral action.

CHAPTER 3
IMPULSE PROPAGATION AND
SYNAPTIC TRANSMISSION

Neurological therapeutics embrace the full range of approaches to treatment employed in general medicine—antimicrobial drugs, anti-inflammatory agents, immunosuppressive drugs, analgesics, vitamins, anticoagulants, vaccines and chelating agents. In addition to these, a rapidly evolving group of new drugs are being developed to produce relatively specific changes in neuronal function by modifying transmission along nerves or across synapses. Such drugs are not unique to neurology—they are employed in psychiatry, in anaesthesiology, in endocrinology and in cardiovascular disease.

Advances in knowledge of the pharmacology of transmission have allowed rational approaches to be developed for the treatment of disease in spite of substantial ignorance of basic aetiological mechanisms. For example, powerful therapeutic agents designed to modify synaptic activity have resulted in amelioration of symptoms and prolongation of life in myasthenia gravis, Parkinsonism and hypertension, without any understanding of the ultimate causes of these conditions.

Most of the important developments in this area have emerged from investigation of peripheral nerves and junctions. It is remarkable that for the majority of mechanisms involved in peripheral impulse propagation and neuromuscular transmission, analogous counterparts have been identified in studies of the brain and spinal cord.

In this Chapter transmission will be reviewed in its widest context, emphasising the similarities which have emanated from studies of both the central and peripheral nervous system. First impulse propagation will be discussed. Then synaptic mechanisms will be considered in the following stages: (1) Morphology of synapses; (2) Identification of transmitters; (3) Synthesis of transmitters; (4) Storage of transmitters; (5) Release of transmitters; (6) Inactivation of transmitters; (7) Receptors; (8) Neuro-endocrine transducers.

Impulse propagation

In mechanistic terms, the nervous system is concerned with receiving, transmitting, analysing and storing information; in response to changing circumstances it formulates an appropriate reaction, which it executes. To fulfil these roles an essential requirement is speed, so that information can be conducted quickly from the periphery to the central nervous system, between different central neurons and back to the periphery. The electrical nerve impulse is, in teleological terms, an ideal solution to the problem of achieving the rapid transmission necessary for making appropriate adjustments in an environment which is undergoing swift alterations.

While many aspects of neural function, such as the storage of information, remain relatively obscure, neurophysiological studies have shed considerable light on the mechanism of propagation of nerve impulses. Excitable membranes (nerve and muscle fibres) are relatively impermeable to sodium. An active transport system extrudes sodium ions from the cell (the sodium pump) so that a gradient is established with the extracellular sodium concentration some ten times higher than that inside the nerve or muscle fibre. There is a consequent difference in electrical charge across the membrane (polarisation)—the resting potential.

The arrival of an impulse (action potential) leads to a sudden increase in sodium conductance, allowing ready penetration of sodium ions across the cell membrane. The influx of sodium results in local transient disappearance of the electrochemical gradient. The resting potential across the membrane, some 90 mV negative inside, disappears to be replaced by a positive potential of around 45 mV within the axon. The electrical field generated by these ionic movements results in depolarisation of adjacent membrane and in this way the impulse is propagated. In myelinated nerve a lipid sheath insulates most of the axon so that these phenomena are confined to the exposed portion of the excitable membrane at the node of Ranvier. This leads to an increased velocity of conduction because the electrical changes 'leap frog' from one node to the next over distances of 1.5–3.0 mm. In addition to augmenting the speed of transmission, restriction of ionic flux to the internodal region reduces energy expenditure and thus increases the efficiency of transmission.

The propagation of action potentials is relatively resistant to drug actions. However, conduction can be blocked by local anaesthetics, which prevent depolarisation by inhibiting the activation of sodium conductance (see Chapter 4).

Synaptic transmission

Synaptic mechanisms make an important contribution to the analytic capacity of the nervous system. They allow neurons to integrate complex fluctuations of excitatory and inhibitory input. Synaptic changes related to impulse traffic may also play a part in the storage of information.

Table 1. Comparison of the properties of axonal and synaptic transmission.

AXON	SYNAPSE
Negligible delay	Delay of 0.1–0.2 ms
Bidirectional transmission can occur (orthodromic and antidromic)	Unidirectional transmission only
Maximum frequency of transmission approximately 1,500/sec.	Maximum frequency of transmission approximately 100/sec.
No temporal summation of subthreshold activation	Temporal summation of subthreshold activation
Relatively resistant to drugs and hypoxia	Relatively sensitive to drugs and hypoxia

Junctional transmission differs from impulse propagation along axons in several respects—see Table 1. Although evidence for chemical mediation across synapses had been accumulating since the beginning of the century, the view that impulses are transmitted electrically from one neuron to another was not categorically refuted until 20 years ago. At that time microelectrode recordings within neurons established that synaptic transmission is chemical in the majority of systems studied (though electrical transmission does occur in certain submammalian synapses). The arrival of an impulse at the presynaptic nerve ending releases a chemical transmitter which diffuses across the synaptic cleft and becomes attached to a receptor on the postsynaptic membrane. This process has theoretical advantages over electrical transmission across synapses, which would be biophysically impossible in many situations where the presynaptic ending is very small in comparison to the postsynaptic membrane.

Chemical mediators can transmit excitation—they increase the permeability of the postsynaptic membrane to sodium by opening 'ion gates', which leads to depolarisation. Chemical mediators can also transmit inhibition, by increasing the permeability of the postsynaptic membrane to chloride, with consequent stabilisation of the resting potential.

Central neurons receive synaptic input from many sources and by utilising different transmitters these inputs can exert antagonistic effects. Recently developed neuropharmacological techniques allow activity to be recorded from central neurons while releasing various transmitters by electrophoresis from multibarrelled micropippettes. Such experiments have shown that many cells in the caudate nucleus respond to acetylcholine with an increased discharge of impulses, but dopamine usually reduces the rate of firing (Bloom *et al* 1965; McLennan and York 1967). In this region, therefore, acetylcholine mediates excitation predominantly; dopamine is mainly concerned with transmitting inhibition.

It is not only the identity of the transmitter that determines whether the information conveyed across a particular synapse is excitatory or inhibitory. Postsynaptic receptors on various neurons may respond quite differently to the same transmitter—although most caudate cells display inhibition when dopamine is released onto them, a minority exhibit excitation. Some neurons, such as *facing p. 34*

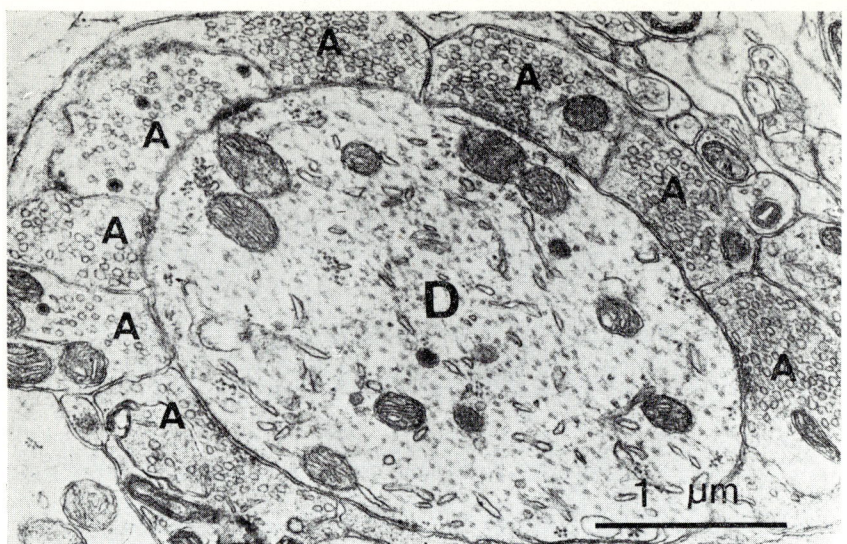

Fig. 12. Electron microscopy of rat's substantia nigra; cross-section of a dendrite (D) completely covered by synaptic contacts with axonal boutons (A). (Bak *et al* 1974, in *Dopaminergic Mechanisms*, Ed. Calne, Chase and Barbeau, Raven Press, New York.)

Fig. 13. (right) Electron microscopy of different types of synapses. (a) Axosomatic junction (cat's oculomotor nucleus). Presynaptic terminal A contains vesicles and mitochondria. Membranes of the synapatic cleft are thickened at I. S is the cell body of the postsynaptic neuron. Magnification 15,000 ×; inset 25,000 ×. (b) Axo-dendritic junction (cat's oculomotor nucleus). The axon A ends at a terminal containing numerous vesicles (ves). D is the dendrite of the postsynaptic neuron, containing mitochondria (m) and microtubules (t). Magnification 16,000 ×. (c) Axo-axonal junctions (monkey's oculomotor nucleus). Axon A_1 is presynaptic with respect to axon A_2 which in turn forms an axo-dendritic synapse with dendrite D_1. At another junction, axon A_3 is presynaptic with respect to axon A_4. A_4 makes an axo-dendritic synapse with dendrite D_2. Magnification 10,500 ×. (These photomicrographs are compiled from illustrations by Pappas and Waxman 1972, in *Structure and function of synapses*, Ed. Pappas and Purpura, Raven Press, New York.)

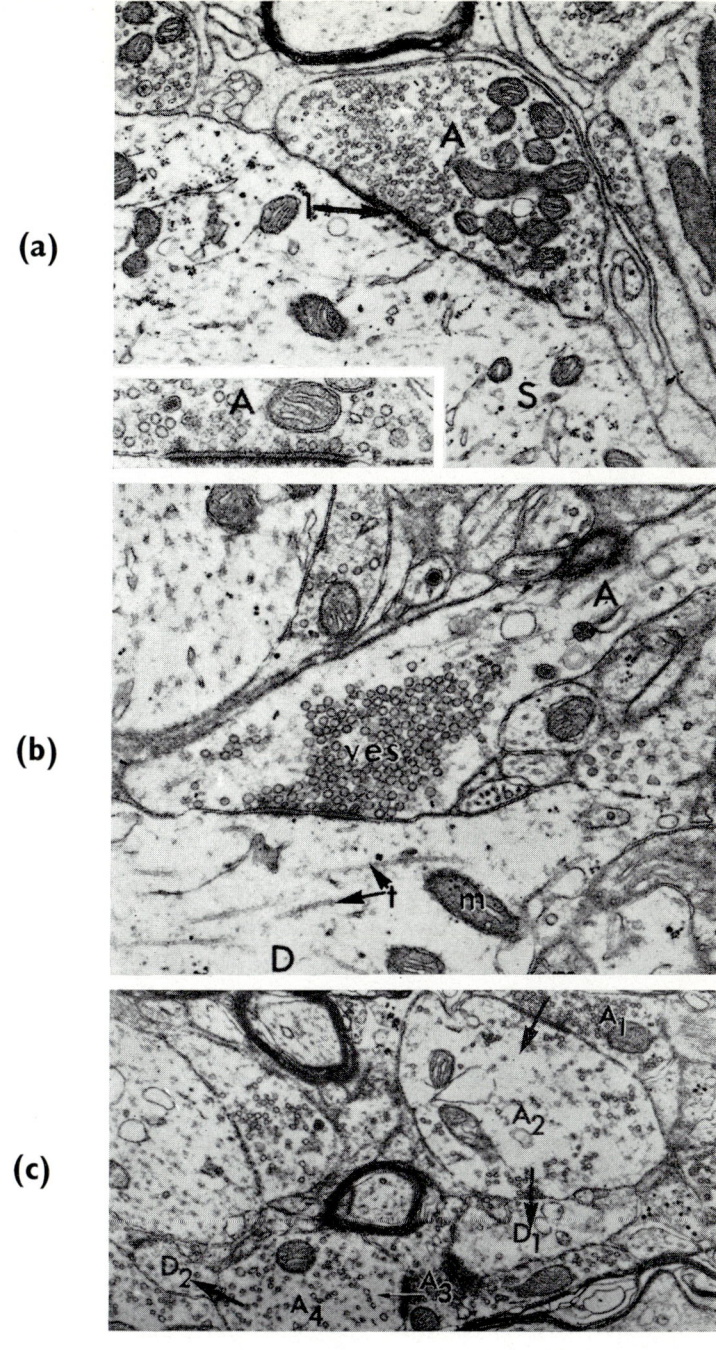

(a)

(b)

(c)

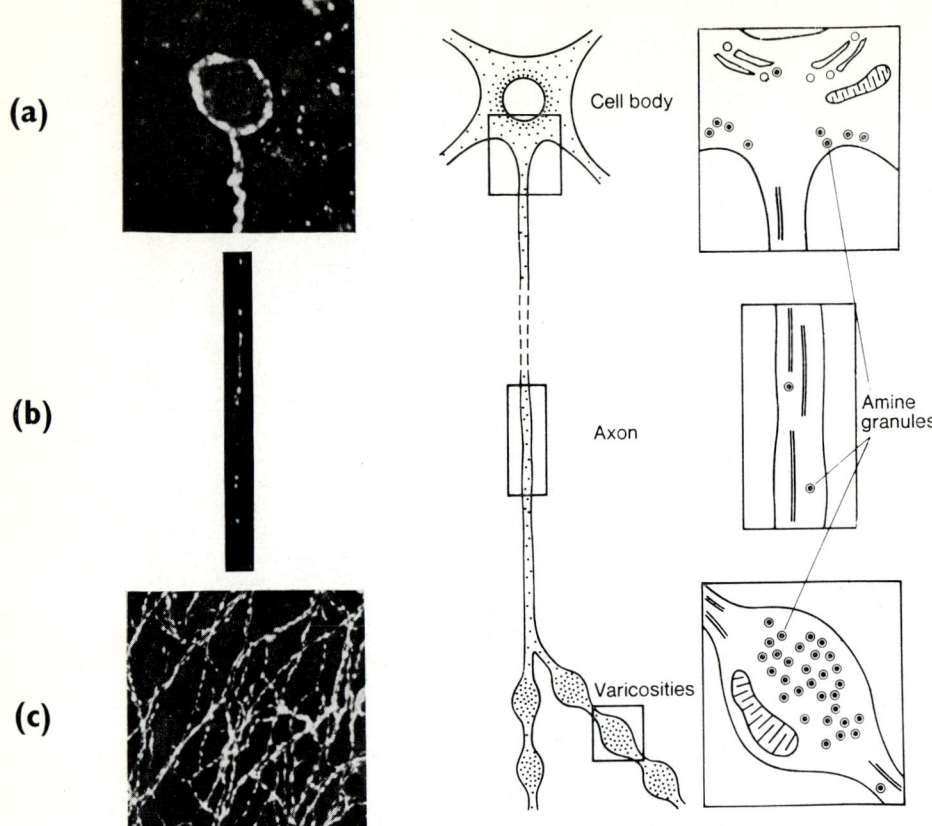

Fig. 14. Composite diagram of the various portions of a monoamine neuron. Fluorescence indicates the presence of amine. (a) Cell bodies containing 10–110 μg/g of amine (from superior cervical ganglion of the rat, magnification 1,450 ×). (b) Axons (from the sciatic nerve of the rat, magnification 200 ×). (c) Axonal terminations, varicosities containing 100–300 μg/g of amine (from the iris of the rat, magnification 200 ×). This figure is compiled from Hökfelt and Ljungdahl 1972, in *Studies of neurotransmitters at the synaptic level*. Ed. Costa, Iversen and Paoletti, Raven Press, New York; Van Orden *et al* 1970, *J. Pharm. Exp. Ther.* **174,** 56; Fuxe and Hökfelt 1971, *Triangle (En.)* **10,** 74.

Renshaw cells, may receive an input from two different excitatory transmitters (Curtis *et al* 1961) while others, such as certain neurons in the cerebral cortex, receive two inhibitory transmitters (Phillis and York 1968). It is even possible for the same cell to respond in two different ways to the same transmitter (Phillis 1970).

These findings illustrate the pharmacological complexity of the nervous system. They also show how chemical mediation at synapses allows much more precise analysis of information than would be possible from electrical transmission—the various inputs are categorised as excitatory or inhibitory according to the transmitter and the postsynaptic receptor. The neuron either fires an impulse or remains silent, depending upon the spatiotemporal summation of excitatory and inhibitory influences.

MORPHOLOGY OF SYNAPSES

The morphology of synaptic contacts is extremely varied. While classical histology established the diversity of junctions at such sites as the cerebellar cortex, new techniques have revealed an unexpected range of complexity throughout the nervous system. Electron microscopy has defined the ultrastructural organisation of synaptic junctions involving almost every possible combination of neuronal element: (1) axo-somatic, (2) axo-dendritic, (3) axo-spinous, (4) axo-axonal, (5) dendro-dendritic (Pappas and Purpura 1972; Bak *et al* 1974). Some examples are illustrated in Figs. 12 and 13.

Histochemical studies of monoamine neurons have demonstrated remarkably elaborate axonal arborisations with multiple varicosities rich in transmitter, each having numerous synaptic contacts, mainly via *boutons en passant* (Fig. 14). A noradrenergic neuron can have 25,000 varicosities which together contain 300 times the quantity of noradrenaline (norepinephrine) found in the cell body, in 1,000 times the concentration (Livett 1973). Similarly in a dopaminergic neuron there may be 500,000 varicosities which together contain 150 times the content of dopamine found in the cell body. In the nigrostriatal pathway of the rat, the arborisations containing dopaminergic varicosities may result in a terminal network 77 cm in length (Andén *et al* 1966b); these morphological characteristics allow extremely diffuse transmission.

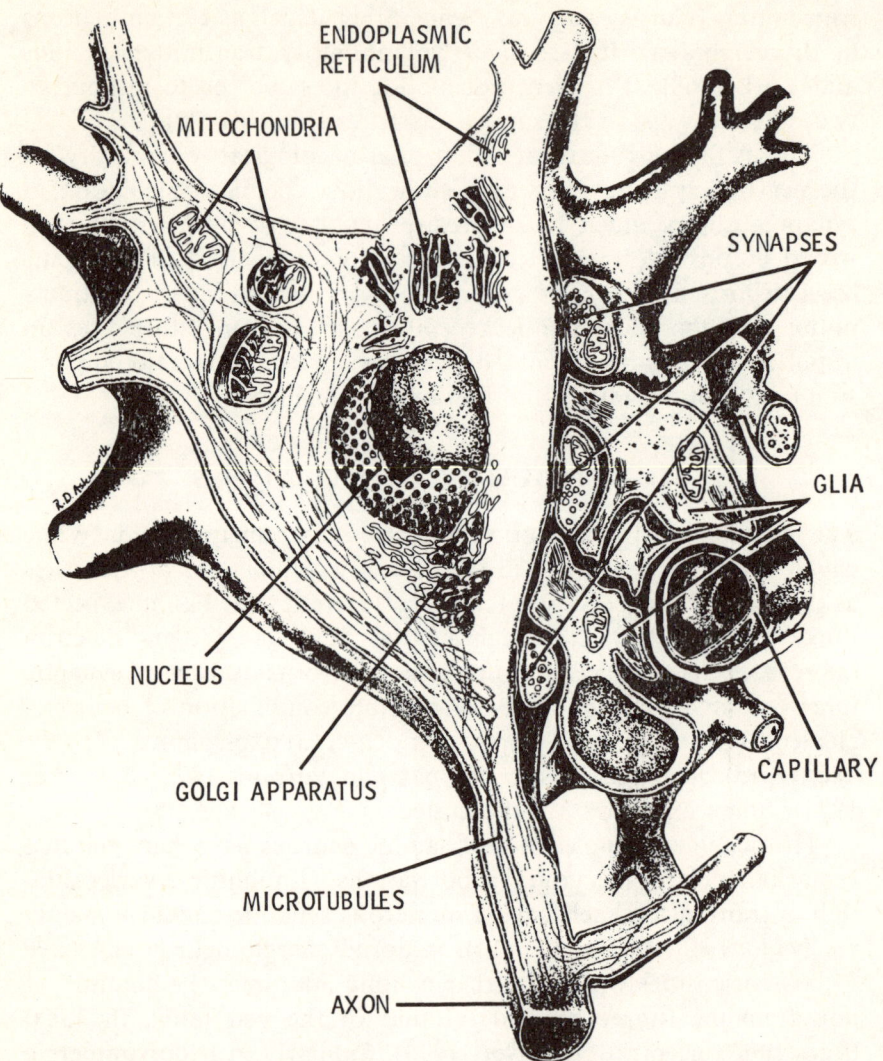

Fig. 15. Diagrammatic representation of the relationship between neurons, glia and capillaries. (From Willis and Grossman 1973, *Medical Neurobiology*, Mosby, St. Louis.)

The general relationships between neuron, synapse, glial cell, capillary and interstitial space are illustrated in Fig. 15. The distribution pattern of synapses is shown diagrammatically in Fig. 16. Both of these figures are naturally crude oversimplifications. Neurons in the cat's spinal cord have been estimated to receive 15,000–30,000 synaptic contacts. Synapses 'clothe the cell surface like a mosaic, the constituent parts of which are separated by a small space presumably occupied by glial cells and their processes' (Illis 1967).

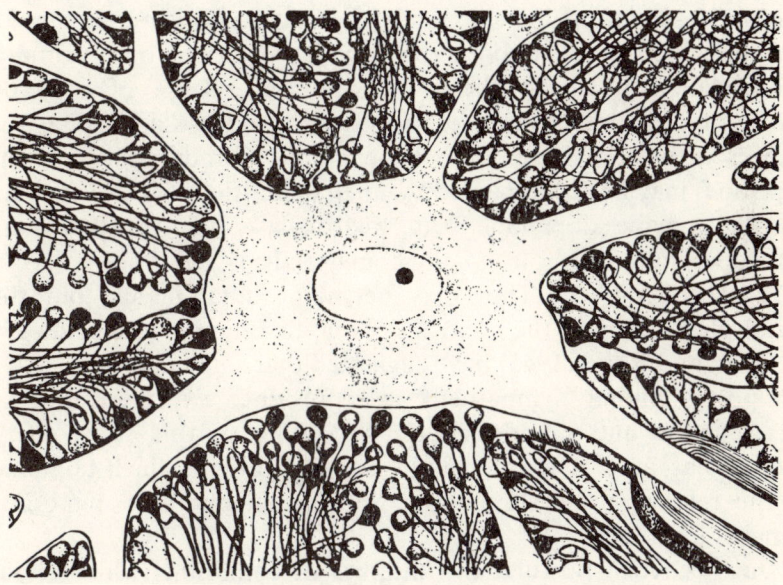

Fig. 16. Diagrammatic representation of the distribution of synapses around a neuron. (From Schadé and Ford 1973, *Basic Neurology*. Elsevier, Amsterdam.)

IDENTIFICATION OF TRANSMITTERS

Acetylcholine, noradrenaline, dopamine, serotonin, glycine and gamma aminobutyric acid (GABA) have been identified as synaptic transmitters. The evidence implicating glutamic acid and aspartic acid (Hebb 1970) is less complete. While acetylcholine and the monoamines (noradrenaline, dopamine and serotonin) are confined to specialised sites in neurons where they are employed solely for transmission, the aminoacids (GABA, glycine, glutamic acid and aspartic acid) are widespread tissue constituents with many roles —this increases the difficulty in establishing their function at synapses.

In 1948, Feldberg and Vogt put forward the challenging hypothesis that neurons release only one transmitter, to which they are themselves insensitive. Neural pathways would then be arranged in chains in which alternate cells employ the same transmitter. Although current observations indicate that the organisation is more complex, present evidence still supports the view that each neuron is primarily concerned with the synthesis, storage and release of only one transmitter. However, certain neurons may release additional substances with their transmitter—for example, noradrenaline (norepinephrine) may be accompanied by small quantities of (1) octopamine, (2) the enzyme dopamine beta hydroxylase, (3) prostaglandins, (4) dopamine. The role of these materials is not known (Kopin 1972; Horton 1973). They may be mere contaminants, but they could play a part in the control of synaptic function (see below).

Burn and Rand (1965) have suggested that some neurons, such as the postganglionic sympathetic cells, produce two transmitters—acetylcholine and noradrenaline. According to this view, acetylcholine has an initial role in the series of events which culminate in the release of noradrenaline; this 'cholinergic link' hypothesis remains unproven.

Just as Koch postulated a number of conditions which should be satisfied before accepting evidence that an organism is pathogenic, a group of criteria have been formulated for establishing the identity of a transmitter with reasonable certainty. These have recently been summarised by Phillis (1970) as follows:

1   The substance must be present in those neurons from which it is thought to be released.

2   The neuron must possess the necessary enzymic mechanisms for the manufacture of the substance.

3   The presence of the various precursors in the synthetic pathway should be demonstrable.

4   There must be mechanisms for inactivation of the substance. These may include an enzyme which destroys the substance and/or

a specific uptake system for reabsorption of the substance into pre- or postsynaptic structures.

5 During stimulation, the substance should be detectable in extracellular fluid collected from the region of the synapse.

6 When applied to the postsynaptic membrane, the substance should reproduce the action of the released transmitter.

7 Pharmacological agents which modify the effects of the released transmitter should influence the actions of the substance in the same way.

SYNTHESIS OF TRANSMITTERS

The synthetic pathways for acetylcholine, noradrenaline, dopamine, serotonin and GABA are shown in Figs. 17–20. The enzymic machinery required for the synthesis of transmitters is present in both the cell body and the nerve ending. Fluorescent histochemical methods can demonstrate monoamine transmitters at a subcellular level (Falck *et al* 1962) and these techniques have shown that following

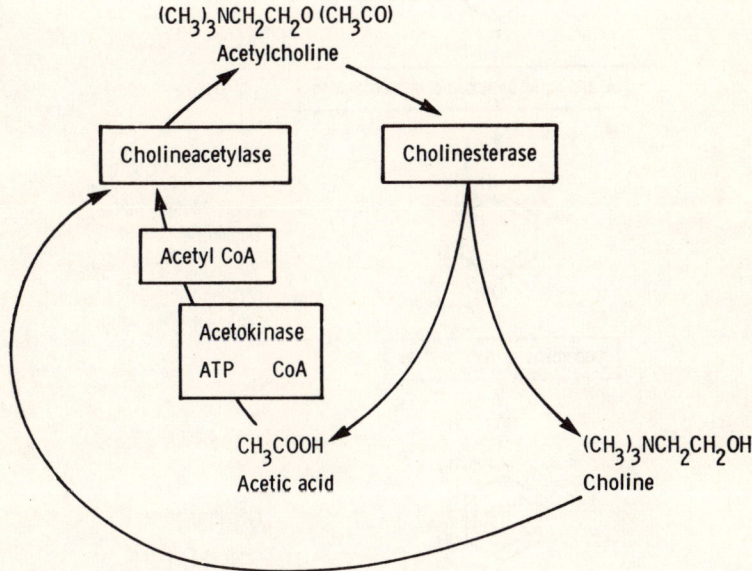

Fig. 17. Synthetic pathway for acetylcholine.

axonotomy, catecholamines (dopamine and noradrenaline) accumulate proximally in the cell body and axon (Dahlström and Fuxe 1964). This suggests that a proportion of transmitter is synthesised at the cell body and transported down the axon to the nerve ending. Recent evidence supports this view—isotopically labelled precursors of dopamine (tyrosine and levodopa) have been found to travel

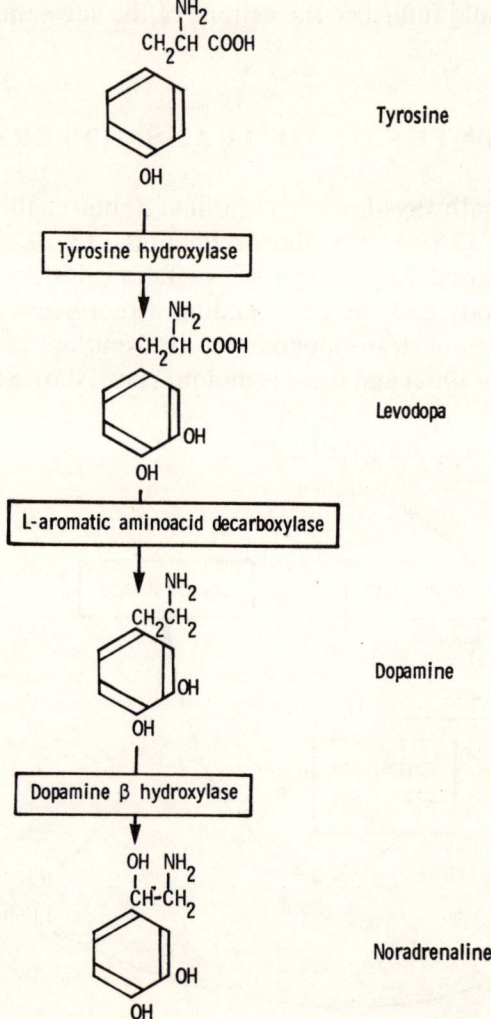

Fig. 18. Synthetic pathway for dopamine and noradrenaline.

along fibres of the nigrostriatal pathway at a rate of 0.8 mm/hour
(Fibiger *et al* 1973). In cholinergic nerves, the synthetic enzyme
choline acetyltransferase (choline acetylase), which accumulates
proximal to a ligature around the nerve, probably undergoes
continuous transport down the axon (Hebb and Waites 1956).

These are particular examples of the general phenomenon of axo-
plasmic flow from cell body to nerve ending, which has been
demonstrated by (1) swelling of nerves proximal to a ligature
(Weiss and Hiscoe 1948), (2) autoradiographic studies (Droz and
Leblond 1963), (3) observations on the movement of labelled protein
following administration of isotopic leucine (Barondes 1964;
Fibiger *et al* 1972).

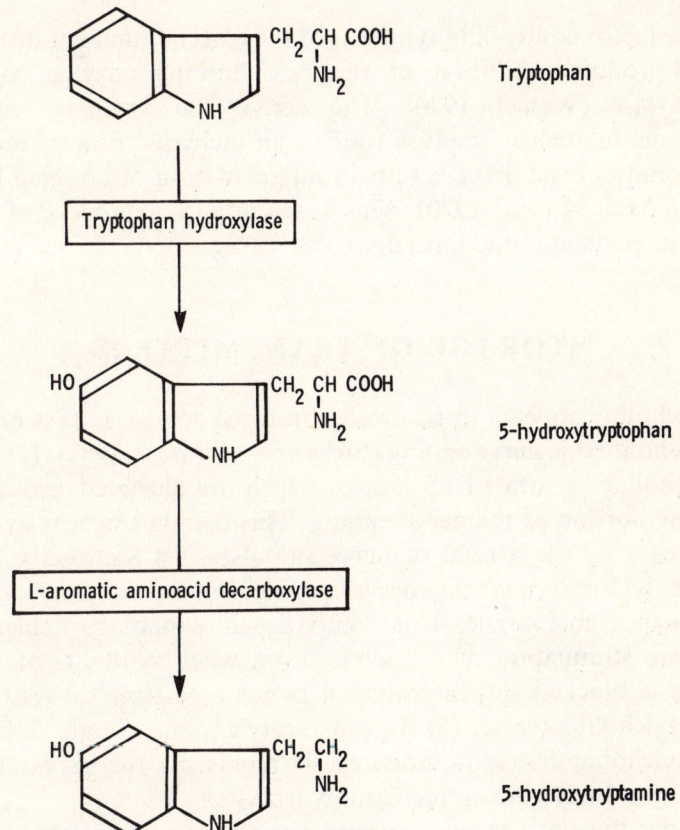

Fig. 19. Synthetic pathway for serotonin.

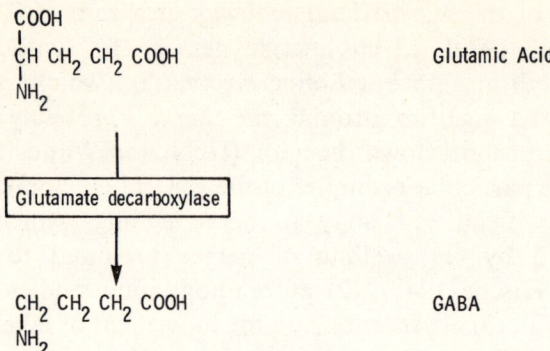

COOH
|
CH CH$_2$ CH$_2$ COOH   Glutamic Acid
|
NH$_2$

Glutamate decarboxylase

CH$_2$ CH$_2$ CH$_2$ COOH   GABA
|
NH$_2$

Fig. 20. Synthetic pathway for gamma aminobutyric acid.

One factor controlling synthesis of the catecholamine transmitters is end-product inhibition of the rate limiting enzyme, tyrosine hydroxylase (Weiner 1970). The activity of synthetic enzymes is also modulated by impulse traffic—an increased flow of impulses in a noradrenergic nerve results in augmentation of tyrosine hydroxylase (Axelrod *et al* 1970). This is essentially a process of trans-synaptic enzyme induction (Blaschko 1973).

STORAGE OF TRANSMITTERS

Acetylcholine appears to be present in three compartments or pools in the cholinergic nerve ending (Birks and McIntosh 1961): (1) Depot acetylcholine is located in vesicles which are clustered around the synaptic portion of the nerve ending. This compartment is available for release by the arrival of nerve impulses. (2) Stationary acetylcholine is located in the nerve ending but some distance from the synaptic membrane. This compartment cannot be depleted by repetitive stimulation of the nerve, even when synthesis of acetylcholine is blocked. Furthermore, it is not accessible to destruction by acetylcholinesterase. (3) Surplus acetylcholine is only detectable if acetylcholinesterase is inhibited. It represents the excess that is normally subjected to immediate hydrolysis.

Under the electron miscroscope, vesicles of acetylcholine appear as translucent structures in the nerve ending (Fig. 21). Analysis of

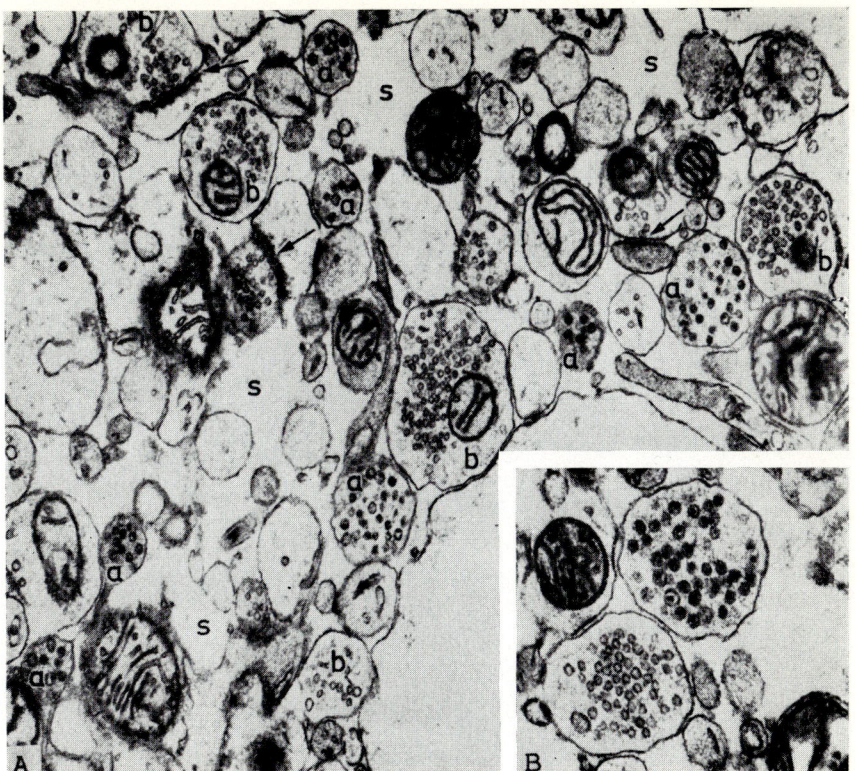

Fig. 21. Electron microscopy of synapses in the rat's caudate nucleus. The small granular vesicles (a) contain dopamine. Indirect evidence suggests that many of the translucent agranular vesciles (b) contain acetylcholine. S is the extracellular space. Arrows indicate synaptic contacts. Magnification 25,000 × ; inset 35,000 × (from Hökfelt 1968, *Z. Zellforsch*, **91**, 1).

these vesicles indicates that in addition to acetylcholine they contain a protein, vesiculin, which probably has a nucleotide (adenosine triphosphate) component (Whittaker 1973).

Noradrenaline also exists in three pools (Glowinski 1972): (1) A functional compartment contains newly synthesised transmitter which is preferentially released by the arrival of a nerve impulse; (2) A much larger main storage compartment with a half-life of 2–3 hours is employed as a reserve source to maintain the level of transmitter in the functional compartment; (3) A reservoir compartment with a half-life of 17 hours seems to correspond to amine in non-terminal regions of the axon. In normal activity depletion of transmitter by nerve impulses can only be demonstrated in the functional compartment.

Morphologically, noradrenaline is stored in vesicles which contain a core that appears dense on electron microscopy. These vesicles also contain adenosine triphosphate and the enzyme dopamine beta hydroxylase. Dopamine is similarly located in dense core vesicles (Fig. 21), though a substantial portion is also present in the cytoplasm (Weil-Malherbe 1959).

RELEASE OF TRANSMITTERS

In 1954 Del Castillo and Katz put forward a quantal theory of transmitter release, based on their studies of the neuromuscular junction in the frog. They suggested that the arrival of an impulse at a nerve terminal led to the release of a number of discrete packages of transmitter. For the amphibian neuromuscular junction some 100 quanta of acetylcholine, out of a total of about 500,000, are likely to be released by each impulse. In addition, there is spontaneous leakage of quanta to produce miniature postsynaptic potentials unrelated to the arrival of nerve impulses. Though the evidence is indirect, it seems probable that the morphological representation of a quantum is a synaptic vesicle. This type of mechanism is likely to operate elsewhere.

It is not easy to deplete nerve endings of transmitter by volleys of impulses at physiological frequencies—synthesis and reuptake (see on) keep pace with release. However, following blockade of synthesis or reuptake, excessive stimulation can lead to depletion and the morphological manifestation is a reduction in the number of synaptic vesicles. Although the mechanism of release is not fully understood, it seems likely that the synaptic vesicle is transported to the cell membrane where exocytosis takes place (Smith 1973). It is not known how the arrival of the nerve impulse sets this system into motion, but there have been speculations that contractile microfilaments may be involved.

INACTIVATION OF TRANSMITTERS

The released transmitter diffuses across the synaptic cleft, reacts with postsynaptic receptors to depolarise (in the case of excitation), or stabilise (in the case of inhibition) the postsynaptic membrane. The reaction between the transmitter and the receptor is reversible; when the transmitter returns from the receptor to the synaptic cleft it must be removed to prevent repetitive transmitter–receptor recombination. One method of inactivation is recapture of trans-mitter into the presynaptic ending by an active uptake system. This has the obvious advantage of conserving material—75 to 80% of released noradrenaline may be recaptured by such means (Iversen 1973). Two pharmacologically distinct mechanisms have been identified for this transmitter (Iversen 1967): (1) uptake$_1$ is a high affinity low capacity system carrying noradrenaline back into the presynaptic nerve ending for retention and further use; (2) uptake$_2$ is a lower affinity but higher capacity mechanism transporting noradrenaline into postsynaptic structures. Whereas uptake$_1$ removes and conserves transmitter, uptake$_2$ seems to be concerned solely with inactivation because after removal from the synaptic cleft by this system, the transmitter is simply metabolised.

Reuptake is a widespread phenomenon. In addition to the mechanisms for noradrenaline, there is evidence that similar systems operate at synapses which employ dopamine, serotonin, GABA and acetylcholine as transmitters (Iversen 1970, 1972).

Enzymes also contribute to inactivation. Catechol-O-methyl-transferase destroys any noradrenaline or dopamine that diffuses away from the synaptic cleft. Within the neuron, unprotected noradrenaline, dopamine and serotonin are destroyed by monoamine oxidase bound to mitochondria.

Acetylcholinesterase is produced in the cell body and passes down the axon to the nerve terminal in a similar way to choline acetyltransferase. However, unlike the transferase, the esterase is present in particularly high concentration in the region of the postsynaptic membrane, a location appropriate for the role of inactivating acetylcholine. Enzymic hydrolysis is followed by active uptake of choline into the presynaptic nerve ending—a mechanism which combines rapid inactivation with efficient recapture.

RECEPTORS

The same transmitter can elicit different types of response which are defined by the nature of the receptor. The separation of cholinergic reactions into muscarinic and nicotinic categories (Table 2) was the first example of this phenomenon to be recognised. In recent years noradrenaline receptors have also been divided into two classes— alpha and beta, the beta receptors undergoing further tentative subclassification (Jenkinson 1973).

Receptors are specific to one transmitter and its structural analogues. Formation of a complex between the transmitter and the receptor initiates a series of linked reactions which result in changes in permeability or conductance of the postsynaptic membrane, that leads to either excitation or inhibition. Receptors are probably all proteins bound to the synaptic membrane. The number of receptors at the rat's neuromuscular junction is about 50×10^6. An impulse only releases about 3×10^6 molecules of acteylcholine (Potter 1970; Miledi and Potter 1971). These findings, together with the observation that the muscle fibres still respond when 90% of their receptors are blocked, indicate that synapses have many spare receptors. Changes in trans-synaptic traffic can modify the number of receptors (Lømo and Rosenthal 1971)—a process which may perhaps contribute to the mechanism of learning.

Chemically, the most clearly defined receptor is that for the cholinergic (nicotinic) synapse, which is a specific membrane protein that seems to undergo an alteration in conformation when it reacts

Table 2. The effects of transmission at various postganglionic autonomic synapses. α = alpha noradrenergic receptor; β = beta noradrenergic receptor; M = muscarinic cholinergic receptor; N = nicotinic cholinergic receptor.

	NORADRENALINE	ACETYLCHOLINE
Cardiovascular system		
Heart rate	Increase (β)	Decrease (M)
Heart force of contraction	Increase (β)	Decrease (M)
Blood vessels	Contraction (α)	—
	Dilatation (β)	—
Respiratory system		
Bronchial muscles	Relaxation (β)	Contraction (M)
Bronchial glands	—	Secretion (M)
Alimentary system		
Salivary glands	Thick secretion (α)	Thin secretion (M)
Peristalsis	Decrease (α and β)	Increase (M)
Sphincters	Contraction (α)	Relaxation (M)
	Dilatation (β)	—
Pupil		
Radial muscle	Contraction (α)	—
Sphincter	—	Contraction (M)
Striated muscle	Contraction (α and β)	Contraction (N)
Autonomic ganglia	—	Excitation (N)

with acetylcholine (Potter and Molinoff 1972). It appears to have a molecular weight of about 252,000 and is made up of subunits, several of which have binding sites for acetylcholine (Potter 1973).

The receptor for dopamine is a protein closely associated with an adenylate cyclase (Kebabian *et al* 1972; McAfee and Greengard 1972); when activated, adenylate cyclase produces an increase in cyclic adenosine monophosphate. It has been suggested that this in turn activates a kinase to phosphorylate a protein constituent of the synaptic membrane, which leads to a change in ion movement across the membrane. Beta adrenergic receptors also utilise an adenylate cyclase in a similar chain of events at noradrenergic synapses (Jenkinson 1973).

Recent evidence suggests that there are presynaptic in addition to postsynaptic receptors. Activation of these receptors on the nerve ending are thought to inhibit the release of transmitter. This constitutes a negative feedback control mechanism (Enero *et al* 1972).

Certain presynaptic receptors may react with materials other than the major transmitter released by the nerve impulse. For example, rapidly repetitive impulse traffic in noradrenergic nerve endings can lead to the release of an increasing proportion of dopamine as the noradrenaline stores become depleted, and dopamine reacts with presynaptic receptors to conserve noradrenaline by inhibiting further release (McCulloch *et al* 1973). Prostaglandin E_2 is also discharged by impulses in noradrenergic nerve endings and this again inhibits further release of noradrenaline (Horton 1973).

The various mechanisms involved in synaptic transmission are summarised in Fig. 22.

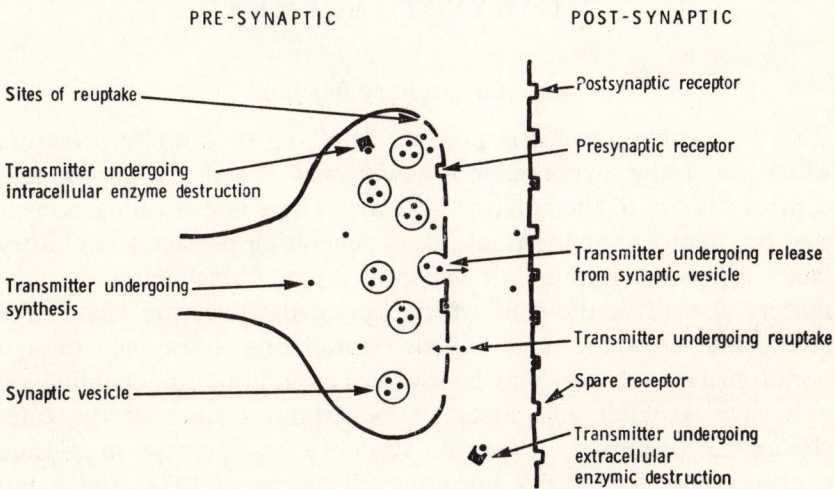

Fig. 22. Diagrammatic summary of the major features of a synapse.

NEURO-ENDOCRINE TRANSDUCERS

Attention has already been drawn to the close similarity in the mechanisms of junctional transmission from neuron to neuron, and from nerve ending to effector organ. Major advances in the analysis of synaptic processes have stemmed from investigation of neural junctions with striated muscle, smooth muscle and cardiac muscle. Many of the early observations on nerve endings in exocrine glands have also contributed to current concepts of synaptic function. In recent years, there has been growing interest in a group of neuro-effector junctions concerned with controlling the secretion of hormones. The term *neuroendocrine transducer* has been coined to describe cells which convert a neuronal input (i.e. transmitter released into a synaptic cleft) to an endocrine output (i.e. a hormone released into the circulation). There are probably many systems of this type but four sites have attracted particular attention (Wurtman 1974): (1) the hypothalamus, (2) the pineal, (3) the adrenal medulla, (4) the juxtaglomerular apparatus.

THE HYPOTHALAMUS

Anterior pituitary function

Cells in the hypothalamus produce releasing or inhibitory factors which enter the hypothalamo-hypophysial portal circulation and control activity of the anterior pituitary. There is general agreement that the neuroendocrine transducers generating prolactin inhibitory factor receive dopaminergic synaptic input. Catecholamine transmitters also drive the cells which secrete the releasing factors for luteinising hormone and follicle stimulating hormone, though noradrenergic synapses may be involved in addition to dopaminergic pathways (Hökfelt and Fuxe 1972). Administration of the catecholamine precursor, levodopa, leads to an increase in plasma concentrations of growth hormone (Sirtori *et al* 1972) and a fall in the level of thyroid stimulating hormone (Spaulding *et al* 1972), but the mechanisms responsible for these changes have not been defined. Accumulating evidence suggests that some anterior pituitary hormones are modulated by both releasing and inhibitory factors (Martin 1973).

Posterior pituitary function

Cells in the supraoptic and paraventricular nuclei receive noradrenergic synaptic input; they control vasopressin and oxytocin.

THE PINEAL

Melatonin is produced by the pineal in response to noradrenergic nerve endings.

THE ADRENAL MEDULLA

Excitation of cholinergic preganglionic sympathetic nerves leads to the secretion of adrenaline (epinephrine) by the adrenal medulla.

THE JUXTAGLOMERULAR APPARATUS

Noradrenergic sympathetic input elicits the release of renin from juxtaglomerular cells in the kidney.

CHAPTER 4
DRUGS WHICH MODIFY IMPULSE PROPAGATION AND SYNAPTIC TRANSMISSION

Drugs which modify transmission along nerves or across synapses are employed therapeutically in many branches of medicine. They are also used as investigative tools for the anatomical mapping of biochemically identifiable pathways in the central nervous system, for the analysis of normal mechanisms of transmission and for the study of abnormal neuronal function. Drugs which influence impulse propagation will be considered in the order: (1) Local anaesthetics; (2) General anaesthetics; (3) Other drugs which influence impulse propagation. Modification of synaptic transmission will be discussed in the following stages: (1) Drugs which increase transmitter function—precursors, releasers, agonists, drugs which block inactivation; (2) Drugs which reduce transmitter function—inhibitors of synthesis, drugs which block storage, inhibitors of release, false transmitters, receptor blockers; (3) Drugs which destroy certain neurons selectively; (4) Denervation supersensitivity.

Drugs influencing impulse propagation

LOCAL ANAESTHETICS

Local anaesthetics were discovered by accident. For centuries the leaves of Erythroxylon coca have been chewed in the Andes mountains because of the sense of well-being which they induce. In 1860 the active alkaloid, cocaine, was isolated; when taken by mouth it was noted that anaesthesia developed over the tongue. Though initially employed for its action upon the central nervous system, cocaine proved to have a far more important peripheral effect—reversible blockade of nerve conduction. After this fortuitous discovery a range of chemical congeners were synthesised of which the most widely used are procaine and lignocaine (lidocaine).

Local anaesthetics block impulse propagation by interfering with the transient increase in sodium conductance normally produced in excitable membranes by low levels of depolarisation (Taylor 1959). Suggested mechanisms include competition with calcium carrier systems, closure of pores, or a general increase in molecular disorder of the membrane (Ritchie *et al* 1970). Local anaesthetics do not depress the metabolism of nerve cells and they do not effect the resting potential (De Jong and Wagman 1963).

There is still confusion concerning the action of local anaesthetics on different types and sizes of nerve fibres. The view that afferent axons are more sensitive than efferents was based upon the observation that injection of local anaesthetic blocks the reflex response to a tendon jerk though the muscle still responds to electrical stimulation of the nerve proximal to the point of infiltration. However, the report that the small motor (fusimotor) fibres are particularly sensitive to local anaesthetics (Matthews and Rushworth 1957) affords a satisfactory explanation in terms of axon size, rather than type, determining the order of loss of function. This interpretation is consonant with the hypothesis that local anaesthetics commonly produce hypalgesia before hypaesthesia because of selective vulnerability of small nerve fibres. The controversy has been reopened by recent evidence casting doubt on the view that axon diameter bears any consistent relationship with the order of blockade or recovery of function in peripheral nerves (Nathan and Sears 1963).

GENERAL ANAESTHETICS

Of all drugs acting upon the nervous system, hypnotics and general anaesthetic agents may perhaps be regarded as having the most profound and obvious effects; yet remarkably little is known of their mechanism of action. The physical and chemical properties of drugs which depress consciousness are so varied that a multiplicity of different actions are probably involved. One property of general anaesthetics which is likely to be of considerable importance is their ability to stabilise cell membranes (Seeman 1972). This effect is not confined to excitable membranes—anaesthetics protect erythrocytes from hypotonic haemolysis. It is also possible that anaesthetics modify junctional transmission (Wall 1967), though their actions at synapses have not been identified with any precision.

OTHER DRUGS WHICH INFLUENCE IMPULSE PROPAGATION

A range of drugs other than local anaesthetics influence impulse propagation along excitable membranes. Procainamide and quinine will be considered when discussing myotonia and muscle cramps in Chapter 17. Alcohol, ether, barbiturates, hydantoins and lithium can also modify the propagation of nerve impulses.

Tetrodotoxin has been used extensively as an experimental tool to separate electrical and chemical events at nerve endings. By selectively blocking the voltage dependent increase in sodium conductance, tetrodotoxin inhibits the development of action potentials, thus facilitating the analysis of presynaptic and post-synaptic events concerned with the release of transmitters.

Drugs influencing synaptic transmission

Depletion of transmitter is likely to occur in many chronic neuro-logical diseases. Profound reduction in the concentration of striatal dopamine has been found in Parkinsonism (Hornykiewicz 1966). Similarly a substantial decrease of striatal GABA has been reported in Huntington's chorea (Perry *et al* 1973); this aminoacid may occur in glia in addition to neurons and it has not been demon-strated that there is a specific loss of the transmitter fraction. It is probable that a fall in the concentration of transmitters occurs in other chronic neurological disorders, such as motoneuron disease and Alzheimer's disease. However, the consequences of reduced transmitter levels may be offset, to a variable extent, by the development of denervation supersensitivity. Experimental studies in animals indicate that this occurs in the central nervous system in addition to the periphery (Ungerstedt and Ljungberg 1974).

In the following discussion it is implicit that the actions of drugs are never completely specific. One of the few generalisations permissible in pharmacology is that all specificity is relative and is usually inversely related to the extent to which the drug has been investigated.

DRUGS WHICH INCREASE TRANSMITTER FUNCTION

PRECURSORS OF TRANSMITTERS

The rate limiting step in the synthesis of the catecholamines (noradrenaline and dopamine) is hydroxylation of tyrosine to form levodopa. Administration of levodopa by-passes tyrosine hydroxylase

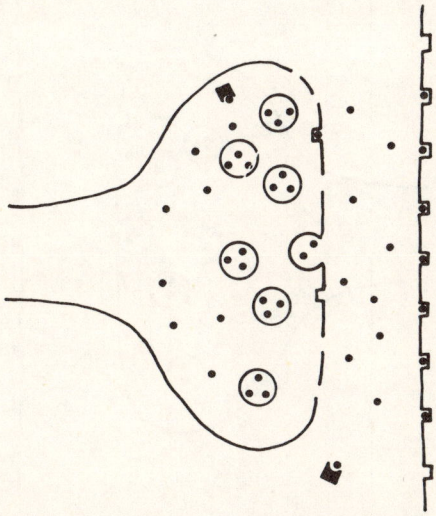

Fig. 23. The effects produced by administering the precursor of a transmitter. There is increased synthesis which leads to a higher concentration of transmitter in the synaptic cleft and more extensive activation of receptors. Symbols are the same as those employed in Figure 22.

and leads to the accumulation of increased concentrations of
dopamine in the central nervous system of experimental animals
(Poirier *et al* 1967). Observations on brains taken post mortem from
Parkinsonian patients indicates that the same phenomenon occurs
in man (Rinne *et al* 1971; Lloyd *et al* 1973). The effects of precursors
are illustrated in Fig. 23.

DRUGS RELEASING TRANSMITTERS

Administration of tyramine leads to the release of noradrenaline
from sympathetic nerve endings. This contributes to the hypertensive
reaction provoked by dietary intake of tyramine in patients receiving
monoamine oxidase inhibitors. Several other drugs have prominent
releasing properties—ephedrine for noradrenaline, amphetamine
for dopamine and carbachol for acetylcholine. The action of
releasing drugs is shown diagramatically in Fig. 24.

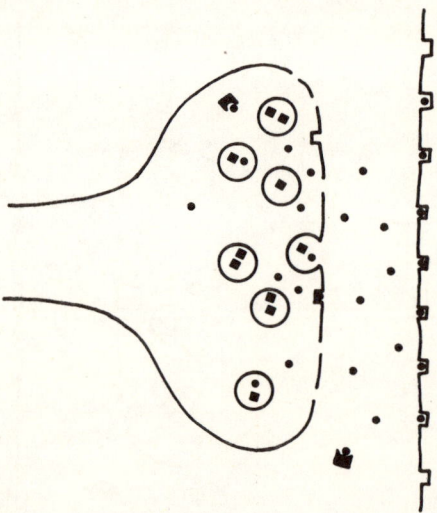

Fig. 24. The effects produced by administering a drug which releases
a transmitter. A higher concentration of transmitter appears in the
synaptic cleft and there is more extensive activation of receptors. The
releaser is represented by ■; other symbols are the same as those
employed in Figure 22.

RECEPTOR AGONISTS

Drugs may reproduce the action of a transmitter by a direct effect on the postsynaptic receptor. Phenylephrine stimulates alpha noradrenergic receptors to produce a rise of blood pressure. Phenylephrine does not readily cross the blood–brain barrier, but a noradrenaline agonist which does enter the brain, clonidine, reduces the blood pressure. Thus the same transmitter can exert different effects at various sites in the peripheral and central nervous system and in some instances these actions may be diametrically opposed to each other.

Numerous other relatively selective agonists have been identified. Isoprenaline acts upon beta noradrenergic receptors to produce such responses as tachycardia and bronchodilatation. Apomorphine is a dopaminergic agonist, which accounts for both its emetic and its therapeutic effect in Parkinsonism. Low concentrations of nicotine selectively activate the autonomic ganglia and neuromuscular

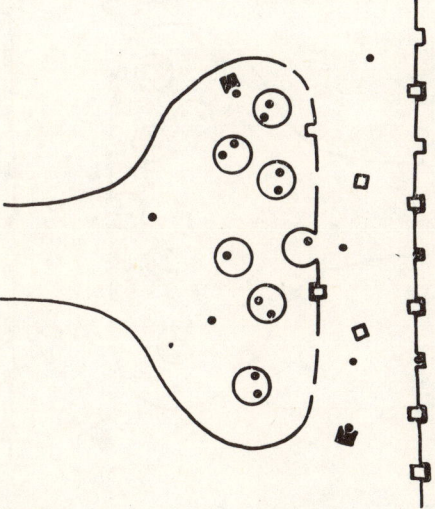

Fig. 25. The effects produced by administering a receptor agonist. The agonist combines with receptors to produce activation. The receptor agonist is represented by □; other symbols are the same as those employed in Figure 22.

junctions (though high concentrations block these synapses). Methacholine elicits parasympathomimetic reactions by behaving as a cholinergic agonist. These effects are illustrated in Fig. 25.

DRUGS BLOCKING INACTIVATION

Certain drugs inhibit the enzymic breakdown of transmitters (Figs. 26 and 27). Neostigmine and pyridostigmine achieve their therapeutic action in myasthenia gravis by blocking acetylcholinesterase, thus increasing acetylcholine concentrations at the neuromuscular junction. Monoamine oxidase inhibitors potentiate the actions of noradrenaline, dopamine and serotonin by decreasing their rate of destruction.

Another method of reducing inactivation is inhibition of the uptake mechanisms responsible for removing certain transmitters from the synaptic cleft (Fig. 28). Imipramine, desipramine and

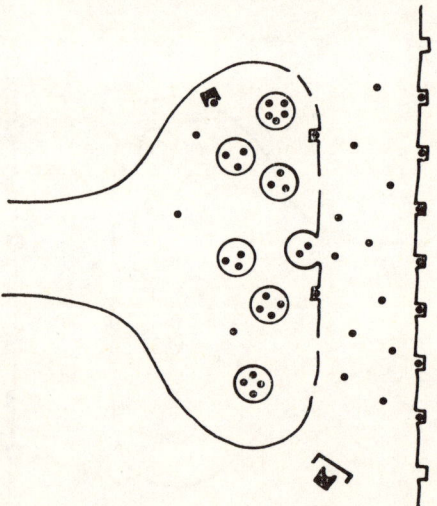

Fig. 26. The effects produced by administering an inhibitor of the extracellular enzymes responsible for destroying transmitter. Increased concentration of transmitter in the synaptic cleft leads to more extensive activation of receptors. The enzyme inhibitor is represented by]; other symbols are the same as those employed in Figure 22.

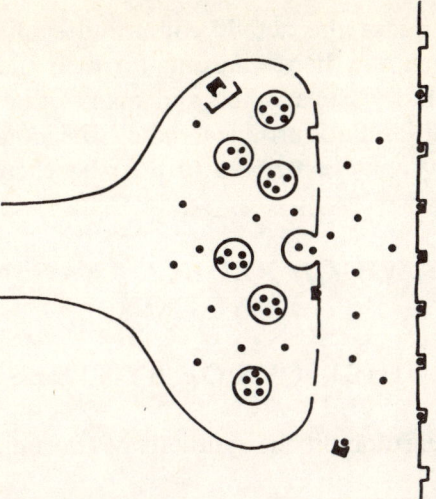

Fig. 27. The effects produced by administering an inhibitor of the intracellular enzymes responsible for destroying transmitter. Increased concentration of transmitter in the synaptic cleft leads to more extensive activation of receptors. The enzyme inhibitor is represented by]; other symbols are the same as those employed in Figure 22.

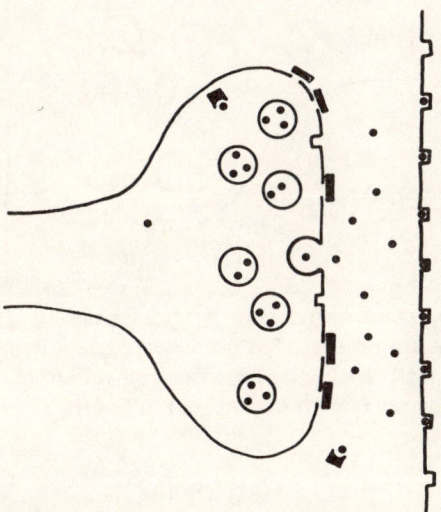

Fig. 28. The effects produced by administering a drug which blocks reuptake of a transmitter. Increased concentration of transmitter in the synaptic cleft leads to more extensive activation of receptors. The reuptake blocker is represented by |; other symbols are the same as those employed in Figure 22.

amitriptyline increase the activity of noradrenaline and serotonin in this way, which may be responsible for their therapeutic effect in depression. Similarly benztropine and many other drugs employed in the treatment of Parkinsonism, block the uptake of dopamine and this property may contribute to their beneficial actions.

DRUGS WHICH REDUCE TRANSMITTER FUNCTION

INHIBITORS OF SYNTHESIS

A number of drugs inhibit the synthesis of transmitters (Fig. 29).

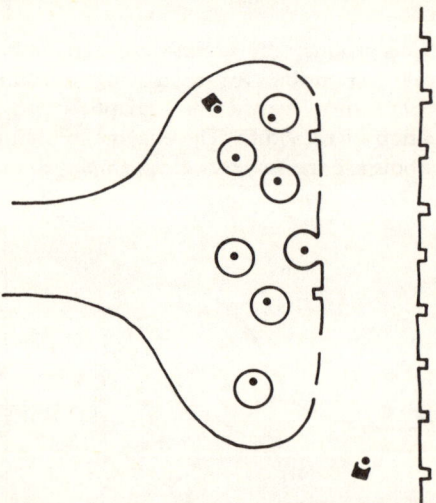

Fig. 29. The effects produced by administering an inhibitor of synthesis of a transmitter. Reduced concentration of transmitter in the synaptic cleft leads to decreased activation of receptors. The symbols are the same as those emplyed in Figure 22.

Acetylcholine

Hemicholinium and triethylcholine reduce the formation of acetylcholine by blocking the transport system responsible for accumulating choline in neurons (Bull and Hemsworth 1963).

Catecholamines

Alpha methyl-p-tyrosine competitively inhibits tyrosine hydroxylase to result in a profound depletion of all the catecholamines. More selective effects can be obtained by blocking dopamine beta hydroxylase which is responsible for the conversion of dopamine to noradrenaline. This enzyme can be inhibited with disulfiram or fusaric acid to achieve an increase in the dopamine/noradrenaline ratio in the nervous system. A more effective blocker is available for experimental studies in animals, FLA 63 (bis-[1-methyl-4-homopiperazinylthiocarbonyl]-disulphide) but this is not suitable for administration to man.

Serotonin

Conversion of tryptophan to 5-hydroxytryptophan is the rate limiting step in the formation of serotonin, so competitive inhibition of this enzyme with p-chlorophenylalanine reduces the concentration of serotonin in the nervous system.

Alpha methyldopa and alpha methyl-m-tyrosine inhibit the enzyme L-aromatic aminoacid decarboxylase, which converts levodopa to dopamine and 5-hydroxytryptophan to serotonin. At one time it was thought that the hypotensive action of alpha methyldopa depended upon this enzymic inhibition, but it now seems that formation of a false transmitter, alpha methylnoradrenaline, is more likely to be responsible.

BLOCKADE OF STORAGE

Reserpine blocks the intraneuronal storage of the monoamines—noradrenaline, dopamine and serotonin. When they cannot be retained in their normal storage sites, these amines are metabolised to result in severe depletion. The consequent reduction in brain monoamines is thought to be responsible for the tranquillising and ultimately depressing action of reserpine. It is now clear that the depletion of striatal dopamine is responsible for the Parkinsonism commonly seen as a dose dependent adverse reaction to reserpine.

The hypotensive effect of reserpine is due in part to reduction of peripherial stores of noradrenaline at sympathetic nerve endings, but central actions may also contribute. Tetrabenazine has pharmacological properties similar to reserpine, but its effects are more prominent in the central, rather than the peripheral nervous system. Blockade of storage is illustrated diagrammatically in Fig. 30.

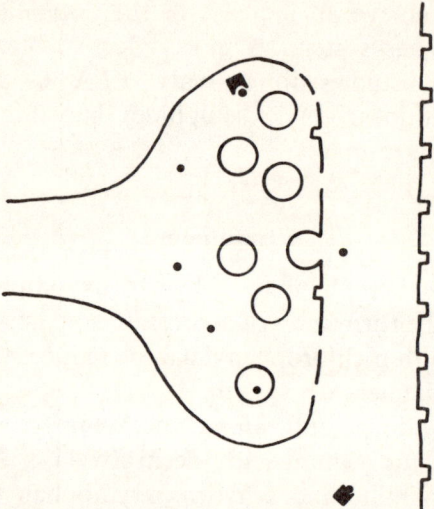

Fig. 30. The effects produced by administering a drug which blocks storage of a transmitter. Reduced concentration of transmitter in the synaptic cleft leads to decreased activation of receptors. The symbols are the same as those employed in Figure 22.

INHIBITION OF RELEASE

Botulinum toxin blocks the release of acetylcholine which normally follows the arrival of nerve impulses at cholinergic terminals. This results in weakness due to decreased neuromuscular transmission which may culminate in death from paralysis of the respiratory muscles.

Other drugs, such as guanethidine and bethanidine, have analogous but reversible effects on noradrenergic nerve endings (Fig. 31). Some of these adrenergic neuron blockers have other actions such as the release of noradrenaline to evoke a transient sympathomimetic effect, which is followed by more sustained depletion of transmitter stores. Several also inhibit monoamine oxidase. Adrenergic neuron blocking agents are concentrated in the nerve terminal by the same transport mechanism that operates the active uptake of noradrenaline. Prolonged administration in high dosage can result in histological damage to noradrenergic neurons. The relative contribution of these various conflicting actions has not been determined, but adrenergic neuron blockers remain useful therapeutic agents in the treatment of hypertension (Laverty 1973).

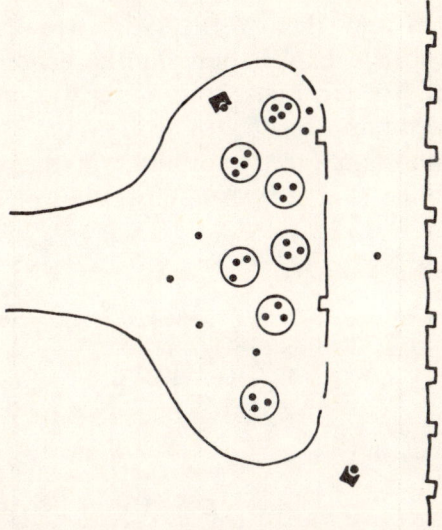

Fig. 31. The effects produced by administration of a drug which blocks the mechanism by which impulses release transmitter. Reduced concentration of transmitter in the synaptic cleft leads to decreased activation of receptors. The symbols are the same as those employed in Figure 22.

FALSE TRANSMITTERS

It is inappropriate to classify false transmitters into drugs which either increase or decrease synaptic function, as they can have either action. They are discussed here because the concept arose historically as an explanation for reduced synaptic transmission. Like many important scientific developments, the concept of a false transmitter was introduced for the wrong reasons. Burgen *et al* (1956) reported that triethylcholine was acetylated in the brain in a similar way to choline. Triethylcholine was then found to inhibit neuromuscular transmission (Bowman and Rand 1961). These observations were interpreted as evidence that triethylacetylcholine was formed and released at the cholinergic nerve ending, but because of its structural differences from acetylcholine, it failed to produce a normal response at the postsynaptic receptors. This idea was rejected when triethylcholine was shown to act by blocking the entry of choline into cholinergic nerves (Bull and Hemsworth 1963). However, the concept affords an appropriate explanation for the action of other drugs at other synapses. The term false transmitter was coined and rapidly became assimilated into neuropharmacology.

The most important false transmitter in therapeutics is alpha methylnoradrenaline (Fig. 32). Administration of alpha methyl-m-

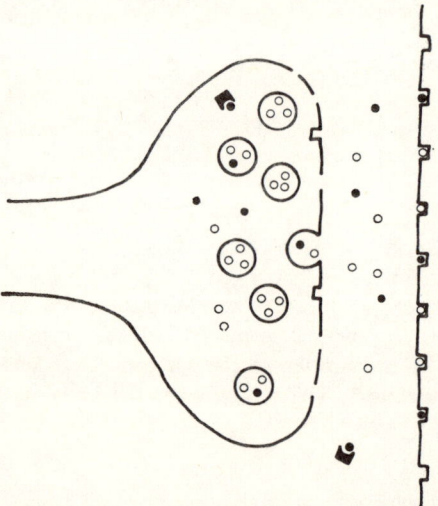

Fig. 32. The effects produced by administration of a partial agonist (or its precursor). The release of false transmitter into the synaptic cleft leads to abnormal activation of receptors, which may be followed by their blockade. The partial agonist is represented by o ; other symbols are the same as those employed in Figure 22.

tyrosine or alpha methyldopa leads to the formation of alpha methyl-noradrenaline and metaraminol because of the limited specificity of the enzymes concerned with catecholamine synthesis (Carlsson and Lindqvist 1962). Alpha methylnoradrenaline and metaraminol are stored in synaptic vesicles (Musacchio *et al* 1965) and released following stimulation of noradrenergic neurons (Muscholl and Maitre 1963). Current evidence favours the view that alpha methyldopa exerts most of its hypotensive effect through an action of alpha methylnoradrenaline in the central nervous system.

Lack of specificity of active uptake mechanisms allows administered monoamines to accumulate at inappropriate nerve endings, from which they can be released as false transmitters (Lichtensteiger *et al* 1967; Kopin 1972). For example, serotonin can be taken up at noradrenergic and dopaminergic terminals. There is also evidence that administration of levodopa leads to high concentrations of dopamine in serotonergic neurons (Butcher *et al* 1970); electrical stimulation can release this dopamine (Ng *et al* 1971).

RECEPTOR BLOCKERS

Acetylcholine receptors

Two types of cholinergic receptor—nicotinic and muscarinic—can each be blocked selectively by drugs which have been known for centuries.

The nicotinic receptors are reversibly blocked by curare, employed on arrow tips by South American Indians to induce paralysis. The purified alkaloid, d-tubocurarine, or its synthetic congener galla-mine, are used to relax muscle during general anaesthesia and to facilitate artificial positive pressure ventilation in patients with respiratory insufficiency due to status epilepticus or tetanus. Irreversible blockade of the nicotinic neuromuscular receptors can be produced with bungarotoxin; the reaction between receptor and toxin is so specific and stable that it can be employed to distinguish the cholinergic receptors from other components of the fractionated postsynaptic membrane.

While the above drugs have a high affinity for the neuromuscular junction, other nicotinic blockers act relatively specifically at the autonomic ganglia. A range of such agents were employed for sympathetic blockade in the treatment of hypertension 20 years ago—hexamethonium, pentolinium, mecamylamine and pempidine. Their main disadvantage was concomitant impairment of parasympathetic function. Patients experienced a dry mouth, difficulty with ocular accommodation, constipation, urinary retention and disturbances of sexual function.

The oldest use for muscarinic blocking drugs was probably assassination, but less toxic doses were employed by Venetian women to produce mydriasis (which was regarded as a sign of beauty rather than a neurological deficit). Because of this early cosmetic practice the muscarinic blocking agents became known as the 'belladonna' alkaloids. A century ago two of these alkaloids, atropine and hyoscine, were introduced for the treatment of Parkinsonism and over the last 30 years a number of similar synthetic drugs have been produced. The newer preparations have the advantage of achieving similar therapeutic results with less prominent features of parasympathetic blockade.

Catecholamine receptors

Phenoxybenzamine, phentolamine and thymoxamine are the most specific alpha adrenergic blocking agents. Other more widely used drugs, such as ergotamine and chlorpromazine, have less selective alpha blocking properties.

Beta adrenergic blockers, such as propranolol and oxprenolol, are employed to alleviate angina, cardiac arrhythmias and hypertension. They are also beneficial in certain types of tremor and they have been claimed to be useful in the prophylactic treatment of migraine.

Haloperidol, pimozide, thiopropazate and chlorpromazine are dopaminergic receptor blockers (Andén *et al* 1970a). These drugs are major tranquillisers but they produce dose dependent Parkinsonism. Because the dopaminergic receptors are rendered unresponsive, levodopa is of no therapeutic value in such cases.

Other receptors

Serotonergic receptors are blocked by lysergic acid diethylamide; this antagonism may be concerned with its hallucinogenic action. Bicuculline blocks GABA receptors. Since bicuculline is a potent convulsant currently employed to produce experimental seizures in animals, it is possible that GABA function may be reduced in some types of epilepsy. The action of receptor blockers is illustrated in Fig. 33.

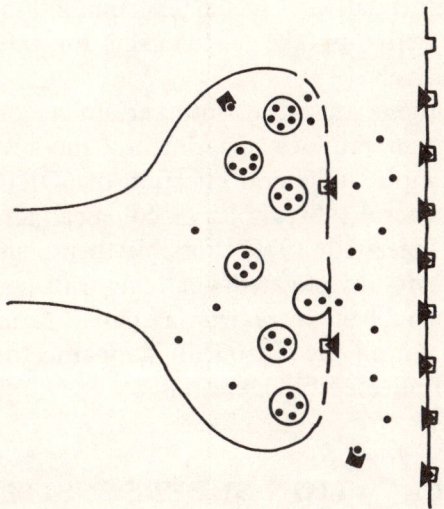

Fig. 33. The effects produced by administration of a receptor blocker. Access of transmitter to the receptors is prevented. Transmission is reduced in spite of a high concentration of transmitter in the synaptic cleft. The receptor blocker is represented by ▶ ; other symbols are the same as those employed in Figure 22.

DRUGS WHICH DESTROY CERTAIN NEURONS SELECTIVELY

In noradrenergic and dopaminergic neurons, 6-hydroxydopamine (6OHDA) produces selective depletion of transmitter followed by degeneration in noradrenergic and dopaminergic neurons. This occurs in either the brain or the periphery, according to the route of administration; 6OHDA does not cross the blood–brain barrier (Tranzer and Thoenen 1968; Bloom *et al* 1969; Ungerstedt 1968; Uretsky and Iversen 1969). Similarly, 5,6-dihydroxytryptamine (5,6DHT) produces degeneration of serotonergic neurons (Baumgarten *et al* 1971). The specificity of the lesions produced by these drugs depends on dose and species, high concentrations in large animals producing less selective changes (Poirier *et al* 1972). 6OHDA and 5,6DHT are extremely reactive chemical agents which damage cells at low tissue concentrations. The localisation of their effect stems from their relatively specific accumulation in monoamine neurons by the active uptake mechanisms for catecholamines and serotonin respectively.

Injection of these substances into certain regions of the central nervous system can produce experimental models of neurological disease. For example, unilateral injection of 6OHDA into the rat's substantia nigra results in a pharmacological analogue to hemi-parkinsonism (Ungerstedt 1971). Possible therapeutic uses for these drugs are also being investigated—patients with peripheral vascular disease have been given intra-arterial 6OHDA in an attempt to achieve vasodilatation by chemical sympathectomy confined to nerve endings of affected blood vessels.

DENERVATION SUPERSENSITIVITY

Drugs which reduce transmitter output, either by depleting storage sites or destroying nerve endings, produce similar synaptic changes to those formulated by Cannon (1939) in his law of denervation: 'When in a series of efferent neurons a unit is destroyed, an increased irritability to chemical stimulating agents develops in the isolated structure.' This concept has been extended to afferent pathways by Drake and Stavraky (1948) and recent evidence indicates that the same phenomenon occurs in the central nervous system (Ungerstedt 1971).

It is likely that several mechanisms contribute to denervation supersensitivity. Postsynaptic changes have been demonstrated at the neuromuscular junction. Denervation results in an extension of the area of sensitivity to acetylcholine on the muscle fibre with a corresponding increase in the number of receptors (Miledi 1960; Miledi and Potter 1971). It has also been suggested that denervation can lead to improved linkage between receptor activation and response (Langer and Trendelenburg 1968). A further postsynaptic factor contributing to supersensitivity may be changes in ionic permeability of the excitable membrane (Nicholls 1956; Klaus *et al* 1960).

Presynaptic consequences of denervation may also be important. Degeneration of the nerve ending results in loss of the active uptake mechanisms normally responsible for removing many transmitters from the synaptic cleft. There is evidence that this sequence of events occurs at denervated sympathetic noradrenergic nerve endings (Trendelenburg 1966) and a similar mechanism may operate for other transmitters at other sites, including the central nervous system.

These various changes, contributing together to increase the response to artificially administered transmitters, may prove to be of considerable therapeutic importance. Denervation supersensitivity should allow substantial responses to be achieved with relatively small increments in the concentration of transmitter at chronically

Table 3. Drugs which increase transmitter function. DA = dopamine; NA = noradrenaline; ACh = acetylcholine; 5HT = serotonin.

MECHANISM	DRUG	TRANSMITTER
Precursor	levodopa	DA, NA
	5-hydroxytryprophan	5HT
Releaser	carbachol	ACh
	tyramine	NA
	amphetamine	DA
Receptor agonist	methacholine	ACh
	phenylephrine	NA(α)
	isoprenaline	NA(β)
	apomorphine	DA
Blockade of inactivating enzyme	neostigmine	ACh
	tranylcypromine	NA, DA, 5HT
Blockade of uptake	amitriptyline	NA
	imipramine	NA
	benztropine	DA

Table 4. Drugs which decrease transmitter function. DA = dopamine; NA = noradrenaline; ACh = acetylcholine; 5HT = serotonin; GABA = gamma aminobutyric acid.

MECHANISM	DRUG	TRANSMITTER
Inhibits entry of precursor	hemicholinium triethylcholine	ACh
Inhibits synthetic enzymes		
(1) tyrosine hydroxylase	alpha methyl-p-tyrosine	NA, DA
(2) tryptophan hydroxylase	pchlorophenylalanine	5HT
(3) dopamine β hydroxylase	disulfiram ⎫ fusaric acid ⎬ FLA 63 ⎭	NA
Inhibits transmitter entry into storage sites	reserpine ⎫ tetrabenazine ⎬	NA, DA 5HT
Inhibits release of transmitter	botulinum toxin	ACh
	bretylium ⎫ bethanidine ⎬ guanethidine ⎭	NA
Forms false transmitters*	alpha methyldopa	NA
Receptor blockade	atropine ⎫ benzhexol ⎬	ACh(M)
	tubocurarine ⎫ hexamethonium ⎬	ACh(N)
	phenoxybenzamine ⎫ phentolamine ⎬ thymoxamine ⎭	NA(α)
	propranolol ⎫ oxprenolol ⎬	NA(β)
	haloperidol ⎫ pimozide ⎬	DA
	lysergic acid diethylamide	5HT
	bicuculline ⎫ picrotoxin ⎬	GABA
	strychnine	glycine
Destroys specific neurons	6OHDA 5,6DHT	NA, DA 5HT

* May be such effective agonists that they increase transmission.

denervated synapses. This may account for some of the more impressive results obtained with levodopa in Parkinsonism in spite of only limited correction of the dopamine depletion (Lloyd *et al* 1973). It is also possible that denervation supersensitivity may be responsible for certain adverse reactions to drugs, such as the dyskinesia produced by levodopa (Carlsson 1970; Klawans *et al* 1970) and phenothiazines (Chase 1972; Klawans 1973).

Tables 3 and 4 are summaries of the mode of action of a number of the drugs which have been discussed in this Chapter, exemplifying the various ways that synaptic transmission can be modified.

TREATMENT FOR CAUSES OF
NEUROLOGICAL DISORDERS

CHAPTER 5
INFECTIONS

The nervous system may be infected by bacteria, viruses, fungi, protozoa or worms. Traditional therapy has at times been bizarre; for example 'the fat of a dragon dried in the sun' (Pliny cited by Juel-Jensen and MacCallum, 1972). The most significant conceptual step forward in the treatment of infection was the realisation, following Erlich's (1909) discovery of salvarsan, that systemically administered agents could be carried by the blood stream to produce selective damage to parasitic organisms without injury to the host. The major advances in the emergence of modern therapy for infective disease have been the introduction of the sulphonamides by Domagk (1935) and of penicillin by Chain, Florey and their colleagues (1940). These developments represent two approaches which have yielded a continuing supply of effective new agents—the synthesis of new drugs based on chemical prediction of their bacteriological properties and the screening of biologically produced materials for possible therapeutic activity.

Antibiotics are substances produced by micro-organisms which are antagonistic, even in high dilution, to the growth or life of other types of micro-organisms. While the term chemotherapeutic agent was at one time restricted to synthetic materials such as the sulphonamides, some of the substances originally discovered as antibiotics are now manufactured chemically, without micro-organisms. The distinction between *antibiotic* and *chemotherapeutic agent* is, therefore, unhelpful. However, in view of the history of semantic separation, the term *antimicrobial agent* is now usually

73

employed to cover both antibiotics and chemotherapeutic substances.

In this Chapter the treatment of infections of the nervous system will be considered in the following stages: (1) Mode of action of antimicrobial drugs; (2) Therapeutic principles; (3) Meningitis; (4) Infective encephalomyelopathies; (5) Focal infection; (6) Infection of peripheral nerves; (7) Tetanus; (8) Diphtheria; (9) Dose regimens and adverse reactions.

MODE OF ACTION OF ANTIMICROBIAL AGENTS

Antimicrobial agents possess the property of selective toxicity to micro-organisms in concentrations which are not harmful to man. They attack pathogens in a number of ways:

Inhibition of cell wall synthesis. Bacteria have a characteristically resilient cell wall which protects them from osmotic damage and affords substantial resistance to mechanical deformation. In Gram-positive organisms this layer is largely made up of a mucopeptide; Gram-negative bacteria have an additional lipoprotein component. There is no comparable structure in mammalian cells so that any substance which specifically inhibits the synthesis of this tough external protection is likely to display selective toxicity to bacteria. Examples of compounds active against the cell wall include the penicillins, cephalosporins, cycloserine and vancomycin.

Inhibition of protein synthesis. A number of antimicrobial agents interfere with the complex series of events whereby messenger ribonucleic acid (RNA) takes the code for aminoacid sequences from desoxyribonucleic acid (DNA) to the ribosome, and transfer RNA picks up aminoacid from the metabolic pool bringing it to the appropriate site for incorporation on the ribosome. Streptomycin blocks the junction of messenger RNA to ribosome; tetracycline interrupts the attachment of aminoacid to ribosome; chloramphenicol inhibits the incorporation of aminoacid into the growing peptide chain. Erythromycin, fusidic acid and lincomycin block the regenerative process essential for repetition of the cycle of reactions at the ribosome (Garrod *et al* 1973).

Inhibition of replication of nucleic acids. Rifampicin inhibits replication of RNA, while nalidixic acid suppresses reproduction of DNA. The antiviral agents cytarabine and idoxuridine impair DNA synthesis.

Folic acid antagonists. Several antimicrobial agents interfere with the synthesis of folinic acid, which, plays an essential role in the manufacture of nucleoprotein. Sulphonamides prevent transformation of para-aminobenzoic acid (to which they are structurally related) into folic acid. Trimethoprim inhibits dihydrofolate reductase, an enzyme concerned with the formation of tetrahydrofolate. Because they act at different stages in the synthesis of folinic acid, sulphonamides and trimethoprim are synergistic. These effects are relatively selective for bacteria; mammalian folate metabolism is not significantly disturbed.

THERAPEUTIC PRINCIPLES

A number of general principles apply to the treatment of infections:
1 Drugs should be administered as early as possible.
2 Dosage must be adequate to reach the site of infection in a therapeutic concentration.
3 Treatment must be continued until the infection is eradicated.
4 When possible, the choice of drug should be determined by bacteriological studies.
5 Combinations of antimicrobial agents can be employed to achieve synergistic effects or to widen the spectrum of activity when treating unidentified or mixed organisms. However, antagonism between drugs can also occur.

Antimicrobial agents fall broadly into two categories (1) those that kill bacteria (bactericidal), (2) those that merely stop bacteria multiplying (bacteristatic) and rely on natural defences to destroy the organism. This distinction may be important because many bactericidal agents are only effective against dividing organisms, so concomitant administration of a bacteristatic drug can reduce therapeutic potency. For example the mortality in a group of patients with meningitis who were treated with benzylpenicillin (bactericidal) alone was 30%; addition of chlortetracycline (bacteristatic) to the same dose of penicillin increased the mortality to 79% (Lepper and Dowling 1951).

Bactericidal agents include the penicillins, aminoglycosides, cotrimoxazole, cephalosporins, polymixin, colistin and isoniazid. Bacteriostatic drugs comprise sulphonamides, tetracyclines, chloramphenicol and para-aminosalicylic acid. From this list it is evident that combinations of bactericidal and bacteristatic agents are not always contraindicated—routine management of tuberculosis involves administration of streptomycin with isoniazid and it has been common practice to combine sulphonamides with penicillins. Experience has failed to reveal any deleterious consequence arising from the use of these therapeutic regimens so there are many exceptions to the generalisation that bacteristatic and bactericidal drugs are incompatible. Furthermore, some drugs which are bacteristatic in low dosage become bactericidal at high tissue concentrations.

Neurological diseases produced by bacteria, viruses, fungi and protozoa are accessible to antimicrobial therapy. The neurological aspects of worm infestations, such as hydatid disease, will not be discussed because when treatable they are attacked surgically.

MENINGITIS

ACUTE PYOGENIC MENINGITIS

The commonest organisms to cause acute pyogenic meningitis are: in children, *Haemophilus influenzae*; in young adults, *Neisseria meningitidis* (meningococcus); in the elderly, *Streptococcus pneumoniae* (pneumonococcus). In spite of the many powerful antimicrobial drugs available, pyogenic meningitis has a high mortality rate-around 11% over the last decade. For *H. influenzae* the figure is 11%, for *N. meningitidis* 2.9% and for *S. pneumoniae* 21% (Garrod *et al* 1973). Neonatal meningitis and secondary adult meningitis have a particularly high mortality owing to the involvement of unusual organisms such as staphylococci, enterobacteria and pseudomonas. Prognosis is substantially better in patients who are treated early. Bacteriological identification of the organism is of crucial importance, but in 12–25% of patients bacteria cannot be recovered from the CSF—sometimes because of previous limited treatment with antimicrobial drugs. The age of the patient offers some guide to the likely organism, the only other clinical clue being the skin eruption often encountered in meningococcal septicaemia. A blood culture and chest X-ray may be helpful.

In patients with severe meningitis, the increased vascular permeability consequent upon meningeal inflammation allows most antimicrobial agents to penetrate the blood–brain and blood–CSF barrier. However, as recovery occurs many drugs are progressively excluded from the central nervous system. Table 5 summarises the

Table 5. Concentration of antimicrobial drugs in CSF, expressed as percentage of concentration in plasma (derived from Garrod *et al* 1973 and Forgan-Smith *et al* 1973).

DRUG	CONCENTRATION
Pyrazinamide	100
Isoniazid	90
Sulphadiazine	40–80
Sulphadimidine	30–80
Chloramphenicol	50
Trimethoprim	50
Sulphamethoxazole	25–33
Tetracycline	10
Rifampicin	10
Benzylpenicillin	10
Ampicillin	10
Cephaloloridine	10
Streptomycin	less than 10
Gentamicin	less than 10

CSF concentrations of a number of antimicrobial agents, expressed as a percentage of their plasma levels. For benzylpenicillin, ampicillin and cephaloridine entry is limited so that high parenteral doses must be given to achieve therapeutic concentrations in the brain and CSF. Streptomycin, gentamicin, kanamycin and polymyxin B penetrate very poorly.

Antimicrobial drugs should be started after samples of CSF and blood have been obtained for examination and culture. If the patient is already unconscious and the CSF is purulent, 10 mg of benzylpenicillin or ampicillin may be injected intrathecally before withdrawing the lumbar puncture needle. In patients who are less severely ill, it is preferable to await microscopy of the CSF before starting treatment. Corticosteroids have no place in the management of acute pyogenic meningitis (deLemos and Haggerty 1969).

The duration of treatment with antimicrobial agents depends upon the clinical course and CSF findings. In the majority of acute infections in which treatment is started early, the CSF becomes sterile over 24 hours and therapy can be stopped in 10–14 days. Persistent fever does not necessarily mean continuing meningitis— it is often caused by drug hypersensitivity (Lambert 1974) or phlebitis consequent upon intravenous therapy (Balagtas *et al* 1970). Other possibilities which should be excluded are brain abscess, paracranial sinus infection and underlying systemic disease such as diabetes mellitus or neoplasia.

Choice of drugs

Meningitis of unknown origin. If examination of the CSF fails to establish the identity of the causal organism, treatment which covers the three common aetiologies should be employed—the most satis-factory drugs have proved to be chloramphenicol or ampicillin. Chloramphenicol is easier to administer, but this advantage must be weighed against the remote risk of marrow depression. The consider-able experience now available with both agents does not reveal any significant difference in their therapeutic efficacy (Garrod *et al* 1973). It is theoretically undesirable to give these drugs together because ampicillin is bactericidal while chloramphenicol is bacteristatic (although combined therapy is often administered without any obviously different result from that obtained with either drug by itself).

Meningococcal meningitis. With the development of many strains of meningococcus resistant to sulphonamides, benzylpenicillin has become the drug of choice.

Pneumococcal meningitis. Benzylpenicillin is also the best antimicrobial agent for pneumococcal meningitis. However, the combination of a potent bactericidal drug and a sensitive pneumococcus is often disappointing. The high mortality is probably attributable to the considerable age and debility of the majority of patients who develop pneumococcal meningitis.

H. Influenzae. The most satisfactory treatment for meningitis due to *H. influenzae* is probably chloramphenicol (Shackelford *et al* 1972); ampicillin is also effective.

Other organisms. Gram-positive. Meningitis due to *Listeria monocytogenes* is becoming recognised more frequently, particularly in the presence of pregnancy, diabetes, alcoholism or lymphoma. The CSF may be predominantly lymphocytic, which can cause confusion with tuberculous meningitis. Ampicillin seems to be the most effective treatment (Garrod *et al* 1973).

Streptococci should be treated with benzylpenicillin. Staphylococci often respond to benzylpenicillin but cloxacillin is also required to cover the possibility of organisms that produce penicillinase.

Gram-negative. Gram-negative bacteria are commonly involved in neonatal meningitis and infection secondary to congenital defects involving the central nervous system. Gentamicin is particularly useful in this setting (Klein *et al* 1971; Newman and Holt 1971) though intrathecal therapy is necessary after acute meningeal inflammation has subsided.

Experience with cotrimoxazole has also been encouraging (Morzaria *et al* 1969)—this combination of sulphamethoxazole and trimethoprim is likely to acquire a firm place in the treatment of meningitis (Boletti and Bertaggia 1971).

Miscellaneous. Leptospiral meningitis is probably not influenced by antimicrobial drugs though penicillins or tetracyclines are sometimes given. There is no specific therapy for aseptic meningitis (viral meningitis, benign lymphocytic meningitis, epidemic serous meningitis).

SUBACUTE AND CHRONIC MENINGITIS

Tuberculous meningitis. Tuberculous meningitis is often difficult to diagnose—delay in starting therapy is probably the most important single factor contributing to its high mortality and morbidity. Patients with either normal CSF or a polymorphonuclear leucocytosis present particular diagnostic problems (Kocen and Parsons 1970). In one recent large series (Freiman and Geefhuysen 1970) some 70% of children with tuberculous meningitis were unconscious on admission to hospital; 40% died and 30% developed sequelae, so that a good recovery was only achieved in 30%. These figures reflect diagnostic difficulties more than therapeutic impotence. Powerful and effective treatment is available and the results are satisfactory if drugs are administered early.

The conventional regimen for tuberculous meningitis has been a combination of streptomycin, para-aminosalicylic acid and isoniazid. The use of intrathecal streptomycin has been controversial; this drug does not readily cross the normal blood–brain and blood–CSF barriers, but it does penetrate inflamed meninges. In the early phase of tuberculous meningitis intramuscular streptomycin is, therefore, effective. Although long term intrathecal streptomycin may be theoretically desirable over the chronic phase, the risk of inducing spinal arachnoiditis renders the ultimate benefit from such treatment difficult to evaluate.

Corticosteroids have been advocated in an attempt to reduce chronic inflammation in patients with tuberculous meningitis. In their critical review of the relevant evidence, Gordon and Parsons (1972) concluded that corticosteroids should be confined to patients with cerebral oedema, spinal block, drug reactions or adrenal failure.

There is no agreement on the use of 'purified protein derivative' (Smith *et al* 1956; Des Prez 1971).

An important new approach to therapy has recently emerged from a careful study of blood and CSF concentrations of anti-tuberculous drugs (Forgan-Smith *et al* 1973). Pyrazinamide achieves excellent penetration into the CSF and there is reasonable entry of rifampicin. With these newer antituberculosis agents available, the routine regimen for managing tuberculous meningitis comprises intramuscular streptomycin with isoniazid, pyrazinamide and rifampicin. Once the acute inflammatory reaction has subsided, the blood–brain and blood–CSF barriers are re-established, so streptomycin can be stopped (provided there is no evidence of tuberculosis outside the central nervous system). Treatment with isoniazid and rifampicin should be continued for the same duration as conventional anti-tuberculous regimens—at least 1 year. Pyridoxine is given to prevent isoniazid induced peripheral neuropathy.

Streptomycin and pyrazinamide are synergistic; it is probably not worth continuing pyrazinamide in long term therapy because it is hepatotoxic and has little antituberculous activity when given without streptomycin.

Over the next few years the value of these new approaches to treatment should become more clearly defined.

Syphilis. The most satisfactory routine treatment for syphilis is procaine penicillin, given by intramuscular injection every day for 20 days. Long acting preparations of benzathine penicillin may be employed if it is considered unlikely that a patient will attend regularly, but the blood levels of benzylpenicillin achieved in this way are lower and more variable. The arguments which have been discussed concerning penetration of the blood–brain and blood–CSF barriers apply to the treatment of neurosyphilis; but because of the increased permeability consequent upon vasculitis and the sensitivity of *Treponema pallidum*, a good response can be obtained in meningo-vascular syphilis and general paresis (general paralysis of the insane). Similar therapy is usually given to patients with tabes dorsalis but the results are less satisfactory, which may be attributable to the relative lack of inflammation and organisms in this condition. The CSF should be re-examined six months after treating neurosyphilis and if there is an excess of leucocytes the course of penicillin should be repeated.

When treatment is started many syphilitic patients develop fever and a transient exacerbation of clinical features (Putkonen *et al* 1966). This *Jarisch-Herxheimer* phenomenon is thought to be an immunological reaction to products released by dying treponemes. It is not related to the dose of penicillin and it is uninfluenced by administration of bismuth and organic arsenicals (Knudson and Aastrup 1965). However, concomitant corticosteroids are reported to reduce its intensity and frequency (De Graciansky and Grupper 1961); a satisfactory regimen is 30–50 mg/day of oral prednisone for 6 days. Syphilitic patients who are allergic to penicillin can be treated effectively with tetracycline for 2 weeks (Garrod *et al* 1973).

Brucellosis. For many years the subacute or chronic meningitis produced by *Brucella* has been treated with tetracyclines. However, recent evidence suggests that cotrimoxazole may be preferable. Therapy is administered over a period of 3 weeks initially and a further 6 weeks if there is a relapse (Garrod *et al* 1973).

Others. Fungal infection of the nervous system caused by *Cryptococcus neoformans* is almost invariably fatal owing to both diagnostic difficulty and therapeutic impotence. However, the latex test for antigen in the CSF has made diagnosis possible even in the absence of viable organisms and recent experience with amphotericin B offers grounds for optimism (Edwards *et al* 1970).

Very limited observations indicate that amphotericin B may also be useful in the amoebic meningitis produced by *Naegleria fowleri* (Apley *et al* 1970).

INFECTIVE ENCEPHALOMYELOPATHY

In the following discussion widespread infection of the brain and spinal cord parenchyma will be reviewed. While some infections are sufficiently acute to produce an inflammatory response and can therefore be described as encephalomyelitis, others are chronic, indolent diseases. To embrace all of these disorders, the term infective encephalomyelopathy will be employed.

Diffuse parenchymal infection of the central nervous system can be caused by many of the organisms which have already been considered—for example *Treponema pallidum* and *Brucella melitensis*. In such diseases, treatment is the same as that used for the corresponding meningitis.

A number of viral and protozoal diseases can also involve the brain and cord. There is current interest in therapy for viral infections such as herpes simplex encephalitis, Creutzfeldt-Jakob disease and poliomyelitis. Allergic reactions of the nervous system to viruses and the controversial status of corticosteroids are discussed later in this Chapter.

Cerebral malaria and trypanosomiasis are treatable protozoal encephalopathies.

VIRAL INFECTIONS

Herpes simplex encephalitis (acute necrotising encephalitis). This condition is fatal in some 55% of cases (Tomlinson and MacCallum 1970) and of the survivors about 50% have serious neurological sequelae. Although uncommon, it is the most frequent cause of severe encephalitis in Great Britain and the United States. In the majority of patients there is no previous history of herpetic lesions and no serum antibody can be found in the early stages. Fever, headache, fits and personality change usually develop acutely. The level of consciousness deteriorates and the clinical picture may closely resemble that of a space occupying lesion in the temporal lobe. Examination of the CSF reveals normal sugar, a predominantly lymphocytic leucocytosis and often an elevated protein concentration. Red cells and xanthochromia may be found. If carotid angiography reveals a mass, this is generally biopsied.

Owing to its sporadic occurrence and the poor documentation of therapeutic regimens, it is difficult to evaluate the results of treating herpes simplex encephalitis (Sarubbi *et al* 1973). Cytarabine is probably the most satisfactory drug available (Farris and Blaw 1972; Juel-Jensen and MacCallum 1972; Oxbury 1974). Diuretics and hypertonic solutions can be employed to decrease cerebral oedema (see Chapter 18). Corticosteroids are widely used for the same purpose—see Chapter 18 (Illis and Merry 1972; Upton 1972). Surgical decompression is sometimes necessary.

Creutzfeldt-Jakob disease (spongiform encephalopathy, Nevin-Jones syndrome). The transfer of Creutzfeldt-Jakob disease to chimpanzees has established its infective aetiology (Gibbs and Gajdusek 1969), which is currently attributed to a slow virus. While no controlled observations are available, it has been reported that the antiviral agent amantadine, currently employed in the treatment of Parkinsonism, may have a therapeutic effect in Creutzfeldt-Jakob disease (Braham 1971; Hamoen 1973; Sanders and Dunn 1973).

Poliomyelitis. There has been a substantial fall in the incidence of poliomyelitis since the introduction of attenuated virus suitable for vaccination—this represents a major therapeutic advance. Once the disease has developed, management is less rewarding; it comprises (1) palliation of symptoms (analgesics for headache and muscle pain), (2) maintenance of respiration (with artificial ventilation if necessary), (3) treatment of secondary infection (pneumonia) or disorders of fluid balance (dehydration).

PROTOZOAL INFECTIONS

Malaria. Cerebral malaria has a poor prognosis, but recently encouraging results have been obtained with a combination of dexamethasone (see Chapter 18) and chloroquine (Woodruff and Dickinson 1968). Quinine can be employed as an alternative to chloroquine. Intravenous heparin (see Chapter 6) has been advocated, but its use should be restricted to cases where there is incontrovertible evidence of disseminated intravascular coagulation (Gilles 1974).

Trypanosomiasis. The most satisfactory drug for cerebral trypanosomiasis is melarsoprol (Gelfand 1973), which has an arsenic content of 20%. Melarsoprol penetrates into the CSF in small but significant quantities. Unfortunately it has prominent adverse effects, but it still achieves a good therapeutic result in the majority of patients.

FOCAL INFECTION

Abscess in the central nervous system. The most important single factor in treating abscesses in the central nervous system is the administration of very large doses of antimicrobial drugs as rapidly as possible—without waiting for the results of bacteriological examination (Garfield 1969). High doses of benzylpenicillin are usually employed pending information on organisms or sensitivities. Since the commonest cause of brain abscess is staphylococcal infection (Beller *et al* 1973), it is reasonable to add cloxacillin to the routine drug regimen.

In a recent study, evidence has been presented that benzyl-penicillin, methicillin and chloramphenicol all penetrate well into abscesses in the central nervous system (Black *et al* 1973). Viable organisms are frequently present in spite of therapeutic concentrations of antimicrobial agents existing within the abscess cavities. These observations indicate that surgical evacuation of pus is always desirable, though direct instillation of antimicrobials is unlikely to improve the outlook and may even have a deleterious effect by increasing the risk of subsequent epilepsy.

Other focal infections. Biopsy evidence is usually required for the diagnosis of tuberculoma or syphiloma (gumma). These focal infections are treated with the drugs employed for tuberculous and syphilitic meningitis respectively. If the lesions are suitably located, medical treatment can be combined with surgical excision.

INFECTION OF PERIPHERAL NERVES

Varicella-Zoster. The varicella-zoster virus infects posterior root ganglia to produce shingles. The virus has been morphologically identified in ganglia, afferent nerves and herpetic skin lesions (Esiri and Tomlinson 1971). Juel-Jensen and MacCallum (1972) advocate local application of idoxuridine. Cytarabine has been claimed to have a useful action if there is involvement of motor nerves or encephalomyelitis. Recent observations suggest that administration of amantadine reduces the incidence of post-herpetic neuralgia (Galbraith 1973). Corticosteroids are generally contraindicated, though it has been proposed that a three week course may be useful for early post-herpetic pain (Juel-Jensen and MacCallum 1972). Other therapeutic regimens for post-herpetic neuralgia are discussed in Chapter 18.

Leprosy. Peripheral nerve involvement is early and extensive in tuberculoid leprosy but it also occurs in lepromatous disease. As there are 10–20 million patients suffering from leprosy, *Mycobacterium leprae* is one of the commonest causes of peripheral neuropathy.

The specific antimicrobial agent for leprosy is dapsone. Where frequent regular treatment is not possible, satisfactory results can be obtained with intramuscular injection of a long acting preparation, acedapsone, which need only be administered once every two months. If patients do not tolerate dapsone or fail to respond, two other drugs have recently been shown to be highly effective. One is rifampicin (Rees *et al* 1970) and the other clofazimine (Karat *et al* 1971). The latter has the advantage of anti-inflammatory properties in addition to an antibacterial action.

Treatment is usually continued until a satisfactory clinical response has been obtained. This generally takes 1–2 years in tuberculoid patients but in lepromatous cases antimicrobial may have to be prolonged for 3–8 years.

Dead *Myco. leprae* bacilli stain irregularly by the Ziehl-Neelsen technique and show degenerative changes on electron microscopy. The proportion of irregularly staining bacilli in a skin biopsy is now taken as an index of therapeutic response (Garrod *et al* 1973). Lepra reactions, such as erythema nodosum leprosum, have been treated with prednisone in the past but recently high doses of clofazimine have been reported to be more effective (Karat 1970).

TETANUS

Tetanus toxin (tetanospasmin) reaches the central nervous system by travelling proximally along peripheral nerves and possibly also via the blood stream (Zacks and Sheff 1966). It inhibits the release of certain transmitters, in particular glycine (Osborne and Bradford 1973). This observation is of considerable interest—glycine has a predominantly inhibitory action at synapses of the spinal cord so loss of inhibition, induced by toxin, could be responsible for the spasms.

Tetanus can be prevented by active immunisation. Once the disease has developed, treatment is directed at (1) *Clostridium tetani*, (2) tetanus toxin, (3) the spasms.

C. tetani. A course of benzylpenicillin or procaine penicillin is given for 10 days and necrotic tissue should be excised from the infected wound if this is identifiable.

Tetanus toxin. Antitoxin is administered to neutralise tetanus toxin. A dose of 10,000 units of horse antitoxin or 3,000 units of human antitoxin is sufficient (Laurence 1973). A small subcutaneous test dose should be given initially to exclude hypersensitivity, though this is very rare with human antitoxin. Provided there is no reaction after 30 minutes, the remaining dose can be administered intravenously. If there is a reaction to the test dose, treatment must be given with considerable caution. Intramuscular injection of the systemic dose of antitoxin is less likely to provoke anaphylaxis, but this route is probably not so effective as intravenous administration. An antihistamine (e.g. diphenhydramine 25 mg by intramuscular injection) or a glucocorticoid (e.g. dexamethasone 8 mg by intravenous injection) may be necessary if hypersensitivity is encountered.

Spasms. Spasms can be localised or generalised. They are often precipitated by non-specific stimuli so disturbances should be minimised. Diazepam (see Chapter 15) is the most satisfactory drug for treating spasms because it induces both sedation and muscle relaxation. It can be given by intramuscular injection or by intravenous infusion, increasing the dose until spasms are alleviated or respiratory depression occurs. If artificial ventilation proves necessary, muscle relaxation is established with pancuronium or tubocurarine (see Chapter 12). Careful surveillance is required to detect pneumonia, electrolyte changes or autonomic disturbances (Corbett *et al* 1973).

In spite of these measures tetanus still has a high mortality rate; drug addicts are a particularly vulnerable section of the population.

DIPHTHERIA

Corynebacterium diphtheriae generates a toxin which induces peripheral neuropathy. Cycloplegia and bulbar palsy are the commonest manifestations but the respiratory muscles and limbs may also be involved.

The only specific treatment is antitoxin, which should be administered as soon as possible after diagnosis. Hypersensitivity must be excluded by skin and eye tests (0.1 ml of 10% antitoxin injected intradermally and dropped in the conjunctival sac). Antitoxin may then be given, 10,000–100,000 units according to the severity of symptoms and signs (half intramuscularly and half intravenously). Effective prophylaxis can be achieved with toxoid.

DOSE REGIMENS AND ADVERSE REACTIONS

The pharmacokinetics, dose regimens and adverse effects of antimicrobial agents will now be reviewed in the following order: (1) Drugs for bacterial infections other than tuberculosis and leprosy; (2) Drugs for tuberculosis; (3) Drugs for leprosy; (4) Drugs for viral infections; (5) Drugs for fungal and protozoal infections.

In the following account the plasma concentrations quoted represent levels which should be exceeded in order to achieve a therapeutic response. Because the plasma half-life is short for many antimicrobial agents, the time relationship of blood sampling to dosage is important; the values discussed derive from plasma taken midway between doses (Garrod 1973).

Drugs for bacterial infections other than tuberculosis and leprosy

Chloramphenicol. Chloramphenicol is readily absorbed from the gut, peak plasma concentrations being reached in about 2 hours. After intramuscular injection the plasma concentration rises more slowly and persists longer. Some 60% is bound to proteins. A large fraction of chloramphenicol is conjugated or reduced in the liver; most of an orally administered dose is excreted in the urine over 6 hours. The plasma concentration should exceed 5 μg/ml for a therapeutic action. In meningitis, a dose of 1.25 g every 6 hours may be given by intramuscular or intravenous injection, changing to oral administration after about 48 hours. Toxic reactions include stomatitis due to *Candida* infections, encephalopathy, optic neuropathy, marrow aplasia and, in infants, the 'grey syndrome' (vomiting, abdominal distension, sweating, pallor). Chloramphenicol has the unusual property of inhibiting protein synthesis in the host—under certain circumstances this may reduce immunological responsiveness (Garrod *et al* 1973).

Cotrimoxazole. This is a combination of trimethoprim (80 mg) and sulphamethoxazole (400 mg) which takes advantage of the synergism that stems from both drugs acting at successive stages in the same metabolic pathway—synthesis of folinic acid. The usual dose is 2 tablets twice daily. This can be increased to 2 tablets thrice daily, but toxic effects become much more frequent. Adverse reactions are those of trimethoprim and sulphamethoxazole.

Gentamicin. Gentamicin is poorly absorbed from the gastro-intestinal tract. Intramuscular injections give peak plasma concentrations after $\frac{1}{2}$–1 hour, with a half-life of $1\frac{1}{2}$ hours. Some 80% is excreted in the urine. The plasma concentration should exceed 2.5 μg/ml. Gentamicin does not penetrate the normal blood–brain barrier to any worthwhile extent. In treating neonatal meningitis an intramuscular dose of 3–6 mg/kg/day can be combined with 1 mg/day by intrathecal injection. For adults, 80 mg is usually given intramuscularly thrice daily, with 2 mg intrathecally every 2–3 days over 2–3 weeks. Adverse reactions include ototoxicity (usually involving the vestibular system but sometimes the auditory division), occasional renal or hepatic damage, convulsions and hypersensitivity. Toxicity is unusual unless kidney function is impaired.

Penicillins. Benzylpenicillin (penicillin G) has been modified to produce a range of antimicrobial agents with more prolonged effects (e.g. benzathine penicillin and procaine penicillin) and different activity spectra (e.g. ampicillin and cloxacillin).

Ampicillin. Ampicillin is readily absorbed from the gastrointestinal tract, peak plasma concentrations being reached 1–2 hours after administration. Some 20% becomes bound to plasma proteins. About 30% of an orally administered dose is excreted in the urine. The concentration of ampicillin in plasma should exceed 5 μg/ml. Because of the blood–brain barrier, high doses are required for infections of the central nervous system. About 2 g by intravenous injection every 4 hours is a satisfactory initial regimen, transferring to intramuscular injections after 2–3 days. The intrathecal dose is 10 mg. Adverse effects are rare; the main problem is hypersensitivity. Patients who are allergic to ampicillin commonly cross react with other penicillins and sometimes to cephalosporins. Excessive intake can induce convulsions.

Benzathine penicillin (*benzathine penicillin G*). An intramuscular injection of 900 mg of benzathine penicillin releases benzylpenicillin in a therapeutic concentration for some 14 days.

Benzylpenicillin (*penicillin G*). Benzylpenicillin is ineffective when given orally because it is rapidly inactivated in the stomach. Peak plasma concentrations occur about 30 minutes after intramuscular injection. Some 60% appears in the urine after 1 hour and 95% after four hours. One mega unit is equivalent to 600 mg. The plasma concentration should exceed 5 μg/ml. Following intramuscular injection 200 mg yields adequate plasma levels for about 5 hours. In view of the concentration gradient between plasma and CSF, infections of the central nervous system should be treated with large doses, initially up to 1.2 g every two hours via an intravenous infusion. After 2–3 days the frequency of administering this dose may be reduced to a 4 hourly regimen and the intramuscular route can be employed. A dose of 10 mg can be given intrathecally.

Adverse reactions include hypersensitivity, convulsions and encephalopathy. High concentrations of benzylpenicillin, encountered in overdosage or renal failure, predispose to neurotoxicity. Encephalopathy is a particular risk in patients undergoing cardiopulmonary bypass, probably because small cerebral emboli lead to increased permeability across the blood–brain barrier, allowing normal plasma concentrations of benzylpenicillin to result in excess brain levels (Dobell *et al* 1966). Intravenous penicillinase protects animals from experimental encephalopathy induced by benzylpenicillin (Gutnick and Prince 1971)—an observation which may have therapeutic implications in man.

Cloxacillin. Cloxacillin is active against those staphylococci which are resistant to benzylpenicillin. There is extensive binding to plasma proteins. In staphylococcal infection of the central nervous system 1 g may be given by intravenous injection every 3 hours. Toxicity resembles that of ampicillin.

Procaine penicillin (*procaine penicillin G*). Intramuscular injections of procaine penicillin are employed where a depot of benzylpenicillin is required to maintain therapeutic concentrations in the plasma for 12–24 hours. The usual dose is 600 mg daily.

Sulphamethoxazole. Sulphamethoxazole is well absorbed, 60% becoming bound to plasma proteins. Some 25% is excreted in the urine over 8 hours, mainly in the form of acetylated derivatives. The initial dose is 2 g followed by 1 g twice daily. An ample fluid intake is desirable to facilitate excretion. Adverse effects comprise anorexia, nausea, lassitude, sedation, fever and methaemoglobin-aemia. Occasionally renal complications result from crystals formed in the urine. Hypothyroidism, vertigo, tinnitus and hypersensitivity also occur.

Tetracycline. Tetracycline is incompletely and irregularly absorbed. The plasma half-life is 8–9 hours; there is variable binding to plasma proteins. Excretion takes place through the bile and the urine. The plasma concentration should exceed 2.5 μg/ml for most organisms against which tetracycline is used. The dose is 1–2 g/day by intravenous infusion or 250–1,000 mg four times daily by mouth. Adverse effects include candidiasis, diarrhoea, staining of teeth in children, renal or hepatic damage and benign intracranial hypertension.

Trimethoprim. Trimethoprim is readily absorbed, peak plasma concentrations occurring after some 3 hours. Some 50% is protein bound. Up to 50% is excreted in the urine over 24 hours. The usual dose is 1.5 g/day. Adverse effects include nausea and diarrhoea, which can be corrected by intramuscular injections of calcium folinate, 3–10 mg daily for 10–15 days.

Drugs for tuberculosis

Isoniazid. Isoniazid is well absorbed from the gut, reaching peak plasma concentrations after 1–3 hours. It is inactivated by acetylation and 50–70% is excreted in the urine in 24 hours. The rate of acetylation is genetically determined. If blood samples are taken 6 hours after oral administration of isoniazid (10 mg/kg), rapid acetylators have a plasma level of 2.5 μg/ml while in slow acetylators the plasma concentration is 3–6 μg/ml. For most strains of *Myco. tuberculosis* a therapeutic effect is achieved at a concentration of 0.2–1 μg/ml. The usual dose for tuberculous meningitis is 100 mg thrice daily, which may be given by intramuscular injection if the patient is unconscious. Adverse reactions include restlessness, anorexia, difficulty with micturition, hypersensitivity reactions, encephalopathy, and optic or peripheral neuropathy. Concomitant administration of pyridoxine 100 mg daily is desirable as prophylaxis against peripheral and optic neuropathy.

Pyrazinamide. Pyrazinamide is readily absorbed after oral administration, peak plasma concentrations occurring at 2 hours; the plasma half-life is 9 hours. Excretion of free drug and metabolites occurs through the kidney. The dose range is 0.5–1 g, twice or thrice daily. Toxic reactions include anorexia, nausea, difficulty in micturition, disturbances in liver function, hyperuricaemia and hypersensitivity.

Rifampicin (rifampin). Rifampicin is well absorbed from the gastrointestinal tract, reaching maximum plasma concentrations in 2 hours; some 75% is bound to plasma proteins. It is acetylated and a major fraction is excreted in the bile. Concentrations of 0.2–0.5 μg/ml are effective against most strains of *Myco. tuberculosis*. The usual dose is 900 mg daily. Adverse effects comprise nausea, thrombocytopenia, red discolouration of body fluids, disturbances of liver function (which are often transient) and hypersensitivity.

Streptomycin. Oral administration of streptomycin is ineffective. Intramuscular injections lead to peak plasma concentrations in 1–2 hours with therapeutic concentrations (in excess of 7 μg/ml) persisting for some 8 hours. About 30% becomes bound to proteins. Up to 70% is excreted in the urine in 24 hours; accumulation can occur in the presence of renal disease. Streptomycin is only detectable in the CSF if the meninges are inflamed. In the early stages of tuberculous meningitis, the dose is 1 g daily. The intrathecal dose is 20–50 mg. Adverse reactions include ototoxicity (usually but not always vestibular), hypersensitivity and impairment of neuro-muscular transmission. Intrathecal administration can lead to arachnoiditis.

Drugs for leprosy

Acedapsone (DADDS). This is a diacetyl derivative of dapsone which is prepared as an intramuscular injection in oil. It undergoes slow hydrolysis to release dapsone. A single administration of 225 mg yields a therapeutic effect for 77 days.

Clofazimine. Clofazimine is absorbed from the gastrointestinal tract and is excreted extremely slowly; unchanged drug is detectable in the urine for several weeks after administration. The normal dose is 100 mg, 2–3 times a week. Clofazimine is particularly effective in controlling lepra reactions such as erythema nodosum leprosum, for which the dose is increased to 200–400 mg daily. Adverse reactions include red discolouration of the skin and urine. Blue-black pigmentation of lesions may occur. Headache, abdominal pain and diarrhoea have also been reported.

Dapsone. Dapsone is well absorbed from the gastrointestinal tract, reaching peak plasma concentrations in 1–3 hours. The drug is still detectable 8–12 days after administration. Some 50% becomes bound to plasma proteins. Enterohepatic recirculation occurs, excretion taking place mainly through the kidney. Treatment is started with 25 mg weekly, slowly increasing to a maximum of 200 mg/week. The commonest adverse reactions are skin eruptions, but other problems that may be encountered include anorexia, nausea, headache, giddiness, tachycardia, haemolytic anaemia, psychosis and hepatic damage. Marrow depression is a rare complication.

Rifampicin. For details see above, in the discussion of drugs for tuberculosis.

Drugs for viral infections

Cytarabine (cytosine arabinoside). Cytarabine is an inhibitor of DNA synthesis, widely used in the treatment of leukaemia and subsequently found to have antiviral actions. It is administered by intravenous infusion; up to 10 mg/kg/day can be given initially. After three days the dose should be reduced so that a total of 2.5–4 g is administered over a week. Adverse reactions include marrow suppression, nausea, vomiting and stomatitis.

Idoxuridine. Idoxuridine, an analogue of thymidine, becomes incorporated into an abnormal DNA. It is very insoluble, which allows high concentrations to be applied topically without producing systemic reactions. It dissolves in dimethylsulphoxide and is usually administered for 4 days in a 40% solution. If the eye is involved in shingles, idoxuridine cream (0.5%) may be applied inside the lower lid, four times daily. Adverse reactions to idoxuridine include leucopenia, stomatitis and alopecia.

Amantadine. The pharmacokinetics, dosage and toxicity of amantadine are discussed in Chapter 13.

Corticosteroids. Current opinions concerning administration of corticosteroids in tuberculous meningitis have already been mentioned.

In encephalomyelitis it is difficult to separate the relative contributions of invasive and immunological damage; from a therapeutic viewpoint, the issue is whether or not to use corticosteroids. While some consider that steroids are generally unhelpful (Illis and Gostling 1972), others (Webb 1969) conclude that they can be useful by the time postinfectious demyelinating encephalomyelitis develops. There is general agreement that corticosteroids are deleterious if taken during the initial infection when viraemia occurs and interferon is being produced. However, administration of corticosteroids at the stage of clinical encephalitis may have a beneficial action on brain swelling and inflammatory infiltration (Upton *et al* 1971; Upton

1972). A suitable starting dose of dexamethasone is 4 mg every 6 hours; this can be reduced over 10–14 days.

Drugs for fungal and protozoal infections

Amphotericin B. Amphotericin B is poorly absorbed from the gut. Following intraveous injection some 10% is bound to plasma proteins. Therapeutic doses give peak plasma concentrations of 0.5–2.0 μg/ml; entry into the CSF is limited unless the meninges are inflamed. Elimination from the body is slow, the plasma half-life being 24 hours. Amphotericin B should be administered intravenously in 0.5–1 litre of 5% dextrose infused over 3–4 hours. An initial dose of 0.25 mg/kg/day may be increased by 0.25 mg each day according to tolerance until 1 mg/kg/day is reached. The concentration injected should never be higher than 0.1 mg/ml and it is desirable to change the site of administration to avoid phlebitis. Intrathecal injections can also be given, starting with 0.025 mg in 5% dextrose, diluted with 5 ml of CSF; this dose can be increased up to 0.5 mg. Intrathecal administration may be repeated 2–3 times a week but a total of 15 mg should not be exceeded by this route. Toxic reactions comprise fever, nausea, vomiting, anaemia, hypokalaemia and a rising blood urea. Severe pyrexia can sometimes be reduced by adding 25–50 mg of hydrocortisone to each infusion. Frequent monitoring of blood biochemistry is necessary during treatment. Renal damage is usually reversible following a total intake of amphotericin B up to 5 g; beyond this, kidney lesions can be permanent.

Chloroquine. Chloroquine is readily absorbed from the gastro-intestinal tract and 50% becomes bound to plasma proteins. Metabolism and excretion are slow, the plasma half-life being 6–7 days. Chloroquine collects in certain tissues. While liver, spleen and kidney may contain chloroquine in 200–700 times the concentration present in plasma, the central nervous system only accumulates 10–30 times the plasma level.

The usual initial dose of chloroquine employed in cerebral malaria is 300 mg (of the base) by intramuscular injection together with 200 mg administered via an intravenous infusion over 45 minutes.

Intramuscular injections of 300 mg should be repeated every 6 hours while the patient remains in coma, converting to oral therapy as consciousness is regained. Treatment is continued until a total dose of 1.5 g has been given. Adverse reactions include convulsions, psychosis, myopathy, pigmentation of the skin, methaemoglobin-aemia and electrocardiographic disturbances. Chronic administration can induce opacification of the cornea and retinopathy. If given too rapidly, intravenous chloroquine may precipitate hypotension and can cause sudden death.

Melarsoprol (melarsen oxide, mel B). Melarsoprol is an organic arsenical. It is administered by slow intravenous injection of a 3.6% solution in propylene glycol. Care must be taken to avoid leakage outside the vein as it is extremely irritant. Courses of treatment for 3 days at a time are employed, gradually building up the dose. In the first series, injections of 2.0, 2.5 and 3.0 ml are given each day. After an interval of 7 days a further 3 day course comprises doses of 3.5, 4.0 and 4.5 ml. Another week is then allowed to elapse before giving 5 ml daily for the last 3 day course. Dosage may have to be reduced if toxicity is encountered. Adverse effects include headache, vomiting, mania, encephalopathy and exfoliative dermatitis. A reaction resembling the *Jarisch-Herxheimer* effect can also occur.

Quinine. Intravenous quinine can be used as an alternative to chloroquine in the initial treatment of cerebral malaria. The dose is 500 mg (of the base) infused in 500 ml of isotonic saline over 30–45 minutes. This can be repeated every 6–8 hours until a response is obtained. Quinine is discussed further in Chapter 17.

CHAPTER 6
VASCULAR DISEASE

Over the nineteenth century, treatment of vascular disease of the nervous system comprised application of ice to the forehead and mustard plasters to the soles of the feet, calves of the legs, or nape of the neck. Therapeutic activity was attributed to arsenic, strychnine, calomel, bromide and croton oil. Leeches and venesection were considered appropriate 'if the heart be hypertrophied and contracting strongly', the purpose being 'to sustain the vital powers and restore, if possible, the cerebral circulation' (Inman 1862). Current treatment is directed to the same ends—some progress has occurred but advances have been limited. In view of the prevalence, morbidity and mortality of cerebrovascular disease, an improvement in its management represents one of the most pressing challenges now facing neurology.

Cerebrovascular disease is responsible for about half the neurological admissions to hospital (Miller Fisher *et al* 1970). Of these, 90% are infarcts and the remainder are haemorrhages; there is, however, some overlap because both pathologies can be present together. The clinical distinction between infarction and haemorrhage is frequently difficult and often impossible. Nevertheless, rational treatment depends upon identification of the cause of the lesion so it may be necessary to perform computerised axial tomography, angiography, measure the cerebral blood flow and examine the cerebrospinal fluid in order to make a diagnosis. After full investigation there still remain many patients in whom the causal pathology cannot be established with certainty.

Therapeutic approaches to cerebrovascular disease will be reviewed by considering: (1) Predisposing factors; (2) Inadequate intracranial perfusion; (3) Intracranial haemorrhage; (4) Hypertensive encephalopathy. Various arteritic pathologies and migraine can lead to infarction of portions of the nervous system, but they are discussed in Chapters 7 and 18. The role of certain drugs in producing vascular lesions is discussed in Chapter 11.

PREDISPOSING FACTORS

HYPERTENSION

Hypertension predisposes to both cerebral infarction (because of the increased incidence of atherosclerosis) and cerebral haermorrhage (by producing microaneurysms). Treatable causes of hypertension include renal disease, phaeochromocytoma, primary aldosteronism, Cushing's syndrome and coarctation of the aorta. However, in over 90% of hypertensive patients no aetiology can be found. Hypotensive therapy is usually undertaken if a diastolic pressure over 100 mm Hg is found on repeated examination. Treatment is directed at maintaining the diastolic pressure at 90–100 mm Hg (Marshall 1973). The benefits deriving from adequate reduction of the blood pressure have recently been demonstrated by Beevers *et al* (1973).

In hypertension the mechanisms of autoregulation of cerebral blood flow operate normally. In consequence, there is no fall in cerebral perfusion when the blood pressure is brought down to normal levels, though there is a risk of ischaemia in the presence of severe extracranial arterial stenoses, or if excessive antihypertensive therapy precipitates hypotension.

A wide range of drugs are available for the treatment of hypertension. In mild cases, a thiazide diuretic (see hydrochlorothiazide, Chapter 12) may afford adequate control. More potent drugs include noradrenergic neuron blockers (adrenergic neuron blockers), beta noradrenergic receptor blockers (beta adrenoceptor blockers) and noradrenergic partial agonists. The choice between drugs depends upon the balance between therapeutic response and toxicity in individual patients.

Adrenergic neuron blockers

Adrenergic neuron blockers inhibit the release of noradrenaline by nerve impulses. In high doses they also deplete stores of noradrenaline at the nerve endings.

Guanethidine. Some 30–50% of an orally administered dose of guanethidine is absorbed; it does not readily cross the blood–brain barrier. Excretion occurs predominantly in the urine, but a proportion is retained in the body for several days. An initial dose of 10–20 mg daily is usually increased by 10 mg at weekly intervals until a satisfactory response is obtained. Dosage is seldom raised beyond 300 mg/day. Dose dependent adverse reactions include diarrhoea, hypotension, lassitude, dyspnoea, oedema, nasal congestion, parotid pain, tremor, failure of ejaculation and frequency of micturition. Uraemia may be precipitated in patients with renal failure; there have also been reports of exacerbation of peptic ulceration. Of these unwanted effects, diarrhoea is particularly common.

Bethanidine. Bethanidine is rapidly absorbed from the gastro-intestinal tract. Most of the drug is excreted in the urine over 12 hours. The starting dose is 10 mg twice daily by mouth, increasing by 5 to 10 mg each day until a satisfactory control of blood pressure occurs or toxicity is encountered. An average maintenance dose is 100 mg/day. Adverse reactions are similar to those occurring with guanethidine but diarrhoea and parotid pain are less troublesome.

Beta adrenoceptor blockers

These drugs reduce the force of contraction of the heart and they also mediate a hypotensive action through the central nervous system.

Propranolol. In the treatment of hypertension (Prichard and Gillam 1969) an initial intake of 10 mg four times daily can be doubled every week, until an adequate response is obtained or unwanted effects develop. The usual maintenance dose is about 480 mg/day. For details of pharmacokinetics and toxicity see Chapter 14.

Oxprenolol. A dose of 80 mg daily is slowly increased until the blood pressure falls to required levels or adverse reactions appear. Oxprenolol is considered in more detail in Chapter 14.

Noradrenergic partial agonists

As discussed in Chapter 4, these drugs may either increase or decrease synaptic transmission, depending upon the balance between their agonist–antagonist activities. Noradrenergic partial agonists may exert their main effect on hypertension by driving noradrenergic hypotensive pathways. Alternatively they may block a noradrenergic pressor system, or modify presynaptic function. Although the significance of their various pharmacological effects remains obscure, it is now generally accepted that their main site of action is the central rather than the peripheral nervous system.

Alpha methyldopa. When the hypotensive action of alpha methyldopa was first discovered it was attributed to inhibition of the enzyme L-aromatic aminoacid decarboxylase, which is involved in the synthesis of noradrenaline. However, subsequent studies have indicated that impaired production of noradrenaline is not an adequate explanation for the reduction of blood pressure. Formation of a partial agonist, alpha methylnoradrenaline, seems to be of more importance.

About 50% of an orally administered dose of alpha methyldopa is absorbed, peak plasma concentrations being reached in 3–6 hours; some 90% is excreted over 48 hours, in urine and faeces. The dose range is 0.5 to 3.0 g/day. Initial drowsiness is not usually sustained. More troublesome adverse effects are depression, nightmares, dryness of the mouth, nasal congestion, nausea, headache, oedema, and hypotension. The direct Coombs test often converts but this seldom leads to haemolytic anaemia. There have been occasional reports of leucopenia and disturbances of liver function.

Clonidine. Clonidine is a relatively new hypotensive drug. It is a noradrenergic partial agonist. The usual dose in hypertension is 0.1 mg thrice daily, slowly increasing up to 4.5 mg/day if necessary. These doses are much larger than those employed in the prophylaxis of migraine. Adverse reactions are listed in Chapter 18.

OTHER PREDISPOSING FACTORS

Cerebrovascular lesions can result from such predisposing conditions as cardiac arrhythmia, myocardial infarction, diabetes mellitus, hyperlipidaemia, anaemia, polycythaemia, syphilis, leukaemia and sickle cell disease. Treatment of these disorders is seldom undertaken by a neurologist and is therefore outside the scope of this book. Vascular surgery may be required for extracranial arterial stenosis.

INADEQUATE INTRACRANIAL PERFUSION

Inadequate cerebral perfusion falls into 4 major categories: (1) Transient ischaemic attacks (TIA)—these are focal neurological deficits of sudden onset (seconds) and brief duration (minutes) followed by complete recovery within 24 hours. (2) Stroke in evolution —progressive deterioration of neurological signs occurring over a minimum of 6 hours. (3) Completed stroke—a stable neurological disability which has persisted for more than 24 hours. (4) Cerebral venous thrombosis—usually associated with serious disease outside the nervous system, in particular infection.

The precise times specified here are somewhat arbitrary and the term *stroke* is also employed for abrupt neurological deficits produced by intracranial haemorrhage. While haemorrhagic lesions usually have a catastrophically sudden onset, they sometimes progress less rapidly, displaying the temporal profile of a stroke in evolution. Nevertheless, the definitions which have been offered provide a useful framework upon which a programme of management can be built.

TRANSIENT ISCHAEMIC ATTACKS

Natural history of transient ischaemic attacks (TIA)

Patients who experience a TIA have a much higher risk of developing a stroke than the rest of the population of comparable age and sex (Acheson and Hutchinson 1964; 1971; Whisnant *et al* 1973a).

The risks are considerably greater for attacks in carotid territory than those involving the vertebrobasilar circulation (Marshall 1973a). From a therapeutic viewpoint the diagnosis is of importance because treatment can reduce the chance of a stroke (Millikan 1971; Whisnant *et al* 1973b).

Mechanism of TIA

Most attacks are produced by emboli arising from atheromatous plaques in the extracranial arteries or the larger intracranial vessels. Clot formed in the heart provides another source. A minority of episodes are caused by a fall in arterial perfusion pressure, particularly if stenotic arterial lesions are present.

Treatment of TIA

HYPERTENSIVE PATIENTS

If the diastolic pressure is above 100 mm Hg, therapy is directed to establishing a level of 90–100 mm Hg. In the occasional patient with hypertension and evidence of an extracranial stenosis (such as a localised bruit in the neck) carotid angiography and if necessary endarterectomy should be performed before introducing hypotensive treatment. This precaution reduces the risk of precipitating cerebral ischaemia when the blood pressure is reduced.

NORMOTENSIVE PATIENTS

Angiography is generally undertaken providing the patient's health would allow endarterectomy if a surgically accessible stenotic lesion is found. Irrespective of whether investigations and operative procedures are pursued, the patient should be given drugs to inhibit either platelet adhesiveness or blood coagulation. Treatment is usually continued for a year, to allow endothelium to grow over areas of atheromatous ulceration. After this time, an attempt is made to stop therapy by gradually reducing dosage. Recent evidence suggests that shorter courses of treatment may be adequate (Whisnant *et al* 1973b). If attacks recur, therapy should be started again

(Marshall 1973a). Table 6 shows Frank's (1971) analysis of published reports on the results of surgical and anticoagulant management in 695 patients followed over an average of 40 months. While it is not entirely satisfactory to compare different forms of treatment unless the selection of patients is carefully controlled, these figures indicate that active management of TIA is worthwhile in relation to morbidity but not mortality.

Table 6. Experience with 695 patients suffering from TIA. Untreated course is compared with anticoagulant therapy and surgery. Pooled results from several centres adjusted for a follow-up period of 40 months (Frank 1971).

	UNTREATED	ANTICOAGULANTS	SURGERY
Patients with TIA	280 (100%)	246 (100%)	169 (100%)
Progressing to stroke	54 (19%)	13 (5%)	18 (11%)
Death rate	57 (20%)	43 (18%)	28 (17%)

Drugs which inhibit platelet aggregation

There has recently been considerable interest in the therapeutic potential of drugs which reduce platelet adhesiveness. The mechanism of action of these agents is not fully understood, though modification of adenine nucleotides may be involved (Zucker 1973).

Aspirin. Aspirin inhibits platelet aggregation and prolonged administration in low dosage (300 mg twice daily) has a prophylactic effect in TIA (Wood 1972). Patients with amaurosis fugax also benefit from aspirin, (Harrison *et al* 1971). Its pharmacokinetics and toxicity are reviewed in Chapter 18.

Sulphinpyrazone. Sulphinpyrazone is a uricosuric agent employed in the treatment of gout. Because it inhibits platelet aggregation, therapeutic studies have recently been undertaken in TIA and amaurosis fugax. Initial results have been encouraging; there is evidence that the frequency of attacks is reduced by sulphinpyrazone, though it has not been established that the incidence of stroke is decreased (Evans 1972).

Sulphinpyrazone is readily absorbed from the gastrointestinal tract. A large fraction becomes bound to plasma proteins; the plasma half-life is about 3 hours. The dose range is 200–800 mg/day according to tolerance. Unwanted effects include nausea, vomiting, abdominal pain and exacerbation of peptic ulcers. There have been reports of leucopenia and thrombocytopenia.

Dipyridamole. Dipyridamole is another drug which reduces platelet aggregation. It has not proved to be effective in unselected cerebral ischaemia (Acheson *et al* 1969) though it has been useful in the more limited context of embolism from prosthetic heart valves (Sullivan *et al* 1968). The dose is 100 mg four times daily; adverse reactions include nausea, vomiting, diarrhoea, headache and dizziness.

Anticoagulants

Oral anticoagulants are commonly employed in the treatment of TIA. They comprise coumarin derivatives such as warfarin or dicoumarol, and indandiones such as phenindione. Oral anticoagulants take 16 to 72 hours to achieve an effect and their activity persists for several days after stopping treatment. They operate by inhibiting the formation of clotting factors II (prothrombin), VII, IX and X. Overdosage can be corrected by vitamin K_1 (phytomenadione), 10 mg given as a slow intravenous injection, which takes 3–5 hours to act.

There is wide variation in the pharmacokinetics of anticoagulants in different individuals. It is therefore necessary to titrate the dose for each patient by regularly estimating the delay in blood clotting by means of the prothrombin time, which should be kept 2–3 times the normal value (this differs from one laboratory to another). An estimate of anticoagulant activity is necessary about 40 hours after the first dose. Over the initial period of treatment, assays should be repeated every 2 weeks; as control becomes stabilised the interval can gradually be extended to 4 weeks (Marshall 1968).

Numerous interactions can occur between anticoagulants and other drugs. Increased effect may be caused by displacement from binding sites on plasma proteins (e.g. by aspirin, phenylbutazone) or competition for metabolising enzymes (e.g. by phenytoin, tolbutamide). Decreased anticoagulant action can follow induction of metabolising enzymes (e.g. by barbiturates, griseofulvin), or accumulation of clotting factors (e.g. by oral contraceptives). Termination of treatment with certain drugs can also present problems in patients receiving anticoagulants; for example stopping barbiturates can precipitate a brisk rise in anticoagulant plasma levels because of reduced enzyme induction.

Anticoagulant therapy is contraindicated in patients with uncontrolled hypertension and other diseases associated with haemorrhage such as peptic ulceration, cirrhosis, leukaemia and bacterial endocarditis.

Warfarin. Warfarin is readily absorbed from the gastrointestinal tract and binds extensively to plasma proteins. The plasma half-life is about 44 hours. It is metabolised in the liver, the products being excreted in the urine. A reasonable loading dose is 40 mg, followed after 48 hours by 3–10 mg daily according to the prothrombin time. The major adverse reaction is haemorrhage, particularly into the renal and gastrointestinal tract.

Dicoumarol (bishydroxycoumarin). The absorption of dicoumarol is erratic. A substantial fraction binds to plasma proteins; the plasma half-life ranges from 25–100 hours. An initial dose of 600 mg should be followed after 48 hours by 25–100 mg daily according to the prothrombin time. Unwanted effects include haemorrhage, nausea, vomiting and diarrhoea.

Phenindione. The rate of absorption of phenindione is unpredictable. A large proportion is bound to plasma proteins; its plasma half-life is 5–6 hours. A suitable starting dose is 200 mg, followed after 24 hours by 100 mg. The daily intake is then adjusted according to the prothrombin time, the usual range being 75–125 mg. While the commonest adverse reaction is haemorrhage, phenindione can cause hypersensitivity reactions involving the skin, marrow, liver or kidney. Because of the risk of hypersensitivity, indandiones are generally regarded as less satisfactory than coumarin derivatives.

STROKE IN EVOLUTION

Stroke in evolution is most commonly caused by progressive intra-cranial ischaemia, but may occasionally be due to extension of a haemorrhage. It is important to establish a precise diagnosis; progressive infarction should be treated with intravenous heparin (Marshall 1968), whereas cerebral haemorrhage may be catastrophic-ally exacerbated by this management.

Although diagnosis is usually correct, a confident distinction between infarction and haemorrhage cannot always be made. Ross Russell and Harrison (1973) have recently reviewed the factors determining diagnosis: the most useful clinical feature in favour of infarction is a history of previous small episodes, while the main clues to haemorrhage are headache, vomiting and neck stiffness. The diagnosis can often be resolved by finding blood at lumbar puncture, though in 10–20% of intracerebral haemorrhages the CSF remains clear. Diagnostic errors are unlikely if facilities are available for skull X-ray, ultrasound, brain scan, computerised axial tomography and angiography. Unfortunately, there always remains an element of risk in the use of anticoagulants because haemorrhage may occur into a cerebral infarct. Nevertheless, anticoagulant therapy is usually bene-ficial in ischaemic stroke in evolution (Carter 1960); anticoagulants are firmly indicated if the cerebral lesion can be attributed to an obvious source of emboli such as a myocardial infarct.

In treating a stroke in evolution, an anticoagulant effect is required as quickly as possible. The optimum action of oral anticoagulants takes many hours to develop (see above), so it is usual to start with intravenous heparin; this is continued until satisfactory oral therapy has been established. Anticoagulants should be restricted to patients with a diastolic blood pressure less than 100 mm Hg (with or without hypotensive therapy).

Heparin. Heparin is a highly ionised acidic mucopolysaccharide which is normally present in mast cells. Its anticoagulant effect is achieved by a rapid reaction with plasma proteins that are involved in the clotting mechanism. Heparin also has slight vasodilating proper-ties and it releases lipoprotein lipase. It is metabolised in the liver and excreted in the urine, the plasma half-life being 50–150 minutes.

Intravenous administration of heparin produces an immediate anticoagulant effect. For a reasonably sustained action, heparin should be given every 4–6 hours or by continuous infusion. The usual dose is 500 mg (50,000 units) daily. An initial bolus injection of 50 mg is generally followed by infusion of 250 mg in 1 litre of isotonic saline or glucose (Marshall 1968). The dose can be adjusted according to the whole blood clotting time. The normal value is 5–7 minutes; a satisfactory therapeutic level of heparin extends this to some 15 minutes.

The main adverse reaction to heparin is haemorrhage; alopecia, osteoporosis and diarrhoea have occasionally been reported. Contraindications are the same as those listed for oral anticoagulants. It is seldom necessary to reverse the effect of heparin because its short half-life results in a rapid return to normal coagulation when treatment is stopped. However, if immediate neutralisation is required, protamine sulphate can be administered by slow intravenous injection. The appropriate dose of protamine falls rapidly as time elapses after the last heparin injection, but within the first half hour 1 mg of protamine is needed for 1 mg of heparin (100 units).

THE COMPLETED STROKE

In patients who have a completed stroke due to ischaemia, anticoagulants are of no proven value and may induce bleeding into the infarct. If the stroke has been caused by haemorrhage, anticoagulants are positively dangerous.

Dexamethasone. The most useful drug in the management of stroke is dexamethasone, which reduces cerebral oedema. The mechanism of action of corticosteroids in this context is not known (see Chapter 18). Although some observations on animal models have failed to reveal therapeutic activity (Plum *et al* 1963; Siegal *et al* 1972), others have been more encouraging and most of the controlled clinical studies have yielded favourable results (Rubinstein 1965; Patten *et al* 1972). A satisfactory regimen is 8–10 mg of dexamethasone intravenously, followed by 4 mg intramuscularly every 6 hours for

10 days. The dose may then be tailed off over about 7 days. Details of the pharmacokinetics and toxicity of corticosteroids are given in Chapter 18.

Glycerol. Glycerol is an alternative drug that reduces cerebral oedema. It acts as an osmotic dehydrating agent for the central nervous system because of its poor penetration across the blood–brain barrier. Intravenous glycerol has been shown to be effective in a controlled study of cerebral infarcts, though patients with cerebral haemorrhage failed to benefit (Matthew *et al* 1972). A dose of 50 g glycerol is infused intravenously in 500 ml of 5% glucose. This procedure is repeated daily for 6 days. Cerebral oedema can also be alleviated with oral glycerol, 1 g/kg thrice daily.

The main advantage of glycerol over dexamethasone is a more rapid action, within 30 minutes. The major problem with osmotic dehydrating agents is the risk that their therapeutic effect may be followed by a compensatory rise in intracranial pressure.

Fibrinolytic agents. Fibrinolytic agents have been studied in cerebrovascular disease but results have been discouraging, largely because of the tendency for these drugs to provoke bleeding into infarcts (Meyer *et al* 1965).

CEREBRAL VENOUS THROMBOSIS

Cerebral venous thrombosis is usually secondary to disease elsewhere. When dehydration is present, this can be corrected by fluid replacement. Infection is a common predisposing factor (Kalbag and Woolf 1972); if an organism is found, for example in blood cultures, appropriate antimicrobial therapy can be selected. Where no organism is identified, broad spectrum treatment is generally given, as in the management of meningitis of unknown aetiology (see Chapter 5). Dexamethasone may be useful in reducing cerebral oedema. Phenytoin (see Chapter 12) is commonly administered to patients with cerebral venous thrombosis because of the high incidence of seizures. The use of anticoagulants is controversial; good results have been claimed in uncontrolled studies (Krayenbuhl 1967).

INTRACRANIAL HAEMORRHAGE

There is no satisfactory medical treatment for intracranial haemorrhage, though efforts to reduce brain oedema—with dexamethasone or glycerol—are often effective in acute episodes of cerebral compression (King 1973). These drugs are also helpful in subarachnoid bleeds where arterial spasm can lead to infarction with considerable cerebral swelling.

Surgery may be indicated for extradural, subdural or subarachnoid haemmorhage, but bleeding into the brain itself is seldom improved by exploration. There are two exceptions: evacuation of and cerebellar subcortical cerebral haematomas can result in substantial benefit (Marshall 1972).

HYPERTENSIVE ENCEPHALOPATHY

Hypertensive encephalopathy is a medical emergency characterised by headache, papilloedema, vomiting and ultimately a deteriorating level of consciousness. Visual defects and seizures are common. In addition to vascular hypertension there may be a rise in the pressure of CSF. In the presence of uraemia, relatively minor elevation of the blood pressure can precipitate encephalopathy.

The transient but often profound neurological disturbances which occur in hypertensive encephalopathy probably result from vasoconstriction and cerebral oedema (Ziegler 1972). However, because of the common experience that improvement occurs when the blood pressure is reduced, efforts are directed at hypotensive measures rather than drugs to relieve intracranial oedema and vascular spasm. Diazoxide is the most satisfactory drug for hypertensive encephalopathy (Merrill 1970); reserpine is also useful (McDowell 1971).

Diazoxide. Diazoxide is a thiazide; it is thought to operate by relaxing smooth muscle of the precapillary resistance vasculature. Intravenous injection of 300 mg over 10–15 seconds produces a fall in blood pressure in about 30 seconds which is sustained from 2–4 hours. The speed of administration is important because avid binding to plasma protein rapidly removes free drug from the blood stream. The hypotensive response does not have a prominent orthostatic component. Diazoxide has potent hyperglycaemic and hypernatraemic properties so both glucose and sodium levels in the blood should be measured if treatment is continued (Finnerty 1968). Extrapyramidal disorders have been reported following administration of diazoxide, raising the possibility that this drug may alter the concentration of catecholamines in the central nervous system (Neary *et al* 1973). Other adverse reactions include flushing, nausea and vomiting.

Reserpine. Reserpine depletes catecholamines and serotonin throughout the central and peripheral nervous system. An intramuscular injection of 1 mg can be repeated every 2 hours up to a total dose of 10 mg. The hypotensive response usually follows about 1½ hours after administration. The maximum effect generally occurs in 3–4 hours and clears after 7–10 hours. This regimen can be repeated, but after two days nasal congestion, flushing and lethargy become prominent (Finnerty 1968); subsequently depression and Parkinsonism may develop.

CHAPTER 7

IMMUNOLOGICAL AND INFLAMMATORY DISEASE

In this Chapter a number of diseases of unknown aetiology will be considered. All have been attributed, at one time or another, to abnormal immunological or inflammatory reactions, though for many it now seems probable that an infective cause will ultimately be found.

The diseases considered here share one common denominator— they are currently treated with anti-inflammatory, immunosuppressive drugs. This therapeutic approach has yielded variable results. In discussing the response to treatment, efficacy cannot be interpreted as evidence that immunological damage plays a causal role because the properties of the drugs involved are not specific. In particular, it is often impossible to separate the relative contributions of treatment to alleviation of cerebral oedema, inhibition of local inflammatory cell infiltration, suppression of circulating lymphocytes and interference with antibody production.

Another common problem in interpreting the significance of immunological abnormalities is difficulty in distinguishing between cause and effect. It is impossible, on current evidence, to decide whether the increased immunoglobulins in the cerebrospinal fluid of patients with multiple sclerosis indicate an allergic aetiology, or merely represent the consequences of a particular pattern of myelin degeneration. Elevated immunoglobulins may even signify both cause and effect—for example infective pathology may release antigens which provoke an autoimmune attack on the neurons.

The use of corticosteroids and other immunosuppressive anti-

111

inflammatory agents, will be reviewed in the following diseases: (1) Multiple sclerosis; (2) Idiopathic polyneuropathy; (3) Idiopathic mononeuropathy; (4) Polymyositis and dermatomyositis; (5) Systemic lupus erythematosus; (6) Polyarteritis nodosa; (7) Giant cell arteritis and polymyalgia rheumatica; (8) Allergic encephalomyelitis; (9) Sarcoidosis. Myasthenia gravis is considered in Chapter 17.

MULTIPLE SCLEROSIS (DISSEMINATED SCLEROSIS)

Differences in criteria for the diagnosis and selection of patients may have contributed to the divergent accounts of the natural history of multiple sclerosis. While one study has suggested that the mean survival time from the onset of symptoms is only 17.4 years (Leibowitz *et al* 1969), another investigation reported that 50% of patients are still alive 35 years after developing the disease (Kurtzke *et al* 1970). Since there is no general agreement on prognosis for untreated patients, it is not possible to comment on whether survival is influenced by treatment.

There are three major views of the aetiology of multiple sclerosis. Epidemiological evidence supports a viral origin, while an immunological cause has been argued on the basis of the elevated globulin, IgG, found in the CSF. A third suggestion is that dietary factors are important—this idea has received renewed interest following a recent claim that linoleic acid, which is present in high concentration in certain vegetable oils, has a therapeutic action. These three concepts may perhaps be united into a single working hypothesis following the observations that (1) there is a high titre of antibody against measles in the CSF of patients with multiple sclerosis (Haire *et al* 1973) and (2) linoleic acid inhibits the mobility of macrophages from multiple sclerotics more than controls (Mertin *et al* 1973). Hence it is possible to speculate that there may be an abnormal immunological response to the measles virus and linoleic acid might exert its therapeutic action by immunosuppression.

Evaluation of therapy in multiple sclerosis is difficult because such wide spontaneous fluctuations occur. Some 44% of patients recover completely from their first attack without any treatment (Poser 1972). In a paper entitled *The evolution of management of multiple sclerosis—wading through fads*, Schumacher (1971) reviews therapeutic claims that have been made for 75 medicaments. Over the last two decades multiple sclerosis has been treated with plasma, blood, dicoumarol, heparin, extracts of pancreas, extracts of heart, extracts of yeast, ergot alkaloids, vaccines, clofibrate, cyanocobalamin, galactose, histamine, androsterone, chloroquine, isoniazid, tolbutamide, tranylcypromine, tetraethylammonium chloride, adenosine monophosphate and intrathecal tuberculin (Sibley 1970). The diversity and length of this list is cogent evidence that no satisfactory treatment is available.

A number of immunosuppressive drugs protect animals from experimental allergic encephalomyelitis but their use in multiple sclerosis has been disappointing. Melphalan, methotrexate, cytarabine, cyclophosphamide and mercaptopurine have all been unrewarding (Poser 1972). Recent studies with azathioprine (Swinburn and Liversedge 1973) and antilymphocytic globulin (MacFadyen *et al* 1973) are similarly discouraging. One problem relevant to these studies is the failure of such agents as azathioprine and antilymphocytic globulin to gain ready access to the central nervous system.

The management of spasticity and urinary incontinence, frequently encountered in multiple sclerosis, are discussed in Chapters 15 and 16. Diplopia can be corrected by wearing an eye patch. Intention tremor often responds well to stereotactic surgery. Critical investigations have only revealed four other forms of treatment that may be useful—corticotrophin, tetracosactrin, corticosteroids and linoleic acid.

Corticotrophin. Short courses of intramuscular corticotrophin gel are beneficial in acute exacerbations of multiple sclerosis (McAlpine *et al* 1965), but long term maintenance therapy is ineffective (Millar *et al* 1967). The first controlled study to demonstrate a therapeutic action employed a 3 week schedule of corticotrophin: 60 units twice daily for the first week, 40 units twice daily for the second, reducing to 60, 40 and 20 units on the 2nd, 4th and 6th day of the third week (Miller *et al* 1961). A shorter regimen using lower doses was found to be effective in a more recent investigation—40 units twice daily for 1 week, followed by 20 units twice daily for 4 days, and then 20 units daily for 3 days (Rose *et al* 1970).

Adverse reactions to corticotrophin include retention of sodium, loss of potassium, oedema, hypertension, gastrointestinal haemorrhage or perforation, hyperglycaemia, impaired resistance to infection, osteoporosis, psychosis, cataracts, glaucoma, myopathy and aseptic necrosis of the hip. If treatment is prolonged, patients may develop moon face, buffalo hump, striae, acne and hirsutism. Hypersensitivity reactions are occasionally encountered. Toxic effects are seldom troublesome in short courses of treatment provided patients with diabetes, hypertension, peptic ulceration, infection and psychosis are excluded. Sodium restriction (not more than 4 g/day NaCl), potassium supplements (6 g/day KCl) and antacids are sometimes employed if electrolyte disturbances or gastrointestinal symptoms occur.

The massive dose of corticotrophin advocated in the treatment of multiple sclerosis is considerably greater than that required to produce maximal corticosteroid release from normal adrenal gland—40 units/day. It has therefore been suggested that the therapeutic action of corticotrophin may stem from effects which do not depend upon adrenal stimulation, but there is no convincing evidence to support this view.

Tetracosactrin. The synthetic congener of corticotrophin, tetracosactrin, is probably more satisfactory for routine use because it carries a lower risk of producing hypersensitivity. In other respects, adverse effects are similar to those of corticotrophin. Plain tetracosactrin has a very short period of action, so the sustained release preparation should be used—1 mg corresponds to 100 units of corticotrophin.

Corticosteroids. Tourtellotte and Haerer (1965) have performed a controlled study with long term administration of methylprednisolone which revealed a statistically significant therapeutic action. The authors interpreted their results with caution and avoided the conclusion that maintenance corticosteroids had a place in the routine management of multiple sclerosis; the advantages of prolonged treatment were not sufficiently impressive to justify the risks of chronic toxicity. However, this demonstration is of importance because it offers support for the view that the action of corticotrophin is achieved by releasing corticosteroids rather than a direct effect on the central nervous system.

Corticosteroids are a satisfactory form of treatment for acute exacerbations of multiple sclerosis. There is little to choose between corticosteroids and corticotrophin, but the former have the advantage of being administered orally and causing less fluid retention.

Prednisone and prednisolone are synthetic glucocorticoids which are interconvertible in the body. They are readily absorbed from the gastrointestinal tract and they bind extensively to plasma proteins. Their plasma half-life is 1–3 hours. Methylprednisolone has a longer plasma half-life than prednisone or prednisolone and is reputed to cause less salt and water retention. Dexamethasone produces even less electrolyte disturbance than methylprednisolone. Corticosteroids are metabolised in the liver and kidney; metabolites and free drug are excreted in the urine. Corticosteroids readily cross the blood–brain barrier. Some 4 mg of methylprednisolone is equivalent to 5 mg of prednisone; the corresponding dose of dexamethasone is 0.75 mg. Adverse reactions are similar to those listed for corticotrophin, but long term therapy also results in pituitary-adrenal suppression.

In treating multiple sclerosis, high doses of corticosteroids are employed for a short time. An equivalent of up to 100 mg/day of prednisone may be given for 1–2 weeks; thereafter the dose is reduced substantially. The total course should last 3–6 weeks. Suppression of pituitary-adrenal function is not a problem with such brief periods of treatment so the high single dose alternate day regimen described in Chapter 17 is not necessary.

Linoleic acid. Linoleic acid is present in high concentration in certain vegetable oils. It is a polyunsaturated fatty acid. Low linoleate concentrations have been reported in the serum of patients with multiple sclerosis (Baker *et al* 1964) and the fraction of unsaturated fatty acids is decreased in their brain lipids (Alling *et al* 1971). Furthermore the dietary intake of polyunsaturated fatty acids is poor in geographical areas where multiple sclerosis is common. For these reasons, Swank (1970) studied the effect of supplementing the diet with unsaturated vegetable oils and restricting saturated animal fats in patients with multiple sclerosis. He considered that these dietary modifications were beneficial. Millar *et al* (1973) have recently completed a controlled study in which linoleic acid was given for two years. An emulsion of sunflower seed oil was administered (30 ml, corresponding to 8.6 g linoleic acid) twice daily. There was a rise in the serum linoleate fraction of total fatty acids from 29% (pretreatment) to 36% (after 9–12 months). Clinical relapses were significantly less severe and of shorter duration in the patients treated with linoleate; no conclusion could be drawn concerning the overall progress of the disease. These initial reports are of interest, but further evidence is required before linoleate therapy can be regarded as having an established place in the management of multiple sclerosis.

IDIOPATHIC POLYNEUROPATHY
(LANDRY–GUILLAIN–BARRÉ SYNDROME)

Idiopathic polyneuropathy has a number of similarities to experimental allergic neuritis—a neuropathy induced by sensitising animals to antigenic components of peripheral nerve. Administration of corticosteroids, antimetabolites or alkylating agents can protect animals from experimental allergic neuritis so it has been suggested that these drugs might have a role in the management of idiopathic polyneuropathy. However, the results in unselected cases have been disappointing (Siegenthaler and Regli 1966). One optimistic report following the use of mercaptopurine (Palmer 1965) must be balanced against the experience of a renal transplant patient who developed idiopathic polyneuropathy (Drachman *et al* 1970) while receiving long term treatment with azathioprine—which is metabolised to mercaptopurine.

The only setting in which corticosteroid efficacy is widely accepted is for severe, chronic, relapsing forms of idiopathic polyneuropathy. Small alterations in dosage can produce striking changes in both the clinical features and the concentration of protein in the cerebrospinal fluid (Austin 1958; Thomas *et al* 1969). An initial dose of glucocorticoid equivalent to about 40 mg/day of prednisone should be titrated against the therapeutic response; frequent adjustments of intake may be necessary. If treatment is prolonged, a single high dose alternate day regimen can be employed to minimise adverse effects (see Chapter 17). Sodium restriction, potassium supplements and antacids may be introduced if electrolyte disturbances or gastro-intestinal symptoms occur.

IDIOPATHIC MONONEUROPATHY

Three forms of mononeuropathy deserve brief mention. It is convenient to consider them here because corticosteroids have been employed in their management. They comprise Bell's palsy, neuralgic amyotrophy and the Tolosa–Hunt syndrome.

BELL'S PALSY

If treatment can be started within a week of the onset of symptoms, corticosteroids reduce the incidence of permanent denervation in patients with Bell's palsy (Adour *et al* 1972). An initial dose of glucocorticoid equivalent to 1 mg/kg/day of prednisone is usually maintained for 5 days and then reduced over about 4 days; this form of therapy appears to be better than corticotrophin (Taverner *et al* 1971).

NEURALGIC AMYOTROPHY (BRACHIAL PLEXUS NEUROPATHY)

There have been controversial reports on the use of corticosteroids in neuralgic amyotrophy (Gathier and Bruyn 1970). In a recent study the long term prognosis was found to be extremely good without any treatment; patients who were given corticotrophin or glucocorticoids did not derive any obvious benefit (Tsairis *et al* 1972).

TOLOSA–HUNT SYNDROME

The Tolosa–Hunt syndrome is characterised by recurrent, unilateral, retro-orbital pain with external ophthalmoplegia and sometimes impairment of visual acuity. It is generally associated with an elevated erythrocyte sedimentation rate; limited evidence suggests that the underlying pathology is a periarteritic inflammatory lesion in the cavernous sinus. The response to corticosteroids is so consistent that such treatment has been regarded as a diagnostic test (Matthew and Chandy 1970). Prednisone 1 mg/kg/day, or an equivalent intake of another glucocorticoid, leads to dramatic improvement in 48–72 hours. The dose can be reduced after 1–2 weeks and treatment is usually stopped after 4–6 weeks. Recurrences are common so further courses may be necessary.

POLYMYOSITIS AND DERMATOMYOSITIS

While the aetiology of polymyositis and dermatomyositis remains unknown, a number of observations suggest that immunological disturbances may play an important role, often in association with neoplasms. Relevant evidence includes the finding that guinea pigs sensitised to rabbit muscle develop a generalised myositis (Dawkins 1965) and rat muscle is destroyed by sensitised lymphocytes in tissue culture (Kakulas 1966 a and b). Clinical evidence of an immunological abnormality derives from an increased incidence of polymyositis in certain diseases which exhibit disordered immuno-globulin reactions, such as systemic lupus erythematosus (Walton and Adams 1958).

The various forms of polymyositis and dermatomyositis may be classified into several subgroups (Pearson 1969), but all are treated with corticosteroids (Walton 1969) and from a therapeutic viewpoint they can be considered together. They will be termed polymyositis without any attempt to discriminate between the different categories.

Optimal therapeutic results are obtained when an early diagnosis allows treatment to be started before the pathology is too advanced.

Initially 1 mg/kg/day of prednisone, or the equivalent intake of another glucocorticoid, is adjusted according to the clinical response, erythrocyte sedimentation rate and plasma creatine phosphokinase. Maintenance dosage of 10–20 mg/day of prednisone is usually required (Yount *et al* 1973), increasing if exacerbations occur. Single dose alternate day therapy (20–40 mg every 2 days) can be employed to minimise adverse effects (see Chapter 17). Potassium supplements, sodium restriction and antacids are sometimes necessary. Corticosteroid therapy must be continued indefinitely in most patients; if an attempt is made to stop treatment, dosage should be reduced gradually over a period of several weeks.

Patients who fail to respond to corticosteroids have been reported to benefit from the addition of more potent immuno-suppressive agents. Azathioprine (Haas 1973); mercaptopurine (Goldstein 1965); thioguanine (Demis *et al* 1964); methotrexate (Malaviya *et al* 1968) and cyclophosphamide (Currie and Walton 1971) have all been claimed to have a therapeutic action, though there are few controlled observations.

Azathioprine and mercaptopurine. The anti-inflammatory immuno-suppressive actions of azathioprine and mercaptopurine stem from disruption of dividing cells. These drugs are purine analogues which become incorporated in the synthetic pathway of nucleic acids. Azathioprine is metabolised to mercaptopurine; the 5-phosphate ribonucleotide of mercaptopurine, thioinosinate, inhibits a number of essential cell processes including the formation of adenylate.

Azathioprine is well absorbed from the gastrointestinal tract but does not readily cross the blood–brain barrier. Its active metabolite, mercaptopurine, gains limited entry to the central nervous system. The plasma half-life of mercaptopurine is about 90 minutes; it is inactivated by oxidation under the influence of xanthine oxidase. This enzyme is blocked by allopurinol, which is widely prescribed as a uricosuric agent. Administration of allopurinol to a patient receiving azathioprine or mercaptopurine therefore leads to a substantial rise in the tissue levels of purine analogues, which may precipitate toxicity.

The dose for both azathioprine and mercaptopurine is 100–300 mg/day. The lower end of the range is employed for long term

administration. Adverse reactions include leucopenia, thrombocytopenia, haemorrhage, nausea, vomiting, diarrhoea, jaundice and
occasionally intestinal ulceration. Experience with immunosuppressive
therapy in renal transplantation suggests that azathioprine produces
fewer toxic effects than comparable doses of mercaptopurine.

Methotrexate. Methotrexate inhibits dihydrofolate reductase, which
is responsible for converting folate and dihydrofolate to tetrahydrofolate. This enzymic block has a major impact on the metabolism
of dividing cells.

Methotrexate is rather poorly absorbed from the gastrointestinal
tract, so it is usually administered by intravenous injection. Some
50% becomes bound to plasma proteins, the half-life being about 1.5
hours. Methotrexate is excreted, mostly unchanged, in the urine. It
does not readily cross the blood–brain barrier. The intravenous dose
is 25–100 mg weekly, according to response and toxicity (Malaviya
et al 1968); alternatively 2.5–10 mg/day can be given orally.

Unwanted effects include nausea, vomiting, diarrhoea, skin
eruptions, marrow depression and alopecia. Gastrointestinal ulcers
and impairment of hepatic function can occur. Toxic reactions may
be treated with calcium folinate, 3–6 mg by intramuscular injection,
but this is unlikely to be effective unless given within 4 hours of the
methotrexate.

Cyclophosphamide. Cyclophosphamide is itself pharmacologically
inert, depending for its effect upon hepatic hydroxylation to form
an alkylating agent. The active metabolite probably achieves
cytotoxicity by reacting with guanine bases of nucleic acids to produce
relatively selective damage to dividing cells.

Cyclophosphamide is incompletely absorbed from the gastrointestinal tract, reaching peak plasma concentrations in about 1 hour.
The oral dose range is 50–20 mg/day; up to 600 mg/day is occasionally tolerated (Currie and Walton 1971). Adverse reactions include
alopecia, nausea, vomiting, diarrhoea, haemorrhagic cystitis and
metaplasia, leucopenia, thrombocytopenia, headache, ulceration of
the mucosae and hepatic damage.

SYSTEMIC LUPUS ERYTHEMATOSUS (DISSEMINATED LUPUS ERYTHEMATOSUS)

Systemic lupus erythematosus runs a very variable course ranging from a few weeks to 20 years. Involvement of the nervous system occurs in the majority of patients. Neurological features include an abnormal mental state, epilepsy, hemiplegia, chorea, cranial nerve lesions, peripheral neuropathy and polymyositis (Johnson and Richardson 1968; Bennett *et al* 1972). While many of these disorders are thought to result from vasculitis, other contributory factors are hypertension, uraemia, electrolyte disturbances and drug toxicity.

In patients with severe manifestations of lupus affecting the central nervous system—for example serial epilepsy or coma—corticosteroids should be given parenterally. Intramuscular dexamethasone, 4 mg every 6 hours, is a suitable initial regimen. The patient can subsequently be transferred to oral dosage, equivalent to 1–2 mg/kg/day of prednisone. For prolonged therapy, a high single dose alternate day schedule has been advocated (Ackerman 1970), but some prefer to give frequent divided doses (Yount *et al* 1973). When a remission is induced the intake of corticosteroids can be decreased. If there is no response to treatment, azathioprine 150 mg/day or cyclophosphamide 200 mg/day may be added though the evidence that these drugs have a significant therapeutic action is not conclusive.

POLYARTERITIS NODOSA

Polyarteritis nodosa can produce a variety of neurological lesions: infarcts and haemorrhages of the brain or spinal cord, multiple mononeuropathy and possibly polymyositis. Although polyarteritis nodosa often improves and occasionally arrests, the prognosis is usually poor. Corticosteroid therapy increases the 5 year survival rate from 13% to 48% (Tumulty 1970). These figures indicate that in spite of early suggestions that corticosteroids can provoke diffuse arteritis with peripheral neuropathy in patients with connective tissue diseases (Kemper *et al* 1957), these drugs are the most satisfactory treatment available for polyarteritis nodosa. Dose regimens are similar to those employed in systemic lupus erythematosus.

GIANT CELL (TEMPORAL) ARTERITIS AND POLYMYALGIA RHEUMATICA

Untreated polymyalgia rheumatica often progresses to typical giant cell arteritis (Hamilton *et al* 1971). Corticosteroid therapy should be started as soon as either diagnosis is made, because early treatment can prevent such catastrophies as blindness, stroke and myocardial infarction. An appropriate initial regimen is 1 mg/kg/day of prednisone, or the equivalent dose of another glucocorticoid. This may subsequently be converted to high single dose alternate day therapy, to minimise adverse effects (see Chapter 17). Treatment should always be maintained for at least 6 months, but the dose may be reduced if clinical features improve and the erythrocyte sedimentation rate falls; conversely, intake must be increased if there is a relapse (Hamilton *et al* 1971). Therapy should not be stopped until symptoms and signs have cleared and the sedimentation rate has reverted to normal.

'ALLERGIC' ENCEPHALOMYELITIS

Encephalitis, myelitis and meningitis can result from systemic viral infections such as measles, mumps or chickenpox. Neurological features follow viraemia after a variable time, which may be as long as 14 days. It was once considered useful to distinguish between (1) *invasive* encephalomyelitis, in which neuronal damage was attributed to the direct effect of viral infection and (2) *allergic* encephalomyelitis, where neuronal damage was thought to arise from an immunological reaction to antigenic material released from the central nervous system by the initial infection. These subdivisions stemmed from the discovery that an animal model of immunological disease of the central nervous system—experimental allergic encephalomyelitis—could be induced by injecting antigenic fractions of brain tissue. However, current evidence does not support the separation of encephalomyelitis into invasive and allergic types because neuronal damage is usually consequent upon a combination of factors which include viral invasion, oedema and inflammatory cell infiltration.

Corticosteroids are deleterious at the time of initial infection and viraemia because they impair normal defensive mechanisms, but when inflammation and cerebral oedema are prominent they can be beneficial. Webb (1969) considers that by the time the clinical features of encephalomyelitis appear it is safe and indeed desirable to administer corticosteroids. A suitable regimen is intramuscular dexamethasone 4 mg every 6 hours for 3 days, followed by a reduced dose for a further 10–14 days. Others are sceptical about the value of such treatment (Bøe *et al* 1965). No firm conclusion is justified until more evidence has been obtained.

SARCOIDOSIS

In reviewing a large series of patients with histologically proven sarcoidosis, Silverstein *et al* (1965) found that ˙4% developed neurological disturbances. The cranial nerves were most commonly involved; in a minority of cases there were lesions in the central nervous system or peripheral nerves. Many patients with neurological manifestations of sarcoidosis have been given corticosteriods, but it is not possible to make an adequate assessment of the value of therapy (Scadding 1967), because of the high rate of spontaneous remission and the lack of controlled observations. Matthews (1965) considers that prednisone is effective in subacute sarcoidosis of the nervous system; chronic disease is reputed to be less responsive (Camp and Frierson 1962). About 15 mg/day of prednisone, or the corresponding dose of another glucocorticoid, have been employed in the past. Treatment is often extended over several months so higher (30 mg) single dose alternate day therapy may prove more satisfactory (see Chapter 17).

CHAPTER 8
NEOPLASIA

Neoplastic disease involving the nervous system is usually treated by radiotherapy or surgery, but there are two situations in which worthwhile palliation can be achieved with drugs—infiltration of the meninges and raised intracranial pressure.

MENINGEAL INFILTRATION

Meningeal infiltration in leukaemia, lymphoma and breast cancer have all been reported to respond to cytotoxic drugs (Olson *et al* 1974; Spiers 1974). Results have been particularly encouraging in leukaemia. In the past, the inexorable progress of disseminated neoplasia culminated in death so rapidly that neurological problems were uncommon. However, the development of improved therapy has extended survival so that neurological disturbances are now becoming more frequent (Aur *et al* 1971).

Neoplastic cells have a relatively privileged opportunity to develop in the central nervous system owing to poor penetration of cytotoxic drugs across the blood–brain and blood–CSF barriers. This pharmacokinetic limitation has two important consequences: (1) The existence of neoplastic cells in a sanctuary where they are exposed to sublethal concentrations of drugs encourages the development of clones which are resistant to treatment and these may subsequently leave the central nervous system to reseed the peripheral tissues. (2) Intrathecal or intraventricular therapy is employed in order to establish therapeutic levels of cytotoxic agents in the central nervous system. The use of these routes of administration leads to high local concentrations in the brain and spinal cord which generate new toxicological problems (see Chapter II).

The risks of neurological involvement are particularly high in acute lymphatic leukaemia of childhood. Spiers (1974) has estimated that 75% of children suffering from this disease have neoplastic cells in their central nervous system without any relevant clinical features; it is therefore current practice to give prophylactic therapy. In other types of leukaemia the prevalence of infiltration of the central nervous system is not so high so prophylaxis is not usually undertaken, treatment being reserved for those patients who develop neurological or CSF abnormalities.

Methotrexate and cytarabine are the most satisfactory drugs. They can be given alternately.

Methotrexate. Direct access to the CSF can be achieved by either intrathecal injection at lumbar puncture, or insertion of an Ommaya reservoir under the scalp with a cannula running into the lateral ventricle of the non-dominant hemisphere. The dose of methotrexate usually employed is 7.5 mg/square metre. Some 10–12 such injections may be given over 40 weeks as a prophylactic regimen. When treating neurological involvement which is clinically manifest, the dosage is adjusted according to toxicity and the cytological response in the CSF. Adverse reactions to intrathecal and intraventricular methotrexate include paraparesis (Bagshawe *et al* 1959), encephalopathy (Shapiro *et al* 1973) and sudden death (Back 1969). The use of intravenous methotrexate is discussed in Chapter 7.

Cytarabine. Cytarabine has been reported to be useful in meningeal infiltration (Wang and Pratt 1970; Broder and Carter 1972) though experience is limited; the dose range is 20–100 mg/square metre intrathecally or via an Ommaya reservoir. The first four doses may be given on alternate days, continuing with a weekly injection thereafter. The optimum duration of treatment has not been established; therapy is commonly continued for 5 months. Cytarabine is discussed further in Chapter 5.

Pharmacotherapy for neurological leukaemia is generally combined with irradiation of the skull and spinal cord (Spiers 1974).

While alopecia often occurs following such treatment, an adequate head of hair is commonly regained in about four months despite continuing cytotoxic therapy.

PALLIATION OF RAISED INTRACRANIAL PRESSURE

One factor contributing to the symptomatology of intracranial tumours is cerebral oedema which may be either localised around the growth, or diffuse throughout the hemispheres. Glucocorticoids alleviate cerebral oedema and they therefore have a palliative therapeutic role in the management of many patients with cerebral neoplasms. In addition to this effect, experimental studies on brain tumours in mice suggest that corticosteroids may retard neoplastic proliferation by inhibiting the incorporation of DNA precursors (Shapiro 1972). However, clinical evidence does not support the view that steroids have any action on tumour growth. In a recent series of observations on patients with cerebral neoplasia, the effect of corticosteroid therapy has been investigated by studying CSF pressure, CSF protein, cerebral angiography and cerebral blood flow (Weinstein *et al* 1973). Improvement in neurological deficits only occurred if the tumour was initially associated with cerebral oedema. It was concluded that oedema led to local, reversible impairment of cerebral blood flow by the following sequence of events: increased tissue pressure compromised the cerebral micro-circulation, inadequate perfusion being exacerbated because the tumour acted as a low pressure shunt and diverted blood away from cerebral tissue. Autoregulatory systems did not operate because of the gross regional distortion of microanatomy. By reducing brain oedema, corticosteroids reversed this vicious circle.

Dexamethasone (see Chapter 18) is the most satisfactory drug for reducing cerebral oedema. An initial intravenous injection of 8–10 mg is usually followed by intramuscular administration of 4 mg every 6 hours. The dose can be decreased as improvement occurs; long term oral treatment with the minimum effective intake of dexamethasone (generally 0.5–1 mg/day) often allows neurological symptoms to be alleviated for several months.

CHAPTER 9
METABOLIC DISEASE

Neurological manifestations of metabolic disorders are treated by correcting the underlying biochemical pathology. Most of this Chapter is therefore concerned with the management of diseases which are outside the usual scope of neurological therapeutics. The following topics will be considered: (1) Encephalopathy—hepatic disease, diabetic coma, hypoglycaemia, hyperosmolar states, hyposmolar states, hypothyroidism, adrenocortical insufficiency, hypercalcaemia, hypocalcaemia, aminoacidaemias, organicacidaemias, other treatable encephalopathic syndromes; (2) Peripheral neuropathy—diabetic neuropathy, porphyria, Refsum's disease, alcoholic neuropathy, renal failure; (3) Myopathies—hypokalaemic paralysis, hyperkalaemic paralysis, normokalaemic paralysis, hyperthyroid myopathy, hypothyroid myopathy, Cushing's syndrome, adrenocortical insufficiency, acromegaly, hypopituitarism, calcium disturbances.

While vitamin deficiencies may reasonably be regarded as metabolic diseases, they represent a distinct group from a therapeutic viewpoint and will be considered separately in Chapter 10. Drug induced disturbances are discussed in Chapter 11. The treatment of Wilson's disease, thyrotoxic chorea and the Lesch–Nyhan syndrome are reviewed in Chapter 14.

Encephalopathy

Encephalopathy is a generalised disturbance of cerebral function—deterioration of intellectual performance leads to a declining level of consciousness often accompanied by widespread involuntary movements and seizures. Encephalopathic syndromes can be produced by biochemical abnormalities, infections, vascular disorders or degenerative diseases. Metabolic causes are common. Hepatic, renal and respiratory failure all give rise to biochemical disturbances which can induce encephalopathic reactions. These may be treated by decreasing the relevant metabolic work load or replacing the role of these organs by artificial means (transplantation, dialysis, mechanical ventilation). Renal and respiratory failure will not be considered here, because neurologists are seldom called upon to undertake dialysis programmes, manage ventilators, or titrate oxygen intake against blood gas tensions and pH. The treatment of other reversible encephalopathies can be a matter of urgency and neurologists may be involved in taking initial decisions, particularly if the patient presents in coma.

HEPATIC DISEASE

Hepatic encephalopathy is usually associated with impaired liver function but it can occur in the presence of normal biochemical findings if there is an extensive portosystemic shunt; presumably such shunting allows neurotoxic materials absorbed from the gut to reach the brain without undergoing metabolic transformation in the liver.

Treatment of hepatic encephalopathy is directed to (1) reducing the metabolic load on the liver by restricting dietary protein, (2) decreasing the formation of toxic products in the gut. Purgation and intestinal washouts may be necessary to remove blood accumulating from gastrointestinal haemorrhage and to clear the colon. Lactulose is given to produce an osmotic diarrhoea and to lower the intestinal pH, thus favouring the growth of innocuous organisms such as *Lactobacilli* (Bircher *et al* 1966). Oral neomycin also suppresses colonic micro-organisms that generate toxic materials.

In acute encephalopathy, nutrition is maintained with 20% solutions of glucose or lactose by mouth or by intravenous infusion. Potassium supplements are given in doses adjusted according to the plasma concentration. Sedatives and diuretics are withheld because they commonly precipitate or exacerbate hepatic encephalopathy. There have been limited reports that levodopa has a therapeutic action in hepatic coma; its introduction was based upon claims that it produces an 'arousal reaction' on the electroencephalogram (Parkes *et al* 1970; Fischer and James 1972).

Lactulose. Lactulose is employed in the treatment of both acute and chronic hepatic encephalopathy (Avery *et al* 1972). It is a disaccharide which undergoes fermentation in the colon to form acetic and lactic acids. It is not absorbed from the gastrointestinal tract. In addition to reducing colonic pH, it has a prominent laxative action. The usual starting dose is about 30 g/day administered orally in a 50% solution. This is increased until the bowels are opened 2–3 times daily, which generally occurs on 45–60 g/day. Up to 100 g/day can be given if necessary. Adverse effects are unusual, though abdominal cramps can occur; there have also been occasional reports of skin eruption, albuminuria and haemoglobinuria.

Neomycin. Some 97% of an orally administered dose of neomycin is excreted unchanged in the faeces. For hepatic encephalopathy, 1 g is given four times daily by mouth. In spite of its limited absorption, neomycin can induce systemic adverse reactions, in particular deafness. Opportunist infections, such as candidiasis, may also occur. For these reasons neomycin is being used less in the treatment of chronic hepatic encephalopathy, though it is still widely employed in acute episodes.

Levodopa. In hepatic coma, levodopa can be administered by nasogastric tube, 3.5–5.0 g/day in divided doses. Therapeutic effects appear to be limited by its erratic action and a tendency to provoke vomiting and gastrointestinal bleeding in patients suffering from hepatic failure.

DIABETIC COMA

Traditional treatment of ketotic diabetic coma has included large doses of insulin and bicarbonate. In recent years this practice has been undergoing reappraisal; there is now a trend to employ smaller doses of insulin and avoid the use of bicarbonate unless the pH is extremely low (Alberti *et al* 1972; Fraser 1974).

There is severe dehydration in ketotic diabetic coma. The deficits often reach 6 litres of water, 500 mEq of sodium and 350 mEq of potassium.

Insulin. Soluble insulin is administered as soon as possible, 80 units by intramuscular injection and 20 units intravenously. Subsequently small frequent intramuscular doses are given, 40–60 units every 4 hours until the blood sugar has fallen to about 200 mg/100 ml.

Intravenous fluids. Over the first $1-1\frac{1}{2}$ hours, 2 litres of isotonic saline should be infused intravenously, adding 10 mEq of potassium chloride to each litre. The rate of infusion is reduced if the jugular venous pressure rises. As the blood sugar falls more potassium chloride can be administered with the intravenous fluid; 20 mEq/litre is satisfactory providing the serum concentration of potassium (or the electrocardiogram) is monitored. A total of 6–8 litres of fluid should be given over the first 12 hours, substituting 5% dextrose for normal saline when the blood sugar has fallen below 300 mg/100 ml.

General management

Important general points in the management of ketotic diabetic coma include:

Nasogastric intubation. The stomach is usually evacuated to prevent aspiration pneumonia; the nasogastric tube is retained until the patient is conscious and nausea has cleared.

Monitoring blood biochemistry. Blood is taken initially for estimation of sugar, electrolytes and pH. A further sample should be analysed

1½ hours after the first injection of insulin and then regularly every 2 hours.

Treatment of infection. A search is undertaken for any infection which may have precipitated the coma. If an organism is found, it is treated with appropriate antimicrobial therapy. When no source of infection can be detected, prolonged diabetic coma is treated with prophylactic benzylpenicillin, 300 mg twice daily (see Chapter 5).

HYPOGLYCAEMIA

Hypoglycaemia produces sweating and light headedness which may progress to seizures and coma. The commonest cause of hypoglycaemia is an incorrect balance between diet and insulin in patients with diabetes mellitus. The symptoms can be corrected by ingestion of sugar, but when consciousness has already been lost 10–40 g of glucose should be administered intravenously in a 50% solution followed by an oral intake of carbohydrate to prevent recurrence. If it is not possible to get a needle into a vein, 1 mg of glucagon can be given by intramuscular injection.

Insulin secreting tumours also cause hypoglycaemia; acute episodes can be managed with intravenous glucose, but the definitive treatment is surgical resection of the neoplasm.

Reactive hypoglycaemia produces faintness 3–4 hours after a meal; consciousness is never lost. Causes include rapid gastric emptying (e.g. partial gastrectomy), leucine hypersensitivity and anxiety states. A reduction of carbohydrate intake is often beneficial.

HYPEROSMOLAR STATES

Occasionally diabetic coma occurs without ketosis—hyperosmolar coma. This responds to intravenous half-isotonic saline and small doses of insulin. Other causes of hyperosmolar states include diabetes insipidus, profuse diarrhoea, severe burns and excessive administration of solutes to patients being fed via a nasogastric tube or an intravenous infusion; these are also reversed by giving half-isotonic saline (intravenously or by mouth). Care must be exercised to avoid overcorrecting the disturbance to produce hyponatraemia.

HYPOSMOLAR STATES

Water intoxication leads to delirium and eventually coma. A relatively frequent cause is compulsive drinking of water, though normal subjects often manage 10 litres/day without any symptoms. Haemodialysis can precipitate water intoxication, sudden removal of plasma urea producing cerebral oedema because of the limited permeability of the blood–brain barrier—this is the opposite osmolar situation to that obtaining when mannitol is administered intra-venously for rapid alleviation of brain swelling. Inadequate salt intake (following dehydration) and excessive 'inappropriate' secretion of antidiuretic hormone (often from a bronchial carcinoma) are sometimes responsible for hyposmolar states. Diuretics can induce water intoxication by selectively increasing sodium excretion.

The normal serum osmolality is 290 ± 5 mOsm/litre. A plasma sodium concentration of 120 mEq/litre is compatible with water intoxication—a value below 110 is firm evidence (Plum and Posner 1966).

Hyposmolar states can usually be corrected by restricting water intake to less than one litre/day; this may be supplemented by infusing 5% sodium chloride until a satisfactory clinical and biochemical response has been achieved.

HYPOTHYROIDISM

Untreated myxoedema proceeds from lethargy and drowsiness to sleep and coma. While hypothermia is often regarded as a character-istic feature of hypothyroid coma, low body temperature is common in any neglected unconscious patient.

The prognosis is poor in hypothyroid coma; it still has a mortality rate of 50–90%. Gradual warming is undertaken, together with administration of hydrocortisone and very low doses of tri-iodothyronine, followed by thyroxine. Assisted ventilation may be necessary if there is carbon dioxide retention. Cardiac monitoring is desirable because the risks of arrhythmia and myocardial infarction are considerable. Therapy should also be directed against any concomitant infection.

Tri-iodothyronine (liothyronine). Tri-iodothyronine is absorbed from the gastrointestinal tract and has a plasma half-life of about 2 days. It is employed in the initial treatment of hypothyroid coma. A starting dose not exceeding 5 μg by intramuscular injection or nasogastric tube is increased by 5 μg each day provided the electrocardiogram does not develop ischaemic features. At 20 μg/day therapy may be changed to thyroxine (20 μg tri-iodothronine is equivalent to 0.1 mg of thyroxine).

Thyroxine. Following absorption, thyroxine becomes bound to plasma proteins and has a plasma half-life of about a week. Its action is slower to develop but more prolonged than that of tri-iodothyronine. Having converted from tri-iodothyronine to thyroxine, the dose of the latter is slowly built up from 0.1 mg/day, adding 0.05 mg every 2–4 weeks until the normal maintenance level of 0.2–0.3 mg/day is reached.

Hydrocortisone (cortisol). In hypothyroid coma, 50 mg of hydrocortisone is given twice daily by intramuscular or intravenous injection. For further details of corticosteroids see Chapter 7.

ADRENOCORTICAL INSUFFICIENCY

Almost all patients with Addison's disease have symptoms of anxiety or a disturbance of mood. Profound metabolic encephalopathy may develop in Addisonian crises; stupor can progress into coma and convulsions.

Once a firm diagnosis has been made, 100–300 mg of hydrocortisone should be given intravenously, followed by 500 ml of isotonic saline over 30 minutes. Thereafter, isotonic saline is infused at a rate of 1–4 litres/day with 100 mg of hydrocortisone by intramuscular injection every 8 hours. If the blood sugar is found to be low, glucose should be administered intravenously (40–60 ml as a 50% solution).

For maintenance therapy 5.0–7.5 mg/day of prednisone (or 20–30 mg/day of hydrocortisone) is given orally, together with fludrocortisone, 0.1–0.2 mg/day. Fludrocortisone has prominent mineralocorticoid properties; the main toxic effects of overdosage are hypertension, oedema and electrolyte disturbances.

HYPOPITUITARISM

Patients with pituitary insufficiency may progress into coma as a result of adrenal insufficiency, which is managed as described above under 'Adrenocortical Insufficiency'.

HYPERCALCAEMIA

Severe hypercalcaemia can lead to headache, nausea, vomiting, delusions and occasionally a deteriorating level of consciousness. The usual causes are carcinomatosis and hyperparathyroidism. Temporary correction of hypercalcaemia can be achieved with a high fluid, low calcium intake which may be supplemented with phosphate.

Phosphate. A suitable phosphate solution contains Na_2HPO_4 (11.5 g/litre) and KH_2PO_4 (2.6 g/litre). Some 500 ml may be administered intravenously over 4 hours. If the serum calcium remains elevated, a further 300 ml is given either orally or intravenously, according to the severity of nausea and vomiting.

HYPOCALCAEMIA

Dementia, papilloedema and convulsions can be induced by hypocalcaemia; tetany is usually present. The commonest causes are hypoparathyroidism and deficiency of vitamin D (see Chapter 10). Hypoparathyroidism may be treated with calciferol, 1.25 mg/day and calcium lactate, 4 g six times daily. If immediate correction of hypocalcaemia is required, calcium gluconate should be administered by intravenous infusion, up to 20 mg/kg over 4 hours.

AMINOACIDAEMIAS

A number of hereditary neurological paediatric diseases are characterised by elevated plasma concentrations of aminoacids. These inborn errors of metabolism are not necessarily caused by an enzymic defect immediately concerned with the transformation of aminoacids. For example in maple syrup urine disease decarboxylation of branched chain ketoacids is impaired but because transamination is reversible, the precursor aminoacids accumulate to become the most obvious biochemical abnormality in the blood. The commonest aminoacidaemias are phenylketonuria, maple syrup urine disease and homocystinuria.

PHENYLKETONURIA

In phenylketonuria there is a high concentration of phenylalanine in the blood. This metabolic disturbance arises from a failure of phenylalanine hydroxylase, which is involved in the conversion of phenylalanine to tyrosine. The outstanding clinical features are poor intellectual performance, increased motor activity, agitated behaviour, hypertonia, tremor and epilepsy. Children with phenylketonuria commonly have blond hair and eczema. Early diagnosis allows dietary treatment to be undertaken before extensive neurological damage has occurred. Phenylalanine should be restricted but must not be excluded from the diet. For the first three years of life phenylketonuric infants need an intake of 50–70 mg/kg/day of phenylalanine; thereafter requirements fall to less than 20 mg/kg/day (Stanbury *et al* 1972).

MAPLE SYRUP URINE DISEASE

As already mentioned, the basic biochemical abnormality is inadequate decarboxylation of branched chain ketoacids. These are transaminated back to leucine, isoleucine and valine. The clinical presentations are failure to thrive, vomiting, hypertonia alternating with hypotonia, and convulsions. Initial management entails exclusion of branched chain aminoacids from the diet until their plasma level has fallen to near normal levels. Milk and other natural sources of protein can then be given in quantities which are controlled by regularly monitoring the plasma concentrations of branched chain aminoacids.

HOMOCYSTINURIA

The inborn error of metabolism in the classical form of homocystinuria is defective cystathionine synthetase. This leads to abnormally low tissue cystathionine, the appearance of homocystine in plasma and urine, and the accumulation of methionine in the blood. The salient clinical manifestations are ectopia lentis, mental retardation, thromboembolic phenomena, osteoporosis and skeletal abnormalities. The most satisfactory treatment is a diet low in methionine, supplemented with cystine (Stanbury *et al* 1972). In some patients large doses of pyridoxine (250–500 mg/day) improve the biochemical disturbances and may influence the clinical course.

ORGANICACIDAEMIAS

The organicacidaemias are a rare group of hereditary metabolic encephalopathies which have only recently become recognised. They present in the initial decade of life (commonly in the first year) as hypotonia with a declining level of consciousness, acidosis and ketosis; deterioration is often triggered off by minor infections. The organicacidaemias are caused by impairment of enzymes concerned with the metabolism of major dietary constituents. The most fully described are isovaleric acidaemia, methylmalonic acidaemia and propionic acidaemia. These conditions cannot be distinguished by clinical examination; their features are very similar to certain disorders of ketone body metabolism. Diagnosis therefore depends upon biochemical identification of an abnormal organic acid in the urine. Rational therapy is not possible until the biochemical defect has been established.

Many patients respond to restricting the intake of dietary precursors of the appropriate organic acids. Some also benefit from large doses of vitamins—thiamine, B_{12} or biotin—which are capable of increasing the activity of certain defective enzymic reactions (Gompertz 1972). The dosage of vitamins is frequently 100–1,000 times the normal adult maintenance requirement; intake does not have to be adjusted once a satisfactory response has been obtained.

OTHER TREATABLE ENCEPHALOPATHIC SYNDROMES

Other treatable encephalopathies occur in certain infective diseases (see Chapter 5), vascular disorders (see Chapter 6) and porphyria (see below). Neurological syndromes which may be clinically indistinguishable from an encephalopathy are encountered in patients with frontal tumours, chronic subdural haematoma or normal pressure hydrocephalus—three conditions which can often be corrected by surgery.

Peripheral neuropathy

Some metabolic peripheral neuropathies can be arrested or even improved by correction of the underlying biochemical abnormality. The progress of others may be delayed by avoiding provocative factors which exacerbate the causal metabolic disturbance.

DIABETIC NEUROPATHY

Neurological complications of diabetes mellitus commonly present as: a multiple mononeuropathy, a symmetrical neuropathy which generally has prominent sensory features, or an autonomic neuropathy. Treatment is directed at controlling the blood sugar by dietary restriction of carbohydrates. It is usually necessary, in addition, to administer hypoglycaemic agents—insulin, sulphonylureas or biguanides.

Insulin

Patients with ketonuria usually need insulin. Mild diabetics can manage on a single daily injection of lente insulin (insulin zinc suspension) or isophane insulin each morning, but if requirements exceed 40 units/day it is generally more satisfactory to give twice daily injections of either soluble insulin alone, or a combination of soluble insulin with isophane insulin in approximately equal quantities. Unstable ('brittle') diabetics may require more than two injections of insulin each day.

The commonest unwanted effect is hypoglycaemia. Repeated injections can cause atrophy of subcutaneous adipose tissue or the development of lipomata; local hypersensitivity reactions are occasionally encountered.

Sulphonylureas

Chlorpropamide. Chlorpropamide is well absorbed and has a plasma half-life around 36 hours, so that only one dose is needed each day. Requirements range from 100–500 mg daily. Chlorpropamide can induce hypoglycaemia, nausea, tinnitus, vertigo, headache, lassitude, paraesthesiae, flushing, jaundice, alcohol intolerance, skin eruptions, marrow depression and weight gain.

Tolbutamide. Tolbutamide is readily absorbed from the gastro-intestinal tract. It becomes bound to plasma proteins and undergoes rapid oxidation in the liver; the plasma half-life is about 5 hours. Two to three doses over the day are necessary to obtain reasonably sustained control of the blood sugar. The usual intake is 0.5–3.0 g daily. Adverse reactions are similar to those of chlorpropamide.

Glibenclamide. Some 50% of an orally administered dose of glibenclamide is absorbed. It becomes bound to plasma proteins;

the plasma half-life is about 5 hours. Some 5 mg of glibenclamide is equivalent to 250 mg of chlorpropamide or 1 g of tolbutamide. Toxic effects resemble those of chlorpropamide.

Biguanides

Phenformin. Phenformin is readily absorbed from the gut. Optimum intake usually lies between 50 and 150 mg/day which is taken in 1–2 doses of the sustained release preparation. Phenformin is often added to the therapeutic regimen of patients already receiving a sulphonylurea. Nausea, diarrhoea, drowsiness and lassitude can occur.

PORPHYRIA

Acute intermittent porphyria commonly starts with abdominal pain, vomiting, autonomic disturbances, restlessness and confusion which progress to epilepsy, coma, or a predominantly motor neuropathy, often involving bulbar and respiratory muscles (Ridley 1969). During an attack porphobilinogen appears in the urine. The disease is usually transmitted as a dominant trait. The outstanding clinical feature of acute intermittent porphyria is precipitation of attacks by certain drugs, such as apronal, barbiturates, chlordiazepoxide, ethylalcohol, glutethimide, griseofulvin, hydantoins, meprobamate, methyldopa, oral contraceptives, sulphonamides, suximides and tolbutamide (Beattie and Goldberg 1972). The most important therapeutic consideration is the withholding of provocative drugs. Diazepam (see Chapter 15) is the safest sedative in porphyria and carbamazepine (see Chapter 12) is usually satisfactory as an anticonvulsant. Artificial ventilation may be required during episodes of bulbar or respiratory weakness. Propranolol (see Chapter 14) is useful if tachycardia or hypertension are prominent (Beattie *et al* 1973).

Variegate porphyria (porphyria cutanea tarda) is characterised by prominent skin lesions; neurological manifestations are similar to those of acute intermittent porphyria. Exacerbations are precipitated by light, and by the drugs mentioned above.

REFSUM'S DISEASE (HEREDOPATHIA ATACTICA POLYNEURITIFORMIS)

Refsum's disease is caused by an autosomal recessive gene. There is impairment of oxidation of phytanic acid (Herndon *et al* 1969), which accumulates in the blood. Improvement has been reported following restriction of the intake of phytanic acid and phytol (Eldjarn *et al* 1966; Quinlan and Martin 1970). Fruit, vegetables and butter are omitted from the diet. Vitamin supplements (A, B_1, B_6, C) are included.

ALCOHOLIC NEUROPATHY

In some countries alcoholism is the commonest cause of peripheral neuropathy. Axonal damage seems to arise from deprivation of the B complex of vitamins rather than a direct neurotoxic action of ethanol (Victor 1974). Treatment therefore entails administration of vitamins B_1 and B_6 (see Chapter 10), in addition to ethanol withdrawal.

RENAL FAILURE

The peripheral neuropathy of renal failure is improved by dialysis or transplantation (Thomas *et al* 1971).

Myopathies

Treatable metabolic myopathies fall into two major categories—periodic paralysis and endocrine myopathies. Muscular weakness is also encountered in patients with prominent elevation or depletion of serum potassium secondary to renal pathology, gastrointestinal disease, excessive administration of diuretics or inadequately controlled intravenous fluid therapy. Myopathies associated with myoglobinuria cannot be alleviated to any significant extent by any drugs (McArdle 1969). Muscular dystrophies present a similarly depressing picture of therapeutic destitution. The treatment of polymyositis is considered in Chapter 7.

PERIODIC PARALYSIS

Hereditary episodic weakness may be associated with low, high or normal concentrations of potassium in the blood. Periodic paralysis occasionally occurs without any detectable genetic origin, particularly in association with thyrotoxicosis.

HYPOKALAEMIC PARALYSIS

Oral potassium chloride may be helpful in episodes of hypokalaemic weakness. An initial dose of 10 g can be followed after an hour by a further 5 g if necessary (McArdle 1969). Prophylactic treatment is disappointing, though some success has been reported with hydrochlorothiazide 25 mg (see Chapter 12) and potassium chloride 1.2 g, administered together twice a day.

HYPERKALAEMIC PARALYSIS (ADYNAMIA EPISODICA HEREDITARIA, PARAMYOTONIA CONGENITA)

While attacks of weakness in this condition are seldom sufficiently disabling to require treatment, there are several measures which can be tried if necessary (McArdle 1969; Beeson and McDermott 1971): intravenous calcium gluconate (10–20 ml as a 10% solution injected over 5 minutes); intravenous chlorothiazide (500 mg); or intravenous insulin and glucose (1 litre of 10% glucose with 30–40 units of soluble insulin).

The frequency and severity of episodes is usually reduced by regular administration of a diuretic such as hydrochlorothiazide 25 mg twice daily or acetazolamide 250 mg twice daily. These drugs are considered in more detail in Chapter 12.

NORMOKALAEMIC PARALYSIS

Sodium chloride may relieve an episode of normokalaemic paresis. An oral dose of 10 g can be followed by 5 g intravenously if weakness persists (1 litre of 2.7% saline). Poskanzer and Kerr (1961) have reported a reduction in the frequency of attacks following a combination of acetazolamide 250 mg/day with fludrocortisone 0.1 mg/day.

ENDOCRINE MYOPATHIES

Myopathies occur in hyperthyroidism, hypothyroidism, Cushing's syndrome, adrenocortical insufficiency, acromegaly, hypopituitarism and calcium disturbances.

HYPERTHYROID MYOPATHY

Thyrotoxicosis can be managed by subtotal thyroidectomy, administration of I^{131}, or the use of antithyroid drugs such as carbimazole, methimazole or propylthiouracil.

Carbimazole. Carbimazole is well absorbed by the gastrointestinal tract and undergoes rapid excretion in the urine. An initial intake of 10 mg thrice daily can be reduced to 5–20 mg a day as thyroid function is brought under control. Adverse reactions include nausea, abdominal pain, skin eruptions, pruritus, fever, arthralgia, alopecia and blood dyscrasias. Excessive dosage produces hypothyroidism.

Methimazole. Methimazole has similar properties to carbimazole. The initial dose is 5–10 mg thrice daily; maintenance intake is 5–10 mg/day.

Propylthiouracil. Propylthiouracil is an alternative antithyroid drug. A starting dose of 50–200 mg thrice daily can be adjusted to a lower level when the patient becomes euthyroid. Toxic effects are the same as those described for carbimazole.

HYPOTHYROID MYOPATHY

Hypothyroid myopathy is rare. It responds to treatment with thyroxine, which has already been discussed in this Chapter.

CUSHING'S SYNDROME

Cushing's syndrome is treated by destruction of the adrenals (bilateral adrenalectomy) or partial pituitary ablation (incomplete hypophysectomy or yttrium implantation). Subsequent replacement therapy is sometimes required with prednisone 5.0–7.5 mg/day or hydrocortisone 20–30 mg/day. If damage to the pituitary has been excessive, it may be necessary to add thyroxine (0.05–0.3 mg/day) and for men, sustained release testosterone propionate (250 mg by intramuscular injection every three weeks). A mineralo-corticoid such as fludrocortisone (0.1–0.2 mg/day by mouth) may also be required after adrenalectomy.

ADRENOCORTICAL INSUFFICIENCY

Hypoadrenalism is treated with prednisone or hydrocortisone, together with fludrocortisone if necessary, as discussed above.

ACROMEGALY

Patients who have undergone hypophysectomy or yttrium implantation for acromegaly sometimes require replacement of adrenal, thyroid and gonadal hormones as outlined when considering management after pituitary ablation for Cushing's syndrome.

HYPOPITUITARISM

Treatment is the same as that described after destruction of the pituitary for Cushing's syndrome.

CALCIUM DISTURBANCES

Severe hypercalcaemia is usually associated with a myopathy; while this may involve a deficiency of vitamin D, initial management is directed to correcting the hypercalcaemia (see above). Osteomalacic myopathy is considered in Chapter 10.

CHAPTER 10
VITAMIN DEFICIENCY

Neurological disease can result from deficiency of vitamins due to either inadequate dietary intake, or the presence of a gastrointestinal disorder which impairs absorption. Deficiencies are often multiple, with complex clinical mainfestations. In the following account it is convenient to consider the individual vitamins separately, but this presentation is not intended to imply that identification and treatment of one deficiency problem renders the pursuit of others unnecessary.

The terms inadequacy, insufficiency and deficiency will be confined to situations where lack of a vitamin produces symptoms or signs, as opposed to the mere finding of a low concentration of vitamin in the plasma or tissues. Vitamins which are required for normal neurological function will be considered in the following order: (1) Cyanocobalamin; (2) Thiamine; (3) Nicotinic acid; (4) Pyridoxine; (5) Calciferol and cholecalciferol; (6) The controversial status of folic acid.

CYANOCOBALAMIN

Cyanocobalamin (vitamin B_{12}) deficiency can lead to a wide spectrum of disease: megaloblastic anaemia, subacute combined degeneration of the spinal cord (posterolateral sclerosis, combined system disease), peripheral neuropathy, optic atrophy and dementia. In spite of the importance of B_{12} in the haemopoietic and nervous

145

systems, only two enzymic reactions have been identified in which its derivatives play an essential role—conversion of L-methyl-malonic coenzyme A to succinyl coenzyme A, and of homocysteine to methionine. Neither of these transformations has been related to the neuropathology of B_{12} insufficiency.

Vitamin B_{12} deficiency can seldom be attributed to inadequate dietary intake. A nutritional aetiology is virtually limited to vegans—extreme vegetarians who eat neither eggs nor milk products. The commonest cause of B_{12} insufficiency is malabsorption, most frequently due to inadequate intrinsic factor consequent upon auto-immune atrophic gastritis (Addisonian pernicious anaemia). Vitamin B_{12} deficiency sufficient to produce neurological problems also occurs in association with total and partial gastrectomy, gastroenterostomy, diverticulosis of the small bowel, intestinal strictures or anastomoses, tuberculous enteritis, distal gut resection, tropical sprue and intestinal helminthiasis.

In a recent critical review Pallis and Lewis (1974) conclude that provided there has not been prior administration of B_{12}, its serum concentration must be less than 100 pg/ml in order to establish a causal relationship with neurological abnormalities.

All patients with neurological or haematological complications of B_{12} deficiency should be treated. The body stores of B_{12} normally range from 1–12 mg. A daily intake of some 2 μg is required to replace loss. Absorption takes place in two ways: an active transport system involving intrinsic factor and a slow, inefficient passive process. Because availability of intrinsic factor limits absorption, it is usual to correct deficiency by parenteral administration. Following injection of cyanocobalamin there is binding to plasma proteins and storage in the liver, but more than 50% is excreted in the urine within 48 hours. Hydroxocobalamin is now being employed more than cyanocobalamin because the former achieves higher and more prolonged plasma levels. An initial replenishment dose of 1,000 μg of hydroxocobalamin is usually given by intramuscular injection and repeated five times. Maintenance treatment of 500 μg is then given every 2–3 months. While hydroxocobalamin therapy is generally continued indefinitely, there are three situations in which treatment need not be sustained as the cause of B_{12} deficiency can be eradicated.

BACTERIAL OVERGROWTH SYNDROME

Abnormal bacterial colonisation of the small bowel (associated with a blind loop, stricture or fistula) probably causes B_{12} deficiency because enteric organisms compete for supplies of the vitamin. Temporary improvement can be obtained with broad spectrum antimicrobial drugs such as tetracycline and ampicillin, which are usually given in alternating courses lasting 10–14 days. Surgical resection of the offending blind loop, stricture or fistula achieves permanent cure.

TROPICAL SPRUE

In tropical sprue, malabsorption leads to an insufficiency of B_{12}. It usually responds to a broad spectrum antimicrobial agent (such as tetracycline 250 mg four times a day) together with folic acid 10 mg daily. After a few weeks the tetracycline can be stopped and the dose of folic acid reduced to a maintenance level of 5 mg/day.

DIPHYLLOBOTHRIUM LATUM INFESTATION

Diphyllobothrium latum probably induces deprivation of B_{12} by avid consumption of the vitamin. This tapeworm can be expelled by dichlorophen or male fern extract (Felix Mas). Dichlorophen should be given in a dose of 6 g which is repeated after 24 hours; it may cause nausea, vomiting, colic and diarrhoea. Alternatively, male fern is administered after fasting and purgation, 3–4 g usually being sufficient. Toxic reactions to male fern include vomiting, diarrhoea, jaundice and proteinuria.

THIAMINE

The neurological manifestations of thiamine (vitamin B_1) deficiency are peripheral neuropathy, Wernicke's encephalopathy and Korsakoff psychosis. Many now regard the latter two conditions as overlapping to such an extent that they can be considered as a unified syndrome (Victor *et al* 1971).

The active form of vitamin B_1 is thiamine pyrophosphate, which serves as the prosthetic group for enzymes involved in the decarboxylation of pyruvic and alpha ketoglutaric acid. Thiamine is therefore essential for the intermediary metabolism of carbohydrates—severe insufficiency leads to accumulation of pyruvic acid.

Thiamine deficiency is usually due to an inadequate diet, particularly if this is associated with alcoholism. Protracted vomiting is a common exacerbating factor. Deprivation is also caused by malabsorption, in particular gastric surgery and untreated coeliac disease.

Daily requirements of thiamine depend upon the metabolic rate and the proportion of carbohydrate in the diet; the usual range is 0.2–0.4 ng/1,000 kcal.

Thiamine is water soluble; it is absorbed from most of the proximal small intestine by an active transport system. About 1 mg is metabolised daily. An oral intake of 40 mg/day results in 8–15 mg being absorbed; higher dosage merely leads to augmented loss in the faeces. There are negligible body stores of thiamine (some 25 mg).

Parenteral thiamine replenishes the body stores quickly; a dose of 25–100 mg can be given by subcutaneous or intramuscular injection. Oral administration of 5 mg daily provides adequate maintenance therapy.

NICOTINIC ACID

Deficiency of nicotinic acid (niacin) causes pellagrous dementia and acute encephalopathy (Jolliffe's syndrome). Nicotinic acid is converted to the coenzymes nicotinamide adenine dinucleotide and nicotinamide adenine dinucleotide phosphate. Attached to appropriate proteins, these function as dehydrogenases.

Nicotinic acid can be formed from tryptophan. Deficiency usually stems from inadequate dietary intake of both nicotinic acid and tryptophan. Occasionally malabsorption can be responsible, in association with obstructive intestinal lesions or jejunal diverticulosis (Tabaqchali and Pallis 1970).

Nicotinic acid is a water soluble vitamin, readily absorbed from all regions of the gastrointestinal tract. Tryptophan is absorbed by an active transport system. The daily requirement of nicotinic acid, expressed in relation to the dietary calorie intake, is about 6 mg/1,000 kcal. Some 60 mg of tryptophan is equivalent to 1 mg of nicotinic acid.

The initial dose of nicotinic acid to correct deficiency is 50–250 mg daily; this can be given parenterally or by mouth. Maintenance oral therapy is continued at 15–30 mg/day. A high intake of nicotinic acid commonly produces flushing which may be accompanied by itching and burning. To avoid these adverse effects a congener of nicotinic acid, nicotinamide, can be given instead. Nicotinamide has the same actions as nicotinic acid (apart from vasodilation), the same mode of absorption and the same potency. It is therefore administered in an identical way to that described for nicotinic acid.

PYRIDOXINE

Pyridoxine (vitamin B_6) deficiency can lead to peripheral neuropathy (the 'burning feet syndrome'), optic neuropathy and convulsions. Pyridoxine, pyridoxal and pyridoxamine are all converted to pyridoxal phosphate which is a coenzyme involved in decarboxylation, transamination and racemisation. Deficiency can result from administration of antagonists (isoniazid, penicillamine), malabsorption (coeliac disease and tropical sprue) or dietary insufficiency.

The usual daily requirement of pyridoxine is 2 mg, which is absorbed by passive diffusion. It is administered in a dose of 50–150 mg daily by mouth. Pyridoxine has been claimed to possess antiemetic properties; it has also been advocated for the alleviation of depression induced by oral contraceptives.

CALCIFEROL AND CHOLECALCIFEROL

Osteomalacia is associated with a myopathy characterised by chronic proximal weakness, wasting and discomfort (Prineas *et al* 1965; Smith and Stern 1968). This myopathy responds to treatment with vitamin D—it does not correlate with abnormal serum concentrations of calcium.

Vitamin D is a collective term for two fat soluble substances—D_2 (calciferol) and D_3 (cholecalciferol)—either of which can prevent the development of rickets. These vitamins are themselves biologically inert; they are converted to metabolites before they achieve any effect. Two active metabolites to have been identified are 25-hydroxy-cholecalciferol and 1,25-dihydroxycholecalciferol.

Vitamin D is normally formed by ultraviolet irradiation of dietary sterols. It promotes absorption of calcium from the gastro-intestinal tract. Large doses mobilise bone stores of calcium and increase its urinary excretion. Vitamin D is also involved in muscle physiology but its precise role has not yet been defined. Myopathy may be associated with osteomalacia induced by dietary deficiency of vitamin D, malabsorption, renal failure or parathyroid disease. Myopathy has also been reported in patients with osteomalacia due to phenytoin (Marsden *et al* 1973). A form of osteomalacia which does not lead to myopathy is type I hypophosphataemic rickets (Williams *et al* 1966); in this condition it is notable that the plasma concentration of vitamin D is normal.

Calciferol is effective treatment for the myopathy of osteomalacia but additional measures may be necessary to correct the metabolic bone disease. The normal daily requirement is about 2.5 μg (100 units). An oral dose of about 1.25 mg/day is usually employed in the treatment of myopathy associated with osteomalacia, though this intake may have to be modified according to the aetiology of the bone disease. Doses as low as 50 μg daily can be adequate in osteomalacic myopathy following gastrectomy whereas 15 mg daily may be required in gluten sensitive enteropathy (Smith and Stern 1967).

Calciferol is absorbed from the gastrointestinal tract without esterification but bile, in particular deoxycholic acid, is essential. The main excretory pathway is the biliary tract. Calciferol differs from the other vitamins which have been discussed because chronic overdosage can produce serious adverse effects. Prolonged adminis-tration of more than 2.5 mg/day may result in lassitude, anorexia, nausea, vomiting, diarrhoea, polyuria, excessive sweating, thirst and headache. Abnormal deposition of calcium can lead to renal failure and hypertension.

FOLIC ACID

For many years controversial views have been expressed on the neurological implications of folic acid deficiency. It has been suggested that there may be a causal relationship between folate insufficiency induced by anticonvulsants and the peripheral neuropathy which occasionally occurs in epileptics on prolonged treatment with phenytoin. No firm conclusion will be possible until it is established that folic acid has a therapeutic effect on this neuropathy. The argument that folate deprivation causes dementia is similarly difficult to substantiate; this problem is likely to remain unresolved until satisfactory evidence is produced that such intellectual impairment responds to administration of folic acid. Recent reports of 'organic brain syndrome', myelopathy and peripheral neuropathy attributable to folate deficiency (Pincus *et al* 1972; Reynolds *et al* 1973) will no doubt generate further studies in this difficult but important area. Meanwhile it would seem justifiable to give folic acid to any patient when there are reasonable grounds to suppose that a shortage of this vitamin might be contributing to a neurological deficit.

The mechanism by which anticonvulsants induce folate deficiency is not known. There is no convincing evidence to support the view that folic acid supplements interfere with the control of seizures. It is therefore appropriate to administer folic acid if a patient receiving anticonvulsants develops a megaloblastic anaemia with low red cell folate, provided the plasma concentration of B_{12} is normal— administration of folic acid to patients with B_{12} deficiency can precipitate subacute combined degeneration of the spinal cord.

Folic acid is a water soluble vitamin which is absorbed by active transport; it becomes bound to plasma proteins. An intake of 0.1 mg/day is normally adequate. Body stores only amount to about 5 mg. The therapeutic dose range is 5–20 mg daily.

CHAPTER 11

DRUG INDUCED NEUROLOGICAL
DISEASE

From a toxicological viewpoint, the central nervous system is relatively privileged when compared to the skin, blood, liver and kidney. The blood–brain barrier seems to play a major role in protection—the peripheral nerves and muscles are more vulnerable.

This Chapter lists a number of neurotoxic reactions. Few explanations are possible because the biochemical mechanisms whereby drugs induce neurological damage are poorly understood. Treatment is generally empirical—withdrawal of the causal agent. Early recognition of unwanted effects will often allow hazardous trends to be reversed or at least arrested.

Despite a progressive increase in the quantities of drugs consumed each year, there has not been a corresponding rise in the mortality from adverse reactions. In England and Wales, the annual death rate attributable to drugs has ranged from 104 to 236 between 1962 and 1967 (Orme 1972). The commonest neurological cause of death was cerebral haemorrhage due to anticoagulants (2.7% of the total drug induced mortality). The most frequent fatal complication of therapy directed against a neurological disease was aplastic anaemia precipitated by phenytoin (1.4% of the total drug induced mortality).

Drugs are capable of a wide range of neurotoxic manifestations, corresponding to lesions at every level of neural organisation. In this Chapter adverse reactions involving the nervous system and muscles will be considered in the following stages: (1) Predisposing factors; (2) Encephalopathies; (3) Focal intracranial lesions; (4) Etxrapyramidal syndromes; (5) Myelopathies; (6) Cranial neuro-

152

pathies; (7) Peripheral neuropathies; (8) Impairment of neuro-muscular transmission; (9) Myopathies.

PREDISPOSING FACTORS

Several factors predispose to drug induced neurological disease:

1   The most common of all causes of drug toxicity is overdosage. This can be deliberately contrived by subjects who are emotionally unstable. Alternatively, excessive intake may result from an accident, the error being made by the physician, the pharmacist or the patient. The management of coma due to acute overdosage has recently been reviewed by Matthew (1972).

2   Pharmacogenetic variation can lead to symptoms of overdosage; e.g. the peripheral neuropathy occurring in slow acetylators of isoniazid.

3   The presence of concomitant disease may underlie toxicity; e.g. administration of sulphonamides can provoke convulsions in porphyria.

4   Dietary factors may determine drug reactions; e.g. cerebral haemorrhage can follow the sudden rise in blood pressure that occurs when patients receiving a monoamine oxidase inhibitor ingest foods with a high tyramine content.

5   Drug interactions can produce adverse effects; e.g. administration of sulthiame to a patient receiving phenytoin may precipitate a toxic cerebellar disturbance by competitive inhibition of drug metabolism.

6   The route of administration can determine toxicity; e.g. intrathecal injection of methotrexate can precipitate myelopathy and encephalo-pathy; the blood–brain barrier protects the central nervous system from adverse reactions when methotrexate is given intravenously.

7   Damage to the blood-brain barrier renders the central nervous system more accessible; e.g. cerebral emboli during cardiopulmonary bypass predispose to penicillin encephalopathy.

8   Age influences the prevalence of drug induced neurological disease; e.g. dementia may follow general anaesthesia in the elderly. Neurotoxic reactions usually become more troublesome as patients grow old. Impaired excretion may be one causal factor; increased

vulnerability of the nervous system might also be related to the progressive loss of neurons which occurs with advancing age.

ENCEPHALOPATHIES

A number of therapeutic agents can cause headache, confusion, deterioration in the level of consciousness and fits. Such encephalopathy may be encountered in patients treated with azaribine, chloramphenicol, colaspase (asparaginase), fluorouracil, indomethacin, lignocaine (lidocaine), lithium, melarsoprol, methotrexate, para-aminosalicylic acid, penicillins, phenytoin, streptomycin, thallium and vaccines (Meyler and Peck 1972; Norell *et al* 1974; Weiss *et al* 1974).

Any of the above drugs may produce epilepsy without other encephalopathic features, as can amantadine, amitriptyline, amphetamine, baclofen, chlorambucil, chloroquine, cycloserine, digoxin, ephedrine, ergotamine, ethionamide, gentamicin, insulin, phenothiazines, prednisone, reserpine and vitamin K (Spillane 1964).

Dementia consequent upon general anaesthesia has already been mentioned in the context of toxicity in elderly patients. Diuretics and opiates can provoke encephalopathy in patients with cirrhosis (Weisberg 1966). Overdosage with hypoglycaemic drugs may also lead to stupor and loss of consciousness. Chlorpropamide, carbamazepine and diuretics have all been implicated in the production of water intoxication (Radó 1973).

Infective encephalopathy can result from the treatment of septicaemia with antimicrobial agents which do not cross the blood-brain barrier, such as cephalothin; these drugs render the central nervous system a particularly favourable site for bacteria to multiply.

Accumulating evidence indicates that benign intracranial hypertension can be induced by tetracycline, nalidixic acid, vitamin A, oral contraceptives, and administration or withdrawal of corticosteroids (Lorentz 1966; Neville and Wilson 1970).

FOCAL INTRACRANIAL LESIONS

The commonest focal lesion to be produced by drugs is cerebral haemorrhage, due to excessive anticoagulant therapy. Cerebral infarcts are occasionally encountered with oral contraceptives and hypotensive agents. Complications of cerebral angiography are usually caused by the arterial puncture rather than the injected material, but excessive volumes can occasionally lead to multiple small embolic infarcts (Traveras and Wood 1964).

An increased incidence of cerebral tumours, in particular microglioma, has been reported in patients on immunosuppressive drugs following renal transplantation (Schneck and Penn 1971).

Focal brainstem and cerebellar disturbances can occur in patients with excessive plasma concentrations of anticonvulsants.

EXTRAPYRAMIDAL SYNDROMES

Extrapyramidal reactions can be precipitated by phenothiazines, butyrophenones, diphenylbutylpiperidines, tricyclic antidepressants, reserpine, tetrabenazine, procaine and diazoxide (see Chapters 13 and 14). Ocasionally anticholinergic drugs induce dyskinesia (Fahn and David 1973). Chorea is a rare but well documented complication of oral contraceptive therapy (Lewis and Harrison 1969).

MYELOPATHIES

Some 20 years ago a new neurological disease became recognised in Japan—subacute myelo-optic neuropathy (SMON). Up to 1970, over 10,000 cases are estimated to have been diagnosed; rare examples were found in Europe, Scandinavia and Australia. Clioquinol became implicated over the last decade and there has been an abrupt fall in the incidence of SMON following the decision of the Japanese Ministry of Health to prohibit the sale of this drug. The neurotoxic predilection of clioquinol for Japan has not been fully explained (Pallis and Lewis 1974), but it may be relevant that the drug was extremely popular there—184 preparations containing clioquinol could be purchased without prescription during the period of peak prevalence of SMON. Furthermore the doses of clioquinol have been higher in Japan than elsewhere (Nakae *et al* 1973). Retrospective analyses indicate that the majority of patients tolerate up to 0.5 g/day of clioquinol indefinitely, without developing neurotoxicity; doses of 1.5–2.0 g/day tend to produce neurological lesions within two weeks. The biochemical cause of the neuropathology has not been identified. Green discolouration of the tongue, urine and faeces can be produced by iron chelates formed with clioquinol. It is of interest that overdosage with ethambutol can induce a clinical picture very similar to SMON (Satoyoshi 1973).

Other myelotoxic agents include rabies vaccine, intrathecal methotrexate and intrathecal streptomycin. Spinal arachnoiditis can be caused by iophendylate, but there is no agreement on the prophylactic value of its removal after myelography.

CRANIAL NEUROPATHIES

CRANIAL NERVE II

As already mentioned, clioquinol and ethambutol may cause optic neuropathy. Other drugs which can damage the optic nerve include isoniazid, penicillamine, chloramphenicol, digoxin, disulfiram, quinine and organic arsenicals. Pyridoxine protects patients from the optic neuropathy of isoniazid and penicillamine. Chloroquine therapy occasionally leads to retinopathy and corneal deposits. Several drugs can induce cataracts—corticosteroids and phenothiazines are the commonest causes. Corticosteroids can also precipitate glaucoma (D'Arcy and Griffin 1972).

CRANIAL NERVES III, IV, VI

External ophthalmoplegia is an unusual complication of anticonvulsant overdosage, io particular with phenytoin (Orth *et al* 1967).

CRANIAL NERVE V

Trichlorethylene can produce multiple cranial neuropathies (Buxton and Hayward 1967), the trigeminal nerve being specially vulnerable

(Feldman *et al* 1970). There is a high incidence of trigeminal neuropathy in patients receiving stilbamidine.

CRANIAL NERVE VIII

Several drugs can induce selective lesions of the VIIIth nerve and its connections. The aminoglycosides are the most important group; streptomycin and gentamicin cause predominant vestibular damage while neomycin, kanamycin, and viomycin are more toxic to the auditory division. Other ototoxic drugs include ethacrynic acid, frusemide, salicylates, quinine, chlorpropamide and ethionamide (D'Arcy and Griffin 1972).

PERIPHERAL NEUROPATHIES

Peripheral neuropathy is the commonest form of neurotoxicity in current therapeutics. Vincristine is probably the most frequent cause. Isoniazid neuropathy can be prevented by concomitant administration of pyridoxine (see Chapter 10). Nitrofurantoin, rabies vaccine, arsenic, lead, mercury, gold and thallium are all capable of producing a polyneuropathy. It is likely that early reports of peripheral neuropathy induced by thalidomide saved many thousands of pregnant women from receiving this drug and hence protected their infants from phocomelia. Recent evidence suggests that another hypnotic, methaqualone, may also cause peripheral neuropathy (Finke and Spiegelberg 1973). Further drugs which can occasionally be responsible include allopurinol, chloramphenicol, clioquinol, disulfiram, ethambutol, ethionamide, ethoglucid, glutethimide, hydrallazine, kanamycin, nitrogen mustard, penicillins, phenytoin, polymixin B, stilbamidine, streptomycin, sulphonamides, trichlorethylene and tricyclic antidepressants (Le Quesne 1970; 1974; Meyler and Peck 1972). Haemorrhage provoked by anticoagulant overdosage can cause an acute mononeuropathy.

Autonomic disturbances induced by drugs can lead to orthostatic hypotension and sphincter disorders resembling a neuropathy. Such effects are encountered with therapeutic agents deliberately employed to modify sympathetic (e.g. guanethidine) or parasympathetic (e.g. atropine) function. In addition, phenothiazines, tricyclic antidepressants and monoamine oxidase inhibitors can produce profound autonomic deficits. The polyneuropathy of porphyria may be precipitated or exacerbated by a number of drugs: apronal, barbiturates, chlordiazepoxide, glutethimide, griseofulvin, hydantoins, meprobamate, methyldopa, oral contraceptives, sulphonamides, suximides and tolbutamide (Beattie and Goldberg 1972).

IMPAIRMENT OF NEUROMUSCULAR TRANSMISSION

Several antimicrobial agents can induce reversible impairment of neuromuscular transmission; occasionally respiratory weakness is severe enough to require artificial ventilation. Many of the causal drugs to have been identified are aminoglycosides—streptomycin, dihydrostreptomycin, neomycin, kanamycin and viomycin. Polymixin B and colistin can also be responsible. While some of these agents produce abnormalities of neuromuscular conduction smiilar to the Lambert–Eaton syndrome others seem to cause depolarisation blockade.

Further drug induced neuromuscular disturbances include (1) the prolonged apnoea encountered in patients who are genetically slow inactivators of suxamethonium, (2) depolarisation blockade resulting from overdosage with anticholinesterase agents, (3) chronic degeneration of the neuromuscular junction consequent upon long term treatment with normal doses of cholinesterase inhibitors (see Chapter 17), (4) rare impairment of neuromuscular conduction by phenytoin, trimethadione, procainamide, quinine and busulphan.

MYOPATHIES

Corticosteroids produce a myopathy characterised by selective atrophy of type II muscle fibres (Cumings *et al* 1973). This is particularly common with fluorinated molecules; over 60% of patients receiving triamcinolone have been reported to become affected (Meyler and Peck 1972). Myopathy is also a well recognised complication of treatment with chloroquine and emetine. The genetically determined myopathic hyperpyrexial reaction to certain anaesthetic agents, such as halothane and suxamethonium, has already been discussed (see Chapter 1). Myotoxic properties have occasionally been attributed to azathioprine, barbiturates, carbenoxalone, colchicine, mithramycin, oral contraceptives, penicillins, phenothiazines, phenylbutazone and vincristine. The osteomalacia produced by phenytoin can be associated with a myopathy which responds to calciferol (see Chapter 10).

TREATMENT FOR CONSEQUENCES OF NEUROLOGICAL DISEASE

CHAPTER 12
EPILEPSY

In many respects the treatment of seizures is an ideal subject for study—epilepsy is common, chronic and readily quantifiable in terms of fit frequency. It is a sad reflection on clinical neuropharmacology that a critical examination of 200 published investigations has revealed only three reports in which a double-blind procedure was employed to assess anticonvulsant efficacy (Coatsworth 1971). Experience is largely anecdotal so in this Chapter most of the statements, other than those relating to experimental or biochemical observations, represent impressions rather than adequately documented facts.

The history of epilepsy is notable for both the futility and the hazards of early treatment. Early therapeutic approaches included the bot fly, mistletoe, human excrement, castration, excision of the clitoris, trephining and ingestion of the blood of gladiators (or beheaded criminals). The first effective drug, introduced just over a century ago, was bromide (Locock 1857). The recognition that sedatives could help epilepsy led to the successful use of phenobarbitone as an anticonvulsant just before the first world war. The realisation that anticonvulsant actions could be separated from sedative properties resulted in the emergence of phenytoin in the years leading up to the second world war (Merritt and Putman 1938).

Treatable causes of epilepsy include intracranial tumours, infarcts, infections, trauma, congenital anomalies, metabolic disturbances and exposure to toxic agents. In many patients, however, no structural or biochemical abnormality can be detected. The under-

163

lying mechanisms responsible for generating a convulsion are not understood (Jasper *et al* 1969); where a lesion is demonstrable, the clinical features of the fit are determined by its anatomical location rather than the nature of its pathology.

While experimental animal models of epilepsy have failed to make any important impact on the analysis of basic mechanisms, they have proved useful in screening new drugs for anticonvulsant activity. The usual methods employed to produce epilepsy in animals are application of electric shocks to the head; systemic administration of substances that induce fits, such as leptazol (pentylenetetrazol), picrotoxin or bicuculline; and intracranial implantation of irritative material, such as benzylpenicillin, alumina or metallic cobalt. In recent years photically induced epilepsy has been studied extensively in the Senegalese baboon (Killam *et al* 1967; Meldrum *et al* 1972; Wada *et al* 1972).

In this Chapter the treatment of epilepsy will be considered in the following stages: (1) Mechanism of action of anticonvulsants; (2) Pharmacokinetics; (3) Drug interactions; (4) Plasma concentrations of anticonvulsants; (5) Therapeutic principles; (6) Treatment of individual epileptic syndromes; (7) Related conditions; (8) Dose regimens and adverse reactions.

MECHANISM OF ACTION OF ANTICONVULSANTS

Knowledge of the mechanism of action of anticonvulsants is very limited. There is no convincing evidence that they inhibit the discharge of pathological neurons constituting a seizure focus. It seems more probable, on neurophysiological grounds, that they prevent the spread of abnormal activity to normal neurons. Thus many anticonvulsants suppress post-tetanic potentiation—enhancement of synaptic transmission which normally occurs after a rapidly repetitive volley of impulses (Esplin 1957). Certain anticonvulsants also stabilise the normal neuronal membrane (Morrell *et al* 1958) and inhibit the increased excitability induced by hypocalcaemia (Korey 1951). In recent years there has been increasing interest in the effects of anticonvulsants on transmitters in the brain. If the role of transmitters in epilepsy can be elucidated in more detail a rational approach to the development of new anticonvulsants might emerge. Current clinical studies with sodium valproate (sodium di-n-propylacetate), a substance recently found to increase brain concentrations of GABA, offer some support for this optimistic outlook.

GAMMA AMINOBUTYRIC ACID

GABA is usually associated with inhibitory transmission in the central nervous system. Drugs which increase cerebral concentrations of GABA, such as phenytoin (Verendakis and Woodbury 1960) or sodium valproate (Godin *et al* 1969) have antiepileptic properties. Conversely, picrotoxin, bicuculline and benzylpenicillin, commonly employed to provoke convulsions in experimental animals, block the inhibitory action of GABA (Curtis *et al* 1970; 1972; Iversen 1972).

MONOAMINES

Indirect evidence suggests that noradrenaline and serotonin have an anticonvulsant action. These monoamines do not readily cross the blood–brain barrier, so their effects have been studied by using precursors and enzyme inhibitors. High doses of monoamine oxidase inhibitors protect baboons from photosensitive epilepsy. Low doses of monoamine oxidase inhibitors require the addition of monoamine precursors (levodopa or L-tryptophan) to achieve this effect (Meldrum *et al* 1972).

Noradrenaline. Inhibitors of dopamine beta hydroxylase (responsible for converting dopamine to noradrenaline) block the contribution of levodopa to seizure control in the above model, so it seems that noradrenaline is more important, in this context, than dopamine (Torchiana *et al* 1973).

Serotonin. L-5-hydroxytryptophan, the immediate precursor of serotonin, suppresses photosensitive epilepsy in baboons. As already mentioned L-tryptophan augments the anticonvulsant action of monoamine oxidase inhibitors. In contrast parachlorophenylalanine, an inhibitor of serotonin synthesis, increases epileptic reactions

(Wada *et al* 1972). These observations indicate that serotonin, like noradrenaline, possesses anticonvulsant properties.

ACETYLCHOLINE

There are conflicting observations on acetylcholine. While many anticonvulsants increase the brain concentration of acetylcholine (Consolo *et al* 1972), there is also evidence that cholinesterase inhibitors can precipitate seizures, so no conclusion can yet be drawn concerning the part played by acetylcholine in epilepsy (Maynert 1969).

PHARMACOKINETICS

In spite of the obscurity surrounding the mechanism of action of anticonvulsants, significant advances have taken place in the management of epilepsy. These stem from developments in clinical pharmacology leading to increased understanding of pharmacokinetics and drug interactions. In addition, techniques for routine estimation of plasma concentrations of anticonvulsants have enabled physicians to manipulate the dosage of drugs with more precision and confidence than has hitherto been possible. Phenytoin, phenobarbitone and ethosuximide are the most widely used anticonvulsants so they will receive particular attention in the following review of antiepileptic drugs.

Pharmacokinetics will be considered in four stages: absorption, distribution, metabolism and excretion.

ABSORPTION

Most anticonvulsants have reasonably high lipid solubility and are absorbed by passive diffusion across the intestinal mucosa. The speed of tablet dissolution in the gastrointestinal tract varies from one pharmaceutical formulation to another and may be the rate limiting factor in absorption; an epidemic of phenytoin toxicity was recently caused by a change of excipient (Tyrer *et al* 1970).

Peak plasma concentrations of phenytoin are reached 6–12 hours after ingestion (Wilder *et al* 1972) and for phenobarbitone maximum plasma levels are attained in 6–18 hours (Lous 1954). Peak plasma concentrations of ethosuximide occur 3–7 hours after oral intake (Buchanan *et al* 1969).

DISTRIBUTION

The distribution pattern of anticonvulsants depends upon the drug, the route of intake and the time interval between administration and observation. For phenytoin, the highest concentrations are generally found in liver and kidney; rather less in muscle, brain and fat; least of all in plasma (Noach *et al* 1958). Within brain cells, a considerable fraction is bound to the endoplasmic reticulum (Woodbury 1969; Woodbury and Kemp 1971). Phenobarbitone and ethosuximide are more evenly distributed through the tissues (Goldbaum and Smith 1954; Chang *et al* 1972).

METABOLISM

The main site of anticonvulsant metabolism is the liver. Phenytoin and phenobarbitone undergo substantial degradation to inactive products. The major pathway for both drugs is hydroxylation at the *para* position of the phenyl group (Butler 1956; 1957) and, as already mentioned, many other drugs share this metabolic pathway so that important interactions can result.

While hydroxylation products of phenytoin and phenobarbitone do not possess anticonvulsant properties, some drugs are transformed to agents which are themselves capable of suppressing fits. For example, primidone is metabolised to phenobarbitone (Butler and Waddell 1956).

Hydroxylation of phenytoin is a saturable transformation, so the plasma half-life depends upon the concentration which is, in turn, related to dosage (Houghton and Richens 1974). For phenytoin the plasma half-life ranges from 7–80 hours and for phenobarbitone 14–53 hours. The value for ethosuximide is 24–49 hours; it is shorter in children than adults (Sherwin and Robb 1972).

EXCRETION

The major metabolites of phenytoin are formed in the liver. These, together with some 10% of unchanged drug, are discharged via the bile into the gut. Reabsorption leads to ultimate excretion in the urine; only a small proportion, 5–10% of an orally administered dose is detectable as phenytoin in the urine (Noach *et al* 1958) and faeces (Dill *et al* 1956). Phenobarbitone also undergoes an entero-hepatic circulation and only some 10–20% is excreted unchanged in the urine (Maynert and Van Dyke 1949), though raising the pH can increase this fraction—forced alkaline diuresis in overdosage can reduce the duration of coma by 60%.

DRUG INTERACTIONS

Interactions between anticonvulsants become apparent within the first 6 weeks of treatment. A number of examples have already been mentioned in Chapter 1. The major categories are: protein binding, competition for enzymes and enzyme induction.

PROTEIN BINDING

Some 90% of the plasma content of phenytoin is bound to proteins by a rapid and reversible reaction (Woodbury and Swinyard 1972). There is less binding of phenobarbitone, the proportion averaging around 40% (Maynert 1972). Other drugs, such as salicylic acid, sulphafurazole and phenylbutazone may all produce a transient rise in free phenytoin or phenobarbitone by displacing anticonvulsant from plasma protein complexes (Lunde *et al* 1970). A negligible fraction of ethosuximide is bound to plasma protein (Chang *et al* 1972).

COMPETITION FOR ENZYMES

A combination of drugs utilising the same enzymes may compete, so that the rate of metabolism is reduced and plasma concentrations can rise to produce toxicity. Drugs which may decrease the rate of metabolism of phenytoin include sulthiame, aminosalicylic acid, cycloserine, methylphenidate, disulfiram and dicoumarol. The plasma phenytoin concentration is increased in some 10 % of patients taking isoniazid (slow acetylators only); this rise appears to be caused by non-competitive inhibition of metabolism.

ENZYME INDUCTION

Repeated administration of phenobarbitone can induce an increase in the enzymes concerned with its own metabolism. The same enzymes are employed for the metabolism of other drugs such as phenytoin. Addition of phenobarbitone to a patient stabilised on phenytoin may therefore lead to accelerated hepatic hydroxylation so that the plasma concentration of the latter falls. Less complete evidence suggests that phenytoin, primidone and carbamazepine can also increase microsomal enzyme activity. There is considerable variation between individuals in their ability to induce enzymes, which is probably genetically determined.

The clinical consequences of drug interactions are difficult to predict. While addition of one anticonvulsant may lower the plasma concentration of another, the control of fits may improve rather than deteriorate because of the antiepileptic activity of the new drug. The complexities are increased still further because the same anticonvulsants can both induce and compete for metabolic enzymes. In this setting there are so many variables that epileptic management can become a major exercise in clinical neuropharmacology.

PLASMA CONCENTRATION OF ANTICONVULSANTS

The usual therapeutic, non-toxic plasma concentration of phenytoin is 10–20 μg/ml (Kutt 1971). For phenobarbitone the desirable range of plasma level is 10–25 μg/ml (Buchthal and Lennox-Buchthal 1972). Optimal fit control with ethosuximide is achieved with plasma concentration over 40 μg/ml (Sherwin and Robb 1972), but

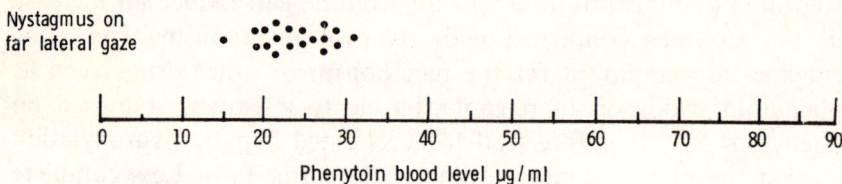

Nystagmus on
straightforward gaze

Nystagmus on 45°
deviation from midline

Nystagmus on
far lateral gaze

0   10   20   30   40   50   60   70   80   90

Phenytoin blood level μg/ml

Fig. 34. The relationship between nystagmus and the plasma concentration of phenytoin. Results of 39 clinico-biochemical correlations on 32 patients (Kutt *et al* 1964, *Arch. Neurol.* **11**, 642).

the values do not correlate well with toxicity; many patients have over 100 μg/ml without any adverse reactions (Buchanan 1972). While estimation of the plasma level has an important place in the management of epilepsy it cannot solve every problem. There remains a substantial variation in the therapeutic response to maximum tolerated intake of anticonvulsants. Furthermore, the relationship between the concentrations of drugs in the blood and brain may not be simple; sometimes the crude clinical titration of anticonvulsant intake against a dose dependent side effect, such as nystagmus, may prove more useful (Fig. 34). However, for phenytoin and phenobarbitone there is a direct linear relationship (Figs. 35 and 36) between concentrations in the brain and plasma (Sherwin *et al* 1973; Vajda *et al* 1974).

Estimation of the concentration of anticonvulsants in the blood has four major applications: obtaining evidence of drug ingestion, establishing genetically determined variation in pharmacokinetics, monitoring interactions, and determining optimum dosage in patients with disease affecting absorption, metabolism or excretion.

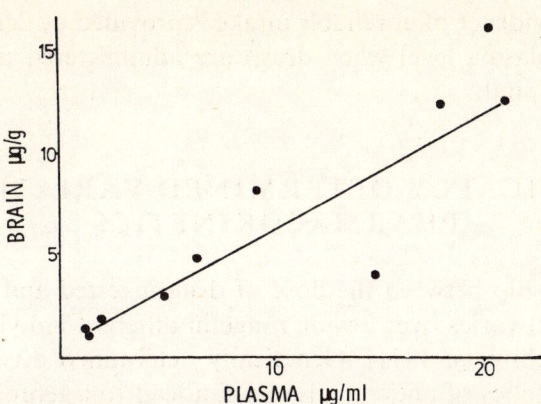

Fig. 35. The relationship between the concentration of phenytoin in the plasma and the brain of patients undergoing temporal lobectomy for epilepsy (Vajda *et al* 1973, *Clin. Pharmacol. Ther.*, **15,** 597).

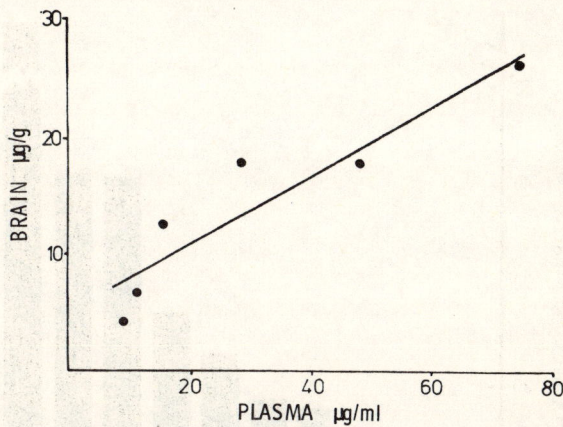

Fig. 36. The relationship between the concentration of phenobarbitone in the plasma and the brain of patients undergoing temporal lobectomy for epilepsy (Vajda *et al* 1973, *Clin. Pharmacol. Ther.*, **15,** 597).

EVIDENCE OF DRUG INGESTION

Estimation of the plasma concentration of drugs may be the only way to establish beyond doubt whether or not patients are taking their anticonvulsants in the prescribed dosage (Gibberd *et al* 1970).

Irrefutable evidence of unreliable intake is provided by demonstration of a rising plasma level when drugs are administered under supervision in hospital.

GENETICALLY DETERMINED VARIATION IN PHARMACOKINETICS

The relationship between the dose of drug ingested and the plasma concentration varies over a wide range in different individuals (Kutt 1971; Morselli *et al* 1971). Genetically determined diversity in the pharmacokinetics of anticonvulsants can lead to a tenfold spread in the plasma levels of phenytoin in patients taking the same dose (Fig. 37), which is a major factor contributing to the poor correlation between anticonvulsant intake and seizure control.

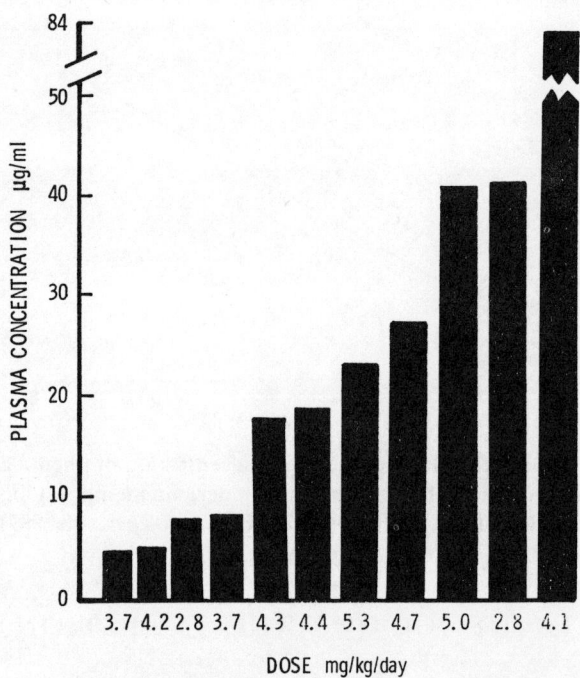

Fig. 37. Variation in the steady state plasma concentrations of phenytoin in different patients (from Morselli *et al* 1971, *Ann. N.Y. Acad. Sci.*, **179**, 88).

MONITORING DRUG REACTIONS

The importance of drug interactions in the care of epileptic patients has already been discussed. Estimation of the plasma concentration of anticonvulsants enables interactions to be managed with far greater confidence and precision than has previously been possible.

ESTABLISHING CORRECT DOSAGE IN PATIENTS WITH DISEASES AFFECTING ABSORPTION, METABOLISM OR EXCRETION

Estimation of plasma concentrations of a drug may be useful when attempting to establish optimal dosage in a patient with severe gastro-intestinal, hepatic or renal disease which distorts normal pharma-cokinetics.

THERAPEUTIC PRINCIPLES

The efficacy of anticonvulsants has not been submitted to the critical methods of evaluation necessary for drawing definite therapeutic conclusions. The antiepileptic potency of most drugs appears to be inversely related to the sophistication of the design employed to investigate them—the more carefully a drug is evaluated, the less active it is found to be. In his review of this subject, Coatsworth (1971) has argued that the predominance of inadequate technique in therapeutic studies means that the overall efficacy of anticonvulsants is probably less than the 70–80% usually cited.

In spite of the paucity of established facts, epileptic patients require treatment so certain principles must be formulated from the admittedly limited evidence that is available:

1 Treatment of epilepsy is directed at reducing the frequency and severity of seizures to an acceptable level, which will depend upon the patient's age, occupation, personality and intelligence. It may sometimes be possible to eliminate fits completely, but this is not necessarily the ultimate aim for every patient. All anticonvulsants produce dose dependent adverse reactions so a compromise is

usually sought between uncontrolled epilepsy on the one hand and drug intoxication on the other.

2　A history of one seizure is an indication for investigation (EEG, skull X-ray and possibly brain scan). It is not usual to start prophylactic therapy unless there is a second fit within a few months, because an isolated convulsion may be precipitated by factors which may never recur.

3　Any treatable cause, such as a metabolic disturbance or intra-cranial infection, should be corrected.

4　Once started, prophylactic therapy should continue until 2–3 years have elapsed without any seizures.

5　A minimum number of drugs should be employed because of the risk of interactions.

6　Alterations in treatment should be undertaken gradually. Anticonvulsants should never be stopped abruptly because sudden cessation of therapy can precipitate major status epilepticus. When antiepileptic drugs are no longer necessary, dosage should be reduced slowly over a period of several weeks.

7　Seizures related to menstruation often respond to a temporary increase in anticonvulsant intake 3 or 4 days before each period. Diuretics such as hydrochlorothiazide may also be helpful at this time.

TREATMENT OF INDIVIDUAL EPILEPTIC SYNDROMES

The use of anticonvulsants in the various forms of epilepsy has been the subject of several recent monographs and reviews (Schmidt and Wilder 1968; Pryce-Phillips 1969; Coatsworth 1971; Pearce 1972; Woodbury *et al* 1972; Brett 1973; Parsonage 1973; Swash 1973). From the therapeutic viewpoint, epilepsy falls into eight categories summarised in Table 7.

GRAND MAL, FOCAL MOTOR EPILEPSY AND FOCAL SENSORY EPILEPSY

These seizure patterns respond to a group of drugs also effective in rare epileptic manifestations such as reflex epilepsy (Whitty *et al* 1964),

Table 7. Summary of drugs commonly employed in the treatment of different forms of epilepsy.

Grand mal, focal motor and focal sensory epilepsy	phenytoin phenobarbitone primidone
Temporal lobe epilepsy	as above plus:— carbamazepine
Petit mal	ethosuximide
Myoclonic and akinetic epilepsy	nitrazepam
Infantile spasms	prednisone corticotrophin nitrazepam
Neonatal epilepsy, febrile convulsions	phenobarbitone phenytoin
Major status epilepticus	diazepam paraldehyde thiopentone phenobarbitone
Minor forms of status epilepticus	diazepam corticotrophin ethosuximide
Epilepsy related to menstruation	hydrochlorothiazide acetazolamide

paroxysmal kinesogenic choreoathetosis (Stevens 1966; Kertesz 1967) and tonic seizures (Matthews 1958).

Because of the extended period of treatment usually involved in managing epileptic patients, long term safety is as important as therapeutic potency in determining the choice of drugs. Phenytoin is usually the most satisfactory anticonvulsant. If toxic reactions are encountered before achieving satisfactory control of seizures, phenobarbitone or primidone can be tried. Carbamazepine is often helpful though the main indication for this drug is temporal lobe epilepsy. Other anticonvulsants which are occasionally prescribed include ethotoin and metharbitone (metharbital). Albutoin (Carter 1971), clonazepam (Birket-Smith and Mikkelsen 1972) and sodium valproate (Harvey 1974) are currently undergoing evaluation.

TEMPORAL LOBE EPILEPSY

All the drugs listed for the treatment of grand mal can also be employed in temporal lobe epilepsy. Carbamazepine is reputed to be particularly effective (Wink 1972); phenytoin and primidone are frequently useful; phenobarbitone is less satisfactory. Pheneturide, phenacemide and sulthiame may be tried in cases of intractable temporal lobe epilepsy but these drugs are relatively toxic. Temporal lobectomy is the treatment of choice for some patients; the criteria for selection of cases for surgery are stringent (Falconer 1970).

PETIT MAL

Ethosuximide is the best drug for petit mal. Encouraging results have recently been reported with clonazepam (Hooshmand 1972a), though the response is not always sustained (Rossi *et al* 1973). Troxidone and paramethadione are often effective but adverse reactions are common. Acetazolamide can be useful but its therapeutic activity seldom persists so it is commonly administered in short courses. Occasionally treatment of petit mal can precipitate grand mal (Lorentz de Haas and Kuilman 1964); if this happens, the grand mal should be managed as already discussed.

MYOCLONIC AND AKINETIC EPILEPSY

Nitrazepam is usually the most satisfactory drug for myoclonic and akinetic epilepsy (Hagberg 1968; Mattson 1972). These types of seizure are commonly refractory to any treatment other than benzodiazepines.

INFANTILE SPASMS (HYPSARRHYTHMIA)

Corticotrophin or corticosteroids ameliorate the fits and the hypsarrhythmic EEG of infantile spasms (Jeavons and Bower 1964).

Nitrazepam (Volske *et al* 1967) and diazepam are often helpful. Unfortunately the long term outlook is poor because mental retardation and hyperkinetic behaviour usually progress (Brett 1973).

NEONATAL EPILEPSY AND FEBRILE CONVULSIONS

Phenobarbitone is generally employed for these conditions. Some children become overactive and aggressive when taking barbiturates —if this occurs, phenytoin should be prescribed instead.

Current evidence indicates that febrile seizures should be treated prophylactically with continuous anticonvulsants (Faerø *et al* 1972); intermittent therapy during episodes of pyrexia is unsatisfactory because of the time required to reach effective plasma concentrations. If a febrile convulsion continues for an hour, admission to hospital is mandatory and the management is that of major status epilepticus.

MAJOR STATUS EPILEPTICUS

Two or more convulsions without regaining consciousness, or a major seizure which lasts more than an hour, constitute major status epilepticus. This is still a grave medical emergency, though the prognosis has been improved by advances in neurological therapeutics and intensive care. Irreversible sequelae are probably caused by a combination of cardiorespiratory factors (Meldrum and Brierley 1973) together with brain damage produced by prolonged excessive electroconvulsive discharges (Epstein and O'Connor 1966).

Intravenous diazepam suppresses epileptic activity (Parsonage and Norris 1967). Recent reports suggest that clonazepam may also be effective (Gastaut *et al* 1971; Bladin 1973). Paraldehyde and phenobarbitone are safe anticonvulsants which can be administered by intravenous or intramuscular injection. Thiopentone is occasionally employed and chlormethiazole may be useful. Phenytoin is not usually given because high dose levels can exacerbate epilepsy (Levy and Fenichel 1965).

In addition to treating the convulsions, the cause of status should be sought, an adequate airway must be established, fluid balance is maintained and hyperpyrexia must be prevented. At the earliest signs of cardiorespiratory complications, positive pressure ventilation should be undertaken. If this becomes necessary, pancuronium or tubocurarine may be given to obtain suitable muscle relaxation. Intramuscular phenobarbitone should be administered to provide sustained control of fits and when this has been achieved conventional oral therapy can be started.

The most important general point in the management of major status epilepticus is that large doses of anticonvulsants must be employed throughout and the switch from parenteral to oral therapy should not be undertaken too early.

MINOR FORMS OF STATUS EPILEPTICUS

Petit mal status is manifested by periods of clouding of consciousness accompanied by a bilateral, regular, 3 Hz spike and wave pattern on the EEG (Lennox 1945). It usually responds to ethosuximide, corticotrophin or intravenous diazepam (Brain and Walton 1969; Gastaut *et al* 1965; Schwartz and Scott 1971).

Minor epileptic status is a syndrome of intermittent mental dullness with frequent small myoclonic jerks and irregular disturbances of the EEG (Brett 1966). Corticotrophin is often beneficial.

Epilepsia partialis continua is characterised by continuous repetition of a movement. It responds poorly to treatment (Schmidt and Wilder 1968), though improvement has been claimed following intravenous administration of diazepam (Gastaut *et al* 1965).

RELATED CONDITIONS—NARCOLEPSY AND CATAPLEXY

Until recently, ephedrine and amphetamine have been the usual drugs employed for narcolepsy and cataplexy (Brain and Walton

1969). However, there is evidence that desipramine is more satisfactory; it is also reputed to alleviate sleep paralysis and hypnagogic attacks (Hishikawa *et al* 1966).

DOSE REGIMENS AND ADVERSE REACTIONS

The dose regimen of anticonvulsants must always be flexible because of the wide variation of pharmacokinetics in different individuals and the extensive range of drug interactions that can occur. Documentation of toxic effects is often inadequate owing to the difficulty in identifying which particular anticonvulsant, out of the several that are usually being taken, is responsible.

In the following summary drugs employed in the treatment of epilepsy are classified according to their structure.

ACETYLUREAS

Phenacemide. The toxic effects of phenacemide usually outweigh its anticonvulsant actions. The dose range is 1.5–2.0 g/day. Phenacemide can induce behavioural disorders, vomiting, fever, skin eruptions, hepatic or renal damage and blood dyscrasias.

Pheneturide. Pheneturide is similar to phenacemide though somewhat less toxic. The dose is 0.6–1.0 g/day.

BARBITURATES

Metharbitone (metharbital). Metharbitone is demethylated to barbitone. Its actions are similar to phenobarbitone and there is no convincing evidence that it has any advantages. The usual dosage is 300–800 mg/day.

Methylphenobarbitone (mephobarbital). This drug is demethylated in the liver to phenobarbitone. The usual dose is 400–600 mg daily. It has not been shown to be superior to phenobarbitone.

Phenobarbitone (phenobarbital). The pharmacokinetics of phenobarbitone have already been discussed. A reasonable starting dose is 30 mg thrice daily, titrating according to seizure control and adverse reactions. In major status epilepticus 200–400 mg can be given intravenously; the transition from intravenous to oral therapy should be managed with 50–100 mg intramuscular phenobarbitone which is repeated as frequently as necessary. Febrile convulsions should be treated with continuous prophylactic phenobarbitone, 3–4 mg/kg/day.

Drowsiness is common over the first few weeks of treatment, but this usually clears spontaneously. Occasionally excitement is induced, particularly in children. Nystagmus and ataxia are dose dependent. Megaloblastic anaemia can develop; this responds to folic acid 15 mg daily (deficiency of vitamin B_{12} should always be excluded). Reynolds (1967; 1970) has claimed that administration of folic acid increases fit frequency but others have failed to confirm this (Grant and Stores 1970; Ralston *et al* 1970). Disturbances in vitamin D metabolism can occur (Hahn *et al* 1972); the causal mechanism is thought to be the same as that responsible for the osteomalacia induced by phenytoin (see below). A morbilliform rash is exceptionally encountered but more serious skin eruptions, blood dyscrasias and hepatic toxicity are all rare. Teratogenic effects have been reported, in particular congenital heart disease, cleft lip, cleft palate and microcephaly (Spiedal and Meadow 1972). There is reputed to be an increased incidence of shoulder–hand syndrome and Dupuytren's contracture in patients receiving long term treatment with phenobarbitone.

Primidone. Primidone, like phenytoin and phenobarbitone, combines potent anticonvulsant actions with a low incidence of serious adverse effects. Peak plasma concentrations are reached 3 hours after oral administration and the half-life is 6–7 hours (Gallagher and Baumel 1972). There is negligible protein binding. Animal studies indicate that primidone is rapidly distributed through the tissues, including the central nervous system. The two major metabolites are phenobarbitone and phenylethlmalonamide, both of which have an anticonvulsant effect. Some 20% of an administered dose of primidone is excreted unchanged in the urine. The therapeutic range of plasma concentrations of primidone has not been established, neither has the relative importance of the two active metabolites pheno-barbitone and phenylethylmalonamide. In routine therapy the plasma concentration is around 8 μg/ml. Adverse reactions are likely to develop if the level rises above 10 μg/ml (Booker 1972).

Occasionally the initial intake of primidone induces profound sedation, with or without ataxia, which can persist for 2 or 3 days. It is therefore common practice to give patients a test dose of 50 mg before starting the usual regimen of 250 mg thrice daily. The dose may be increased according to seizure control and toxicity, but few patients tolerate more than 1.5 g/day. Toxic effects are similar to those already discussed when considering phenobarbitone.

Thiopentone. In major status epilepticus 25–100 mg of thiopentone is administered by slow intravenous injection. Subsequently an infusion of 1 g of thiopentone can be given in 500 ml of isotonic saline, at the minimal rate required for the control of convulsions. The risks of respiratory depression are low with this regimen but facilities should be available for tracheal intubation and positive pressure ventilation.

BENZODIAZEPINES

Clonazepam. This new anticonvulsant is still undergoing evaluation. Initial results are encouraging in both adult and childhood epilepsy (Aarli 1973; Birket-Smith *et al* 1973; Dumermuth and Kovacs 1973; Eeg-Olofsson 1973; Lund and Trolle 1973; Mikkelsen and Birket-Smith 1973; Munthe-Kaas and Strandjord 1973). Oral administration can be started at 1 mg/day increasing by 0.5 mg daily until attacks are controlled or unwanted effects, particularly drowsiness, occur. Usually an anticonvulsant action is achieved on 2–10 mg/day though doses up to 12 mg/day have been employed. Therapeutic plasma levels range from 20–50 ng/ml (Naestoft *et al* 1973).

For major status epilepticus, intravenous injection of 1.0–4.0 mg (at a rate of 0.1 mg/second) is often sufficient to stop seizures for several hours. This can be followed, if necessary, by continuous infusion of 4 mg in 500 ml of isotonic saline, given at the minimum rate necessary to control fits (Ponce 1972).

Diazepam. The pharmacokinetics of diazepam are discussed in Chapter 15. A dose of 10 mg is given intravenously in the treatment of major status epilepticus. Subsequently an intravenous infusion (100 mg in 500 ml of isotonic saline) may be administered at a rate just sufficient to stop convulsions. Facilities for tracheal intubation should be available and care is necessary to avoid lingual respiratory obstruction caused by the muscle relaxant action of diazepam.

Nitrazepam. The pharmacokinetics of nitrazepam are discussed in Chapter 20. In the treatment of myoclonic epilepsy, akinetic attacks and infantile spasms, dosage is in the region of 1 mg/kg/day. Adjustments are made to achieve the maximal therapeutic effect compatible with adverse reactions. High doses of nitrazepam can induce sedation, ataxia and increased secretion of mucus or saliva.

CORTICOSTEROIDS

Dexamethasone. For infantile spasms the dose is 0.3 mg/kg/day. Toxicity is reviewed in Chapter 7.

Prednisone. The dose is 2 mg/kg/day for infantile spasms. Adverse reactions are discussed in Chapter 7.

HYDANTOINS

Albutoin. A recent study (Carter 1971) suggests that albutoin may be as effective as phenytoin in suppressing fits. However, experience with this drug is limited. The dose range is 300–500 mg/day.

Ethotoin. The usual dose of ethotoin is 0.5–3.0 g/day. Adverse reactions are similar to those of phenytoin, but hirsutism and hyperplasia of the gums are reputed to be less common.

Methetoin. This drug has not been demonstrated to be superior to phenytoin. The dose range is 200–400 mg/day. Adverse reactions are similar to those of other hydantoins.

Methoin (mephenytoin). Methoin is more toxic than phenytoin and often less potent as an anticonvulsant. The dose is 100–600 mg/day.

Phenytoin (diphenylhydantoin). Consideration has already been given to the pharmacokinetics of phenytoin. The average dose is 100 mg thrice daily which is adjusted to obtain the maximum therapeutic action with minimal unwanted effects. There is a poor correlation between changes in dosage and corresponding alterations of plasma concentration (Bouchner *et al* 1972); small increments of intake sometimes provoke considerable toxicity.

Ataxia is the usual dose limiting factor in phenytoin therapy. Nystagmus is generally present and overdosage may precipitate an acute posterior fossa syndrome with intention tremor and diplopia. Though usually reversible, cerebellar signs are occasionally permanent. There has been considerable controversy on whether phenytoin induces loss of Purkinje cells; a recent extensive investigation of this problem (Dam 1972) indicates that atrophy of the Purkinje cell layer is a consequence of seizures rather than their treatment. Ophthalmoplegia can occur and an encephalopathic picture may develop with mental impairment, drowsiness, asterixis, choreoathetosis and increased seizure frequency (Levy and Fenichel 1965; Engel *et al* 1971; Kooiker and Sumi 1974); diffuse slow activity can dominate the electroencephalogram (Roseman 1961). There have also been reports of peripheral neuropathy induced by phenytoin (Lovelace and Horowitz 1968) and neuromuscular transmission may deteriorate in patients with myasthenia gravis.

Connective tissue proliferation is common. Some 40% of patients taking phenytoin develop gum hypertrophy, which is exacerbated by poor dental hygiene; though not dose related, it regresses when treatment is stopped. The facial features may thicken and Dupuytren's contractures can occur. The mechanism responsible for these disorders is not understood, both increased fibroblast activity and decreased collagenolysis have been suggested.

Other problems include gastrointestinal symptoms—anorexia, nausea, vomiting and abdominal pain—which can usually be eliminated by taking phenytoin in relatively small frequent doses after meals. Prolonged therapy leads to hirsutism. Occasionally glucose tolerance is disturbed. Osteomalacia can be produced (Kruse 1968; Richens and Rowe 1970), probably by induction of an increase in the microsomal hepatic enzymes concerned with metabolism of vitamin D (Dent *ct al* 1970). This osteomalacia is occasionally associated with a myopathy (Marsden *et al* 1973). Reduction of serum calcium and an increase in alkaline phosphatase are much commoner than clinically detectable bone disease or myopathy. These metabolic disturbances can be alleviated by calciferol 50 μg–2.5 mg (2,000–100,000 units)/day (Richens and Rowe 1970; Christiansen *et al* 1973) or 25-hydroxycholecalciferol, 10–45 μg/day (Stamp *et al* 1972).

Haematological reactions occur; megaloblastic anaemia is related to a low serum and red cell concentration of folate, as discussed when considering phenobarbitone. Exceptionally, aplastic anaemia and agranulocytosis can develop. Lymphadenopathy may arise acutely to resemble glandular fever, or chronically like a malignant lymphoma (Anthony 1970). Fever, skin eruptions, Stevens–Johnson syndrome, systemic lupus erythematosus, hepatitis and thyroiditis have all been reported. It has recently been suggested that phenytoin exerts teratogenic effects similar to those attributed to phenobarbitone (Spiedal and Meadow 1972; Loughnan *et al* 1973). There is no evidence of oncogenic activity (Clemmesen *et al* 1974).

This list of adverse reactions is long because phenytoin is used so extensively. However, it should be emphasised that phenytoin, together with phenobarbitone and ethosuximide, are the safest anticonvulsants at dose levels which achieve a therapeutic effect in the common forms of epilepsy.

OXAZOLIDINEDIONES

Paramethadione. This drug is generally regarded as less effective' but better tolerated, than troxidone. Paramethadione is demethylated and it is possible that certain metabolites may have antiepileptic properties. The dose range is 300–900 mg/day for children with petit mal. Adverse reactions include hemeralopia, skin eruptions and sedation. Blood dyscrasias and renal damage occasionally occur.

Troxidone (trimethadione). Troxidone is rapidly absorbed and metabolised. Demethylation leads to the formation of dimethadione, which also has an anticonvulsant action (Withrow and Woodbury 1972). The serum contains about 20 times more dimethadione than troxidone, so the former may be of greater importance than the latter in the control of fits. Less than 5% of a dose of troxidone can be recovered as unchanged drug in the urine.

The dose range for treating children with petit mal is 300–900 mg/day. Toxicity is relatively frequent. Reactions similar to those described for paramethadione occur, but in addition there may be nausea, vertigo, lassitude, headache and alopecia. Regular examination of the blood and urine are desirable because serious haematological, renal and hepatic damage has been reported.

SULPHONAMIDE DERIVATIVES

Acetazolamide. The usual dose of acetazolamide is 250 mg thrice daily, an effective plasma concentration being 10–14 μg/ml. Some 95% of the drug is bound to plasma protein. Rapid absorption leads to peak plasma concentrations in 2–3 hours. The plasma decay curve displays two components, one with a half-life of about 2 hours and another which is slower, due to drug bound to carbonic anhydrase. Acetazolamide is not metabolised; it is excreted unchanged in the urine (Woodbury *et al* 1972).

Toxic effects are unusual. Occasionally drowsiness and paraesthesia are troublesome. Teratogenicity has been reported in animals, so acetazolamide should not be given during pregnancy.

Sulthiame. When sulthiame is administered with other anticonvulsants extensive interactions occur (see above). No adequately controlled studies have been performed with sulthiame alone. In this setting, it is not possible to draw any firm conclusions about its efficacy, though many are convinced that it is a useful anticonvulsant.

The usual dose is 600 mg/day, but a much lower intake is desirable when starting sulthiame in patients already taking other anticonvulsants. Reactions attributed to sulthiame include anorexia, lassitude, hyperpnoea, paraesthesiae, headache, metabolic acidosis, psychiatric disturbances, blood dyscrasias and exacerbation of seizures.

OTHERS

Amphetamine. For narcolepsy, an initial dose of 5 mg twice daily may be increased up to 40 mg/day. It is inadvisable to exceed 20 mg in a single dose; administration late in the day may lead to insomnia.

Adverse effects include dryness of the mouth, nausea, constipation and difficulty with micturition. Amphetamine dependence, tremor, agitation, depression, psychosis, dyskinesia and convulsions can occur. While there is commonly a rise in blood pressure, extreme overdosage can cause hypotension. Cardiac arrhythmias may precipitate angina in patients with ischaemic heart disease.

Beclamide. A dose of 3–4 g/day is generally employed. Adverse reactions are seldom troublesome, but dizziness, agitation and gastrointestinal symptoms have been reported. Although available for over a decade, beclamide has not been widely used.

Carbamazepine. The desirable range of plasma concentration is 1–6 μg/ml (Meinardi 1972; Parsonage 1972; Cereghino *et al* 1973). A dose of 200 mg taken 3–6 times a day is generally satisfactory. The usual adverse reactions are dizziness, ataxia, diplopia and nystagmus. Skin eruptions are relatively common. Psychotic behaviour (Dalby 1971) and water intoxication (Radó 1973) are occasionally encountered.

Chlormethiazole. For major status epilepticus, chlormethiazole is administered by intravenous infusion at the minimum rate required to control convulsions; 1.2–1.6 g can be given in 0.8% solution (Laxenaire 1966).

Corticotrophin. In the treatment of infantile spasms, 20–30 units of corticotrophin gel can be injected daily for the first 3 or 4 weeks, reducing the dose thereafter because of toxicity. Hypersensitivity is less common if the synthetic preparation, tetracosactrin, is used. Dose equivalents and adverse reactions are discussed in Chapter 7.

Desipramine. The dose range of desipramine is 25–150 mg daily for the treatment of narcolepsy, cataplexy, sleep paralysis and hypnagogic attacks. Unwanted effects include dryness of the mouth, nausea, constipation, difficulty with micturition, hypotension, tachycardia, blurred vision, insomnia, sweating and tremor. Severe overdosage can produce hyperpyrexia, hypomania, convulsions and cardiac arrhythmia. Rarely skin eruptions, blood dyscrasias and hepatitis have been reported.

Ephedrine. In the treatment of narcolepsy, the dose range of ephedrine is 8–60 mg thrice daily. Tachyphylaxis often develops, but the therapeutic response is usually restored after stopping treatment for a few days. Adverse reactions are similar to those described for amphetamine.

Ethosuximide. The pharmacokinetics of ethosuximide have already been considered. For children with petit mal, an initial dose of 250 mg thrice daily should be adjusted according to response and toxicity. The maintenance dose range is 0.5–1.75 g/day. Ethosuximide is usually tolerated extremely well. Drowsiness, dizziness and nausea are the commonest unwanted effects. There have been occasional reports of ataxia, headache, restlessness, photophobia, skin eruptions, leucopenia, elevation of serum transaminase and systemic lupus erythematosus.

Hydrochlorothiazide. Hydrochlorothiazide is well absorbed and widely distributed. Metabolism is not an important mechanism of inactivation. Some 70% of an administered dose is excreted in the urine (Young *et al* 1959), most of this loss occurring over about 12 hours. The dose range is 25–100 mg daily, an adequate response being achieved with 50 mg in the majority of patients. In the management of epilepsy, hydrochlorothiazide is only of use when fits are related to menstruation; a 5 day course of treatment is usually adequate each month, starting 3 days before every period. Adverse reactions include nausea, dizziness, paraesthesiae, skin eruptions and photosensitivity. Prolonged treatment can lead to hypokalaemia, hyponatraemia, diabetes mellitus and gout, but these are very unlikely to be encountered when treatment is limited to short courses.

Pancuronium. Pancuronium is a neuromuscular blocking agent employed to achieve muscle relaxation during artificial ventilation. In the context of neurological therapeutics, its main use arises from cardiorespiratory complications of major status epilepticus, tetanus, myasthenia gravis or poliomyelitis. Its effects are similar to tubocurarine, but it has less ganglion blocking and histamine releasing activity. An initial intravenous dose of pancuronium 1–2 mg produces satisfactory relaxation in most patients. The same dose is repeated at intervals determined by the extent and duration of the response. Muscle relaxation induced by pancuronium can be reversed with intravenous neostigmine 2.5 mg, usually given with atropine 1.2 mg.

Paraldehyde. Paraldehyde is usually administered by deep intramuscular injection of 5–10 ml. Glass syringes should be used, because plastic may be dissolved. Paraldehyde causes local irritation which can lead to formation of sterile abscesses and ultimately sloughing of tissue. If volumes over 5 ml are injected, it is desirable to distribute the dose to more than one site. Paraldehyde may also be given intravenously, 3–6 ml over 30–60 minutes via a fast running infusion of isotonic saline.

Sodium valproate. Sodium valproate is a new drug currently undergoing evaluation as an anticonvulsant. It is of some interest because chemically, as the salt of a branched chain fatty acid, it is quite unlike any other antiepileptic agent. Sodium valproate increases the brain concentration of GABA—a transmitter predominantly employed at inhibitory synapses. A wide spectrum of anticonvulsant activity has been claimed (Förster 1972; Harvey 1974; Jeavons and Clark 1974.)

Sodium valproate is readily absorbed. Excretion occurs rapidly in the urine, mainly as conjugates. The usual dose range is 0.8–2.0 g/day. More experience is required to define its therapeutic value.

Tubocurarine. Tubocurarine is employed for the same purposes as pancuronium. Distribution is rapid after intravenous injection, with particularly high concentrations at the neuromuscular junction and some binding to plasma proteins. Tubocurarine does not readily cross the blood–brain barrier. Some 50% is excreted unchanged in the urine over 3–6 hours; metabolism also contributes to inactivation.

An initial intravenous dose of 7 mg usually allows artificial ventilation to be performed. The dose is then titrated according to the response. Blockade of sympathetic ganglia can lead to hypotension and release of histamine may induce bronchospasm. Tubocurarine can be given by intramuscular injection but distribution by this route is slow and unpredictable.

CHAPTER 13
PARKINSONISM

No effective treatment for Parkinsonism was available until Charcot introduced the belladonna alkaloids 100 years ago. Early therapeutic inadequacy was reflected by the number of useless putative medicaments prescribed, the compendium including arsenic, strychnine, mercury, turpentine and cannabis.

The salient clinical features of Parkinsonism are tremor, rigidity and hypokinesia. Several causes have been established. These include (1) drugs (reserpine, tetrabenazine, phenothiazines such as chlorpromazine, butyrophenones such as haloperidól, diphenylbutylpiperidines such as pimozide, tricyclic antidepressants, procaine and diazoxide), (2) toxic agents (manganese, carbon monoxide), (3) infections (encephalitis lethargica, syphilis), (4) tumours, (5) infarcts, (6) genetic predisposition. However, in the majority of patients no aetiology can be identified (idiopathic Parkinsonism, Parkinson's disease or paralysis agitans). The pathology may be widespread but almost always involves the substantia nigra and basal ganglia (Greenfield 1955). In idiopathic Parkinsonism characteristic neuronal inclusions—Lewy bodies—can usually be found, but their significance is not known.

PHYSIOLOGY

Attempts to analyse the physiological disturbances in Parkinsonism have not achieved any notable success. A number of techniques

190

have been employed to detect changes in the balance of activity in alpha motoneurons and fusimotor neurons. However, studies on the silent period, the H reflex, Jendrassik's manoeuvre and the response to tonic vibration reflexes have all failed to produce any coherent explanation of the neurological deficits at motoneuron level (Angel *et al* 1966; Ward 1970; Dietrichson 1971 a and b; Andrews and Burke 1973; McLellan 1973a).

Changes in supraspinal physiology are shrouded in even more obscurity. Evidence obtained from animal models of Parkinsonism (Steg 1964; Arvidsson *et al* 1966; Morrison and Webster 1973) and observations derived from stereotactic procedures in man afford sufficient material for a number of general speculations (Calne 1970), but until the neurophysiology of normal motor control is better understood it is unlikely that any satisfactory interpretation of the consequences of intracranial pathology will emerge.

PHARMACOLOGY

The outstanding pharmacological abnormality in Parkinsonism is reduced dopaminergic transmission in the nigrostriatal pathway (Ehringer and Hornykiewicz 1960; Hornykiewicz 1966). This may be caused by striatal depletion of dopamine (Fig. 38, as in Parkinsonism which is idiopathic, postencephalitic, or induced by drugs such as reserpine and tetrabenazine. Alternatively, blockade of striatal dopamine receptors may be responsible, as in Parkinsonism due to phenothiazines, butyrophenones or diphenylbutylpiperidines.

In addition to having the highest concentration of dopamine in the central nervous system, the striatum contains large quantities of acetylcholine. Selective impairment of the dopaminergic pathway in Parkinsonism results in relatively excessive cholinergic activity which ultimately disrupts the integration of motor performance to culminate in the clinical features of tremor, rigidity and hypokinesia.

The two major therapeutic approaches to the management of Parkinsonism (Fig. 39) are: (1) *Increasing dopaminergic function.* Since dopamine does not readily cross the blood–brain barrier its immediate precursor, levodopa, is administered to augment transmission. Certain adverse reactions to levodopa can be alleviated by

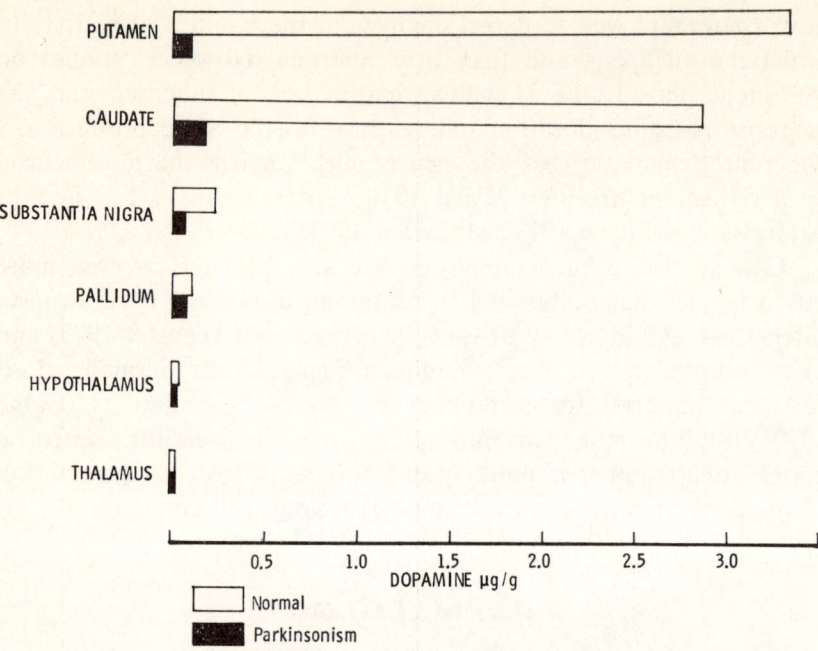

Fig. 38. Concentrations of dopamine in various regions of the brain. Material taken post mortem from 15 normal subjects (open bars) and 12 patients with Parkinsonism (closed bars). (from Bernheimer *et al* 1961, *Klin. Wschr.*, **41**, 465.)

concomitant administration of an extracerebral decarboxylase inhibitor. (2) *Decreasing cholinergic activity*. The central cholinergic synapses in the striatum have muscarinic receptors which can be blocked by belladonna alkaloids or their synthetic congeners.

TREATMENT

The treatment of Parkinsonism will be considered in the following stages: (1) Levodopa; (2) Extracerebral decarboxylase inhibitors; (3) Anticholinergic drugs; (4) Amantadine; (5) Antihistamines; (6) Combinations of drugs; (7) Management of the newly diagnosed patient. Surgery has undergone a somewhat critical reappraisal (Hoehn and Yahr 1969) and in consequence stereotactic thalamotomy is now seldom performed.

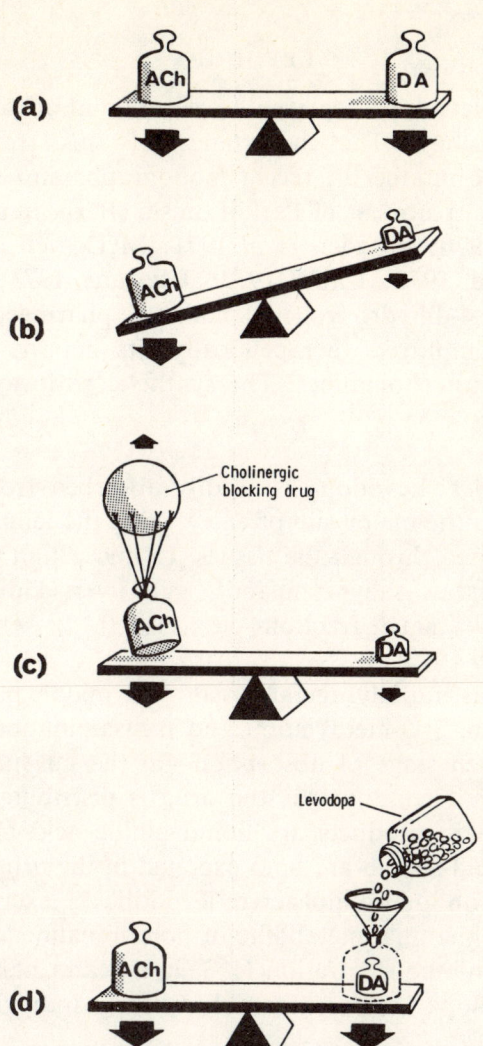

Fig. 39. Diagrammatic representation of dopamine (DA) and acetyl-choline (ACh) acting as antagonistic transmitters in the corpus striatum. (a) Normally there is a balance. (b) In Parkinsonism dopaminergic function is reduced, so that the balance is disturbed in the direction of cholinergic dominance. (c) This disturbance may be corrected by reducing the effect of acetylcholine with cholinergic (muscarinic) blocking drugs such as atropine or benzhexol. (d) Alternatively, the balance may be restored by administering the immediate precursor of dopamine, levodopa (Calne 1971, *Brit. Med. J.*, **3**, 693).

LEVODOPA

The advent of levodopa represents a substantial advance in clinical neuropharmacology. The importance of this step forward is reflected by the number of recent monographs and symposia concerned with the treatment of Parkinsonism (Barbeau and McDowell 1970; Calne 1970; Brogden *et al* 1971; McDowell and Markham 1971; Siegfried 1972; Calne 1973; Klawans 1973; Yahr 1973). Levodopa (L-3,4-dihydroxyphenylalanine) is pharmacologically inert in the doses employed therapeutically; its actions depend upon conversion to catecholamines. The synthetic pathway is illustrated in Fig. 18.

Pharmacokinetics. Levodopa is readily absorbed from the gastro-intestinal tract, the major site of entry being the jejunum. It is then widely distributed through the tissues. In mice, high concentrations occur in pancreas, salivary glands, gut, liver, kidneys and skin (Fig. 40). Only a small fraction—less than 0.1%—enters the brain (Wurtman *et al* 1970).

Levodopa is rapidly metabolised, the major pathways being decarboxylation, 3-O-methylation and transamination. Metabolism proceeds at each stage of absorption—in the gut lumen, intestinal wall and liver; it continues as the drug is distributed through the tissues. The main products are homovanillic acid and dihydroxy-phenylacetic acid, which are both excreted in the urine. Only a very small proportion of administered levodopa is excreted as vanil-mandelic acid, the final metabolite of noradrenaline and adrenaline. The peak plasma concentration (1–3 μg/ml) and half-life (0.75–1.5 hours) of levodopa vary considerably between individuals.

Therapeutic actions. Levodopa is the most powerful therapeutic agent available for the treatment of Parkinsonism. All the clinical features are alleviated (Barbeau 1961; Birkmayer and Hornykiewicz 1961; Cotzias *et al* 1967; Yahr *et al* 1968).

Disabilities attributable to hypokinesia improve to a greater extent than rigidity or tremor (Fig. 41). This is particularly useful because hypokinesia is the most incapacitating, though often clinically the least obvious motor deficit. It is responsible for the clumsi-

PANCREAS KIDNEY LIVER

CAUDATE

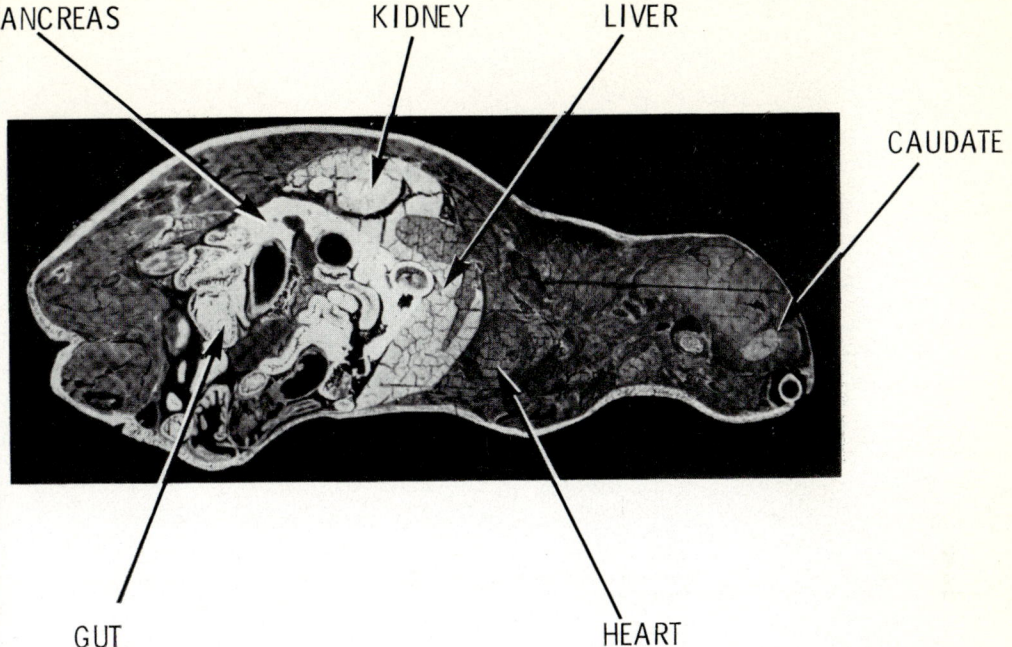

GUT HEART

Fig. 40. Autoradiogram of a mouse injected intravenously with 1 mg of L-dopa 45 minutes before death. Radioactivity appears white. 20 μ section. 100 μc, C^{14} in position 2 of the side chain (R.F. Long, 1969, unpublished).

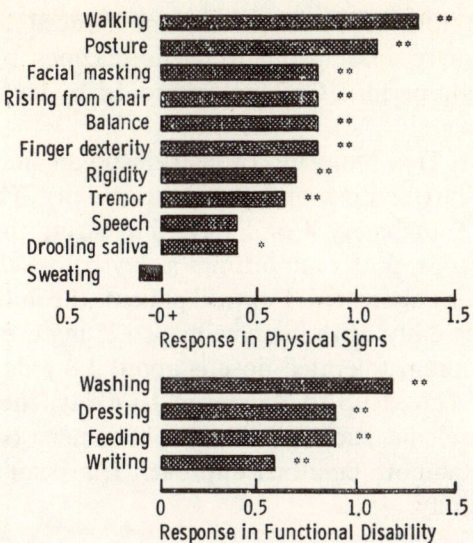

Fig. 41. Actions of levodopa in 20 patients with idiopathic Parkinsonism. These results are derived from a double blind study employing a simple clinical scoring protocol. Positive values denote improvement; negative figures represent deterioration. * indicates significance at the 5% level. ** indicates significance at the 1% level (Calne *et al* 1969 *Lancet*, **2,** 973).

ness, dysphagia, dysphonia and disturbances of gait which limit and ultimately stop work, hobbies and routine procedures such as dressing and washing—upon which independent existence depends. Unfortunately, a satisfactory response is not achieved in all patients. Of those with idiopathic Parkinsonism, a substantial therapeutic effect is obtained in about one third, with moderate results in a further third. The remainder are unable to take levodopa, because of adverse reactions or inability to persevere and cooperate reliably over the difficult period of building up the dose to maximum tolerated intake (see below). A small minority of patients fail to respond in spite of high dosage and satisfactory plasma concentrations (Mones 1973).

The inexorable advance of the pathology of idiopathic Parkinsonism does not appear to be influenced by treatment (Hunter *et al* 1973). Toxicity is more prominent in postencephalitic patients (Calne *et al* 1969b; Hunter 1973). Parkinsonism induced by blockade of striatal dopamine receptors—due to phenothiazines, butyrophenones or diphenylbutylpiperidines—is not improved by levodopa.

Dose regimens. The majority of Parkinsonian patients tolerate levodopa at a starting dose of 250 mg thrice daily. This can usually be raised by 250 mg every 4 or 5 days, increasing the frequency of administration to 4, 5 or even 6 times a day before the size of each individual dose is augmented. For frail patients the initial dose should be 125 mg thrice daily, with increments of 125 mg every 4 or 5 days. The mean maximum tolerated dose is about 3.0 g/day. While some patients have received up to 8 or even 10 g/day, the emergence of late toxicity problems, such as 'on–off' phenomena (see below), has recently led to a more cautious approach (Barbeau 1974), seldom exceeding 5.0 g/day.

Adverse reactions. Adverse reactions to levodopa are prominent, dose dependent and reversible. They can be reduced by avoiding administration on an empty stomach. In the first few weeks of treatment, the commonest problems are anorexia, nausea and occasionally vomiting. These effects are probably generated centrally by dopamine formed in the region of the emetic centre (see Chapter 19).

A fall in blood pressure is often detectable during the phase of building up the dose of levodopa, but it is uncommon for symptoms to be troublesome. This hypotension appears to result from combined central and peripheral mechanisms (Henning and Rubenson 1970; Reid *et al* 1972a; Dhasmana and Spilker 1973); the central action is mediated by noradrenaline and involves a lowering of the set of the blood pressure while the peripheral effect, probably elicited by dopamine, impairs the baroceptor reflexes.

The usual dose limiting adverse reaction to levodopa is dyskinesia —involuntary movements which are generally of a choreoathetoid nature. They frequently start in the face, tongue or neck, but they may begin in a limb or even present as tachypnoea. Their mechanism is not fully understood, though they are likely to be dopaminergic rather than noradrenergic because they can also be produced by administration of dopamine agonists such as apomorphine (Cotzias *et al* 1970), piribedil (Vakil *et al* 1973) and 2-brom-alpha-ergocryptine (bromocriptin) (Claveria *et al* 1974). Since dyskinesia is seldom precipitated by giving levodopa to patients who do not have Parkinsonism, it has been suggested to be a manifestation of supersensitivity (Klawans *et al* 1970a) due to degeneration of the nigrostriatal pathway. Klawans (1973) has argued that dyskinesia induced by levodopa results from overactivity of the relatively few, but perhaps important, excitatory dopaminergic synapses in the striatum. Dyskinesia usually clears within hours or days of stopping levodopa but exceptionally it may persist for several weeks (Weiss *et al* 1971).

Mild psychiatric reactions such as restlessness and insomnia are common. Paradoxically, sedation and depression can also occur. Occasionally, more severe disturbances develop such as hallucinations, delusions and hypomania—a clinical picture reminiscent of the psychosis induced by amphetamine. The mechanism of production of psychiatric reactions to levodopa has not been established. Dopaminergic projections to the cerebral cortex may be relevant (Andén *et al* 1966a; Thierry *et al* 1973). Alternatively or in addition, noradrenergic cerebral synapses may be involved.

Other adverse effects of levodopa are unusual. Cardiac arrhythmias are overdiagnosed because of the difficulty in palpating the radial pulse in the presence of coarse tremor and the prominent arefact which shaking imposes on the electrocardiogram. Levodopa induced cardiac arrhythmias are caused by increased catecholamine formation at the periphery (Parks *et al* 1970); they are uncommon, even in the presence of established heart disease (Hunter *et al* 1971; Jenkins *et al* 1972).

Angina and myocardial infarction are rare complications of levodopa therapy. While there is a high incidence of ischaemic heart disease in the Parkinsonian age group, it is probable that levodopa confers a slightly increased hazard because of (1) sudden increased mobility due to its therapeutic action, (2) hypotension when starting treatment, (3) the possible precipitation of cardiac arrhythmias.

Transient exacerbations of hypokinesia—'on–off' attacks, akinesia paradoxica, oscillations in performance—have been described in patients taking levodopa. They may be associated with dyskinesia and they often cause considerable distress (Barbeau 1972). 'On–off' attacks are most likely to develop in patients who have been taking high doses for at least 18 months (Damásio *et al* 1973); their pharmacology is not understood. In some patients they seem to be related to high plasma concentrations of levodopa (Claveria *et al* 1973) whereas in others, low levels have been reported (Yahr *et al* 1974). More frequent administration of smaller doses can be helpful, but if the episodes persist treatment may have to be decreased or stopped. After a period without levodopa, a favourable result can sometimes be obtained by starting therapy again at a lower dose (Sweet *et al* 1972).

Levodopa occasionally precipitates gout (Honda and Gindin 1972); this responds to probenecid or allopurinol but in addition it may be necessary to reduce the dose of levodopa. Pain in the joints can also arise from the increased mobility which is achieved by levodopa—features of osteoarthropathy may emerge, X-rays revealing chronic joint disease which had previously been clinically silent because movement was prevented by Parkinsonian rigidity and akinesia. Patients often display excessive enthusiasm as their gait improves when starting therapy; this leads to an increased incidence of falls and femoral neck fractures.

Other miscellaneous problems which may be induced by levodopa include hot flushes, distortion of the sense of smell and brown discolouration of body fluids (saliva, urine and vaginal secretions). Pupillary dilation can occur and this predisposes to glaucoma.

There have been rare reports of patients becoming stuporose while taking levodopa and in two cases (Andén *et al* 1970b; Wolf and Davis 1973) this has been followed by irreversible dementia. On the limited evidence that is currently available, it is not possible to be sure of a causal relationship between levodopa and these encephalo-pathic phenomena.

Transient disturbances of transaminases, blood urea, alkaline phosphatase, haemoglobin and haematocrit have been encountered but none seem to have been of significance. Coombs conversion is also recorded. Of greater importance is a rising serum uric acid, although this can be misleading (Cawein 1969) because colorimetric methods of estimation give incorrect values in patients receiving levodopa. Increases in growth hormone have been reported although there has been no experience of acromegaly and the insulin requirement does not usually change in diabetics.

Titration of dosage. Nausea is generally alleviated if dosage is temporarily reduced; intake may subsequently be increased again, at a somewhat slower rate. Occasionally antiemetic drugs may be required, for example cyclizine 50 mg orally.

Hypotension can also be managed by a temporary decrease in dosage; elastic stockings may be necessary for a short time. Where hypotension is prolonged, etilephrine 5 mg thrice daily has proved useful (Miller *et al* 1973).

Dyskinesia and psychiatric problems demand a sustained reduction of the intake of levodopa. If a major tranquilliser is required, thioridazine is the least likely to exacerbate Parkinsonism.

Disturbances of cardiac rhythm should be treated by conventional methods; a decrease or even cessation of levodopa therapy may also be necessary. Myocardial infarction should be managed according to its severity, stopping levodopa temporarily if there has been extensive cardiac damage.

A number of interactions can occur with other drugs. Levodopa should not be administered with monoamine oxidase inhibitors because this combination can lead to potentially dangerous elevation of the blood pressure. Pyridoxine blocks the therapeutic action of levodopa, probably by increasing its peripheral metabolism. Unexpected changes in blood pressure—elevation or reduction—have been encountered in patients undergoing general anaesthesia while receiving levodopa; as a precaution, treatment is usually withheld a day or two before surgery.

EXTRACEREBRAL DECARBOXYLASE INHIBITORS

As already mentioned, levodopa itself is pharmacologically inert at the dose levels employed in treating Parkinsonism; its actions depend on metabolites formed by decarboxylation. Drugs are available which inhibit the relevant enzyme, L-aromatic aminoacid decarboxylase, and some of these agents do not cross the blood–brain barrier. In 1967, Batholini *et al* suggested that such drugs might be of therapeutic use if administered together with levodopa; in particular, extracerebral decarboxylase inhibitors should eliminate adverse reactions caused by conversion of levodopa to catecholamines at the periphery (Fig. 42).

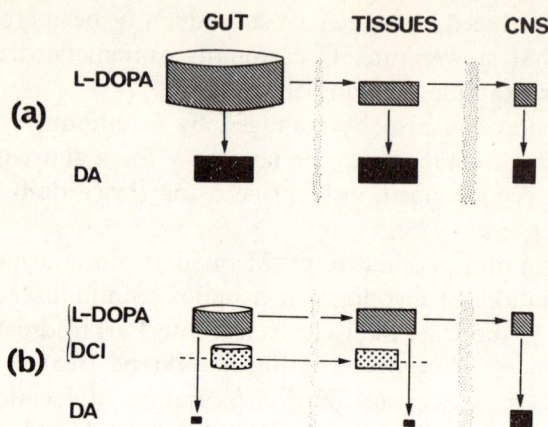

Fig. 42. (a) Diagrammatic illustration of the distribution of levodopa and dopamine after oral administration of levodopa alone. In the gut and extracerebral tissues levodopa (L-dopa) is rapidly decarboxylated to dopamine (DA) which does not readily penetrate the blood–brain barrier. (b) When an extracerebral decarboxylase inhibitor (DCI) is added, conversion of levodopa to dopamine is reduced in the gut and peripheral tissues. Decarboxylation occurs normally in the central nervous system (CNS) because the DCI does not penetrate the blood–brain barrier.

Two extracerebral decarboxylase inhibitors have been studied in man—carbidopa (L-alpha methyldopahydrazine) and Ro 44602 (seryltrihydroxybenzylhydrazine). Because of certain toxic effects encountered with Ro 44602 in animals, most clinical investigators have concentrated their attention on carbidopa (Yahr 1973). Decarboxylase inhibitors which are less completely excluded from the central nervous system have also been studied—notably alpha methyldopa (Sweet *et al* 1971) and brocresine (Howse and Matthews 1973), but these drugs have not been widely used in the treatment of Parkinsonism.

By reducing the peripheral metabolism of levodopa, extracerebral decarboxylase inhibitors allow the dose to be decreased by some

80% without any fall in the plasma level (Reid *et al* 1972b). More important advantages derive from the alleviation of adverse reactions. Nausea is diminished, probably by blockade of catecholamine formation in the area postrema—a region of the brain close to the emetic centre; decarboxylase inhibitors gain access because there is no significant blood–brain barrier at this site. The decrease in nausea enables the dose of levodopa to be built up to maximum tolerated levels in days rather than weeks. Other problems which can be expected to improve following inhibition of extracerebral decarboxylase include cardiac arrhythmias, postural hypotension, pupillary dilatation and hot flushes.

Dose regimen. Carbidopa can be given in a single preparation combined with levodopa. The usual form contains 25 mg of carbidopa and 250 mg of levodopa (marketed under the proprietary name Sinemet). Each of these tablets corresponds to about 1 g of levodopa. A reasonable starting dose is therefore $\frac{1}{2}$ tablet twice daily. Since nausea is generally alleviated by carbidopa, it is often possible to increase the combined preparation at a rate of $\frac{1}{2}$ tablet every two or three days until a satisfactory response is obtained or toxicity develops. Dosage is limited by centrally induced adverse reactions to levodopa, of which dyskinesia is the commonest. When unwanted effects are encountered, the dose of the combined preparation should be reduced by about 20%. The usual stabilised intake is 3–5 tablets daily.

Carbidopa itself has not been found to have any toxic properties, but experience is still somewhat limited (Chase and Watanabe 1972).

The optimum ratio of carbidopa to levodopa varies between different individuals (Calne *et al* 1971) so the above regimen is not satisfactory for all patients. In those who do not respond well, it may be necessary to increase the proportion of carbidopa to levodopa by giving supplements of carbidopa, for example 25 mg thrice daily.

ANTICHOLINERGIC DRUGS

For a century the belladonna alkaloids have been used extensively in the treatment of Parkinsonism. They block the muscarinic receptors for acetylcholine in both the central and peripheral nervous system.

Following the second world war a number of synthetic congeners were developed which are reputed to have the advantage of acting more selectively upon central cholinergic receptors. Two explanations have been proposed for the therapeutic effect of cholinergic blockade in Parkinsonism; they are not mutually exclusive, so they could complement each other: (1) It is possible that dopamine and acteylcholine exert antagonistic actions in the striatum; in Parkinsonism, the selective impairment of dopaminergic function would lead to cholinergic dominance. Anticholinergic drugs should restore the balance (see Fig. 38). (2) Most of the anticholinergic agents employed to treat Parkinsonism inhibit the active reuptake of dopamine from the synaptic cleft (Coyle and Snyder 1969; Farnebo *et al* 1970). In this way they potentiate the pharmacological activity of whatever dopamine remains in the depleted Parkinsonian striatum.

Pharmacokinetic information on anticholinergic agents is very limited because most were introduced before recognition of the importance of drug absorption, distribution, metabolism and excretion.

Therapeutic action. Anticholinergic drugs improve tremor and rigidity but they do not have any worthwhile effect on hypokinesia. When patients have been taking anticholinergic agents for more than a few months, sudden withdrawal of therapy may precipitate a florid exacerbation of the full Parkinsonian syndrome, out of all proportion to the limited benefit attained by treatment.

Patients often claim that one anticholinergic drug suits them better than another. They sometimes prefer to take several together but it is difficult to justify giving more than two at the same time. Although many anticholinergic agents are available (Yahr and Duvoisin 1968; 1972), no clear relationship has been established between the administration of any particular drug and the amelioration of any one clinical feature.

Dose regimen. Anticholinergic drugs are usually administered 3–4 times daily. The dose is gradually increased until an adequate response is achieved or adverse reactions are encountered. Benzhexol (trihexy-phenidyl), for example, can be started at 2 mg thrice daily, with increments of 2 mg every 4–5 days. Table 8 summarises the doses for the most widely prescribed anticholinergic agents.

Table 8. Anticholinergic drugs employed by Parkinsonism.

DRUG	INITIAL DOSE mg/day	MAINTENANCE DOSE RANGE mg/day
Benapryzine	150	150–300
Benzhexol (trihexyphenidyl)	4	6–30
Benztropine	2	4–8
Biperiden	2	3–12
Chlorphenoxamine	150	200–600
Cycrimine	2.5	5–20
Ethopropazine	50	200–500
Methixene	7.5	15–20
Orphenadrine	150	200–400
Procyclidine	7.5	20–60

Adverse reactions. These drugs frequently produce adverse reactions by parasympathetic blockade. The usual problems are impaired ocular accommodation, dilatation of the pupil, reduced salivation, constipation and retention of urine. Central effects are also common —most often confusion, but also hallucinations and delusions; psychiatric disturbances can persist for two weeks after stopping therapy. It has recently been reported that dyskinesia, similar to that induced by levodopa, occasionally occurs in patients receiving anticholinergic agents (Fahn and David 1973).

Antihistamines are reputed to be useful in the treatment of Parkinsonism. There is no good evidence that their antihistaminic actions are relevant—therapeutic efficacy could be explained in terms of the anticholinergic properties which these drugs possess.

AMANTADINE

The introduction of amantadine into neurology stems from a chance observation on a Parkinsonian patient who improved following its use as an antiviral agent for influenza (Schwab *et al* 1969).

The mode of action of amantadine in Parkinsonism is not known; no relevant pharmacological effect has been demonstrated at doses comparable to those employed therapeutically. However, it has been found that high concentrations (1) augment the synthesis of dopamine (Scatton *et al* 1970), (2) increase the release of dopamine (Scatton *et al* 1970; Heikkila and Cohen 1972), (3) inhibit active reuptake of dopamine (Fletcher and Redfern 1970; Heikkila and Cohen 1972; Baldessarini *et al* 1972; Heimans *et al* 1972). All these properties could contribute to potentiation of dopaminergic function.

Pharmacokinetics. Amantadine is rapidly absorbed, peak plasma concentrations being reached 1–4 hours after ingestion. The plasma half-life is 2–4 hours. Metabolic transformation is negligible—86% of the administered drug is excreted unchanged in the urine (Bleidner *et al* 1965).

Therapeutic actions. Numerous controlled studies, reviewed by Birdwood *et al* (1971), have shown that amantadine improves the hypokinesia, tremor and rigidity of Parkinsonism. However, its therapeutic activity is considerably less than that of levodopa.

Dose regimen. The usual dose is 100 mg twice daily. Amantadine is generally administered after morning and midday meals, to avoid insomnia.

Adverse reactions. Adverse reactions are uncommon. They include restlessness, dizziness, confusion, hallucinations, mood changes, nausea, abdominal discomfort, headache, pruritus, cardiac arrhythmias, livedo reticularis and oedema. Excessive dosage can precipitate convulsions. All these unwanted effects can be corrected by reducing or stopping amantadine.

COMBINATIONS OF DIFFERENT DRUGS

Levodopa, amantadine and anticholinergic drugs can be given together. While there have been controversial reports on whether amantadine helps patients who are already taking levodopa in maximum tolerated dosage, there is no doubt that anticholinergic agents are capable of providing additional benefit (Hughes *et al* 1971). A combination of levodopa with anticholinergic drugs may offer maximum alleviation of Parkinsonian features, but certain adverse reactions, such as confusion, can also be increased.

MANAGEMENT OF THE NEWLY DIAGNOSED PATIENT

There is no general agreement on the management of newly diagnosed patients. Opinions differ on the order in which the various therapeutic agents should be offered. Some physicians advocate starting treatment with levodopa as soon as possible, because they consider that early administration delays the development of striatal denervation supersensitivity, which may be a factor contributing to drug induced dyskinesia (Klawans 1973). Others prefer to begin treatment with amantadine or an anticholinergic agent; they argue that prolonged levodopa therapy can produce toxic problems such as 'on–off' reactions, so they reserve it until motor deficits are prominent.

This controversy cannot be resolved on current evidence. Conclusions must await a comparison between the long term experiences of patients managed in these different ways.

CHAPTER 14
DYSKINESIA

Over the last 20 years the foundation upon which the concept of an extrapyramidal system was built has become eroded and much has crumbled away. Many of the original anatomical and physiological tenets have proved false, but there remain a number of established correlations between involuntary movements and degeneration of regions of the central nervous system other than the corticospinal (pyramidal) or cerebellar pathways. The relationship between the site of a lesion and the type of abnormal movement is more obscure. Some clinicopathological correlations comprise syndromes for which there are several causes (such as Parkinsonism) while others are specific diseases (such as Huntington's chorea). It is still useful to group all these disorders together and the term *extrapyramidal disease* persists in spite of the disrepute into which the *extrapyramidal system* has fallen.

Dyskinesia is commonly employed as a non-specific term for extrapyramidal involuntary movement. It does not carry any implications concerning clinical form, aetiology or pathology. It embraces chorea, athetosis, dystonia, torticollis and even tremor, which are merely descriptive subdivisions that similarly lack specific nosological inferences (Duvoisin 1972).

The most important theme to emerge from recent developments in this area is the view that choreoathetosis and Parkinsonism represent two opposite poles in a range of extrapyramidal syndromes characterised by either excessive or inadequate dopaminergic function. Motor deficits can be switched from choreoathetosis to

Parkinsonism by decreasing dopaminergic transmission with drugs such as pimozide, just as they can be changed from Parkinsonism to choreoathetosis by administering the precursor of dopamine— levodopa.

The neuropharmacology of involuntary movements will now be reviewed, excluding Parkinsonian tremor which is discussed in Chapter 13. Dyskinesias will be considered in the following order: (1) Hepatocerebral degeneration; (2) Drug induced dyskinesia; (3) Chorea; (4) Torticollis; (5) Tremor; (6) Other dyskinetic disorders; (7) Dose regimens and adverse reactions.

Dystonia musculorum deformans, dystonic cerebral palsy and occupational cramps are not influenced by any drugs currently available (Marsden 1973).

HEPATOCEREBRAL DEGENERATION

WILSON'S DISEASE

Wilson's disease (hepatolenticular degeneration) is a genetically determined disturbance of copper metabolism, which is transmitted as an autosomal recessive trait. Biochemically, the outstanding finding is reduced serum concentration of the copper binding protein, caeruloplasmin. This leads to high plasma concentrations of freely available copper; tissue levels of copper are increased, up to 100 times their normal content, with consequent damage to the nervous system and liver. There is augmented urinary excretion of copper and renal toxicity results in aminoaciduria.

The most effective drug in the treatment of Wilson's disease is penicillamine—a chelating agent which forms a ring complex with copper. In most patients, penicillamine retards the progress of the disease and there is often neurological improvement. Therapy should be started as soon as possible, so biochemical screening tests must be performed on the siblings of index cases at regular intervals. Triethylenetetramine dihydrochloride is probably the best drug for patients who develop serious toxic reactions to penicillamine (Walshe 1973).

Occasional symptomatic improvement has been reported following administration of levodopa for the hypokinetic and rigid elements of the clinical picture of Wilson's disease (Barbeau and Friesen 1970).

ACQUIRED HEPATOCEREBRAL DEGENERATION

Acquired hepatocerebral degeneration usually presents as choreoathetoid movements involving the face and tongue. Other features include dementia, tremor, rigidity and ataxia. Widespread neuronal degeneration and astrocytosis may occur (Adams 1968); there is cirrhosis with portosystemic shunting. While acquired hepatocerebral degeneration is generally associated with hepatic encephalopathy, the severity of choreoathetosis correlates with neither the level of consciousness nor the extent of asterixis.

The involuntary movements of acquired hepatocerebral degeneration are clinically similar to those induced by levodopa. This observation, together with the reports of gliosis in the striatum, has led Klawans (1973) to suggest that the choreoathetoid movements of acquired hepatocerebral degeneration are caused by denervation supersensitivity of the relatively small population of excitatory dopaminergic neurons. He and his coworkers therefore treated 4 patients with haloperidol, a dopaminergic receptor blocker, and in every case they considered that the involuntary movements improved.

DRUG INDUCED DYSKINESIA

In the context of drug induced involuntary movements, the terms acute and tardive dyskinesia are usually employed to describe relatively well defined clinical entities. Drug induced Parkinsonism (see Chapter 13) and akathisia (see later in this Chapter) are quite separate extrapyramidal reactions.

The commonest cause of drug induced dyskinesia is administration of phenothiazines. Occasionally amphetamines and anticholinergic agents may be responsible. The dyskinesia produced by levodopa is considered in more detail in Chapter 13.

ACUTE DRUG INDUCED DYSKINESIA (ACUTE DYSKINESIA, ACUTE DYSTONIA)

The first few doses of a phenothiazine may precipitate involuntary movement. Acute dyskinesia is characterised by paroxysmal or sustained movements which are often violent. If trismus, retrocollis or opisthotonus are prominent an erroneous diagnosis of tetanus or even meningitis may be made. While almost all acute dyskinesias subside spontaneously when phenothiazines are stopped, rare persistent cases have been recorded (Chateau *et al* 1966; Angle and McIntire 1968), and there have been occasional experiences of hyperpyrexia, electrolyte disturbances and death (Haan and Tilsner 1966).

The pharmacological basis of acute dyskinesia is not understood. In the majority of patients, involuntary movements can be arrested by injection of anticholinergic drugs (Ayd 1961; Lader 1970) such as intravenous benztropine 2 mg; intravenous or intramuscular biperiden 2–5 mg; intramuscular diphenhydramine 5 mg. Alternatively diazepam, 10 mg intravenously, has a rapid therapeutic action (Korczyn and Goldberg 1972). Movements may recur after a few hours so it is usual to follow up parenteral treatment with a few oral doses.

TARDIVE DRUG INDUCED DYSKINESIA (TARDIVE DYSKINESIA, PERSISTENT DYSKINESIA)

Over the last twenty years it has been estimated that 250 million people have received major tranquillising drugs. Many patients have continued on treatment for several months and in such cases the prevalence tardive dyskinesia is about 15%. This disorder therefore represents a serious problem, the dimensions of which have only recently been recognised (Crane 1973 a and b; Baldessarini and Lipinski 1973).

In tardive dyskinesia the involuntary movements assume a choreoathetoid form, usually involving the lingual, buccal or facial muscles but also seen in the neck, trunk, limb girdles and extremities. Tardive dyskinesia differs from the acute syndrome and is recognisable as a distinct clinical entity because (1) it develops as a late complication of therapy, for example after 1 kg of chlorpromazine, (2) it is commoner in elderly patients, (3) it may undergo exacerbation rather than remission when phenothiazines are stopped, (4) it often persists for years, (5) it may be increased, rather than decreased, by administration of anticholinergic drugs.

The pharmacology of tardive dyskinesia has not been adequately explained but three views have been put forward on the basis of current observations. They all propose that phenothiazines induce relatively irreversible augmentation of dopaminergic function, in addition to the well established reversible, dose dependent blockade of dopaminergic receptors.

(a) Klawans (1973) has suggested that prolonged administration of phenothiazines leads to denervation supersensitivity of excitatory dopaminergic synapses, so that normal concentrations of dopamine induce movements analogous to those evoked by levodopa in Parkinsonism. Implicit in this hypothesis is the concept that drug induced denervation supersensitivity can be irreversible, or at least persist long after drug administration has been stopped.

(b) Korczyn (1972) has argued that tardive dyskinesia stems from increased synthesis of dopamine and decreased reuptake at the synapse which leads to augmented dopaminergic function. He does not suggest that the relatively small fraction of excitatory dopaminergic synapses in the striatum has any special role in tardive dyskinesia; he emphasises that inhibitory pathways could be responsible because increased motor activity can be explained in terms of 'inhibition of inhibition'. As with Klawans' hypothesis, it is necessary to postulate that these events persist after phenothiazine withdrawal, in contrast to receptor blockade.

(c) Chase (1972) has independently proposed that a combination of denervation supersensitivity, increased synthesis of dopamine and decreased reuptake all contribute to the production of tardive dyskinesia. This view embraces the elements of both Klawans' and Korczyn's hypotheses. Chase does not speculate on whether excitatory or inhibitory receptors are involved.

Support of the premise upon which all three hypotheses agree—

that tardive dyskinesia is due to increased dopaminergic function—derives from the following findings:

1 As already mentioned, when long term phenothiazine therapy is reduced or stopped, tardive dyskinesia is often exacerbated, or may even present for the first time (Crane and Paulson 1967; Klawans *et al* 1970b). This can be interpreted in terms of disturbing a balance between an irreversible increase in dopaminergic function on the one hand and a dose-dependent, reversible blockade of receptors on the other.

2 Administration of dopaminergic receptor blocking drugs and dopamine depletors can alleviate tardive dyskinesia (Delay and Deniker 1968; Villeneuve and Böszörményi 1970; MacCollum 1970; Roxburgh 1970; Singer and Cheng 1971; Godwin-Austen and Clark 1971; Kazamatsuri *et al* 1972 a and b; Calne *et al* 1974).

3 Levodopa, the precursor of dopamine, exacerbates tardive dyskinesia (Hippius and Logeman 1970; Klawans and McKendall 1971).

Therapeutic implications

From these observations it is evident that tardive dyskinesia may be treated with drugs which reduce dopaminergic function, such as pimozide, haloperidol or tetrabenazine, but these agents can themselves induce extrapyramidal reactions and a satisfactory balance between therapeutic and toxic effects is often unattainable. Treatment, therefore, is often disappointing in spite of the pharmacological advances in analysing the origin of dyskinesia. A proportion of patients undergo spontaneous remission months or years after stopping the causal drug (Lader 1970). It is therefore common practice to reduce or withdraw whatever agent has been implicated, even though this manoeuvre may initially precipitate an exacerbation. The most important conclusion to be drawn from recent developments in the documentation of tardive dyskinesia is that phenothiazines carry a high risk of inducing persistent involuntary movements so they should not be administered for prolonged, continuous periods unless this is essential in the management of psychosis.

CHOREA

HUNTINGTON'S CHOREA

Huntington's chorea is a progressive disease which is inherited as an autosomal dominant trait. The salient features are dementia and chorea, but rigidity, akinesia, tremor and psychosis can all occur. There is profound loss of small neurons in the striatum with prominent gliosis; atrophy of the cerebral cortex is also common.

The outstanding biochemical disturbance in the brains of patients with Huntington's chorea is depletion of GABA (Perry *et al* 1973) and the enzyme concerned with its formation, glutamic acid decarboxylase (Bird *et al* 1973). Beyond the general comment that GABA receptors are usually concerned with inhibition, it is difficult to extrapolate from these findings. GABA is not readily accessible to investigation because there are no plasma or urinary metabolites that can be studied.

Other pharmacological approaches have yielded some interesting observations with therapeutic implications (Barbeau *et al* 1973); in many respects the findings are analogous to those discussed when considering tardive dyskinesia.

1 Drugs which augment dopaminergic function, such as levodopa, exacerbate the involuntary movements of Huntington's chorea (Gerstenbrand *et al* 1963; Bruck *et al* 1965) and may even precipitate chorea in relatives of Huntingtonian patients (Klawans *et al* 1970).

2 Agents which reduce dopaminergic transmission ameliorate the involuntary movements of Huntington's chorea. Such drugs include alpha methyl-p-tyrosine (Birkmayer 1969), reserpine (Bruyn 1968a), tetrabenazine (Dalby 1969; Swash *et al* 1972; McLellan *et al* 1974), perphenazine (Fahn 1973), thiopropazate (Matthews 1958; Bruyn 1962; Lyon 1962), haloperidol (Divry *et al* 1959) and pimozide (Fog and Pakkenberg 1970).

3 Drugs which antagonise acetylcholine, such as benztropine, are claimed to increase the movements of Huntington's chorea (Klawans and Rubovits 1972).

4 Agents which raise the level of striatal acetylcholine, such as

physostigmine, are reported to decrease the severity of chorea (Klawans and Rubovits 1972).

From these observations, together with the established background of antagonism between dopamine and acetylcholine in the striatum, Klawans (1973) has argued that denervation supersensitivity of excitatory dopaminergic receptors occurs in Huntington's chorea.

Therapeutic implications

Dopaminergic function should be reduced with tetrabenazine, thiopropazate, perphenazine, haloperidol or pinozide; dosage can be titrated up to the maximum tolerated level of intake.

Drugs which increase central cholinergic activity produce adverse reactions which preclude their use.

It has been mentioned that administration of levodopa can precipitate involuntary movements in symptom free relatives of patients with Huntington's chorea (Klawans *et al* 1970). Although this may prove to be an effective predictive test for indentification of those asymptomatic relatives who will subsequently develop the disease, the implications of a positive result must be viewed with caution. It is impossible to conceal the result of the test from the patient, so deleterious psychological consequences may exceed the benefits deriving from accurate prognosis.

SYDENHAM'S CHOREA

Sydenham's chorea is a reaction to streptococcal infection. Since the condition usually clears spontaneously, there are few pathological reports. Widespread inflammatory, vascular and degenerative lesions of the central nervous system occur but these may all be caused by the toxic septicaemia that is responsible for death (Thiebaut 1968). Haloperidol is reputed to be beneficial (Nick and Nicholle 1964; Thiebaut 1968), which implies that the pharmacological basis may be similar to that of Huntington's chorea.

THYROTOXIC CHOREA

Choreoathetosis is an uncommon but well documented feature of hyperthyroidism. Studies in animal models of thyroid disease prompted Prange *et al* (1970) to formulate the general hypothesis that catecholamine receptor sensitivity is increased in hyper-thyroidism and decreased in hypothyroidism. Thyrotoxic chorea has, therefore, been attributed to excessive dopaminergic function in the striatum. In support of this view, Klawans (1973) has reported improvement following blockade of dopaminergic receptors with haloperidol. He has also found a reduction in the concentration of homovanillic acid in the CSF of hyperthyroid patients. Decreased homovanillic acid in the CSF is generally regarded as evidence of either degeneration of dopaminergic neurons, or impaired synthesis of transmitter due to increased activation of dopaminergic receptors. The latter explanation seems more plausible in hyperthyroidism because the chorea is reversible by correction of the thyrotoxicosis (Heffron and Eaton 1970).

CHOREA INDUCED BY ORAL CONTRACEPTIVES OR PREGNANCY

Chorea gravidarum is rare, but chorea caused by oral contraceptives is being recognised with increasing frequency (Lewis and Harrison 1969). This form of chorea rapidly clears when contraceptive therapy is stopped, so there are no pathological or pharmacological observations to form the basis of an explanation.

SENILE CHOREA

Chorea in the elderly can be generalised or localised; it may be clinically indistinguishable from dyskinesia produced by drugs. There is neuronal loss and gliosis in the striatum. Reserpine, tetra-benazine and haloperidol have all been claimed to improve senile chorea (Pakkenberg 1968; Fog and Pakkenberg 1970; MacCollum

1970; Klawans 1973)—here again there appears to be a disturbance of striatal transmitters such that dopaminergic function predominates.

IDIOPATHIC CHOREOATHETOSIS

Occasionally involuntary movements which are clinically indistinguishable from tardive dyskinesia develop in patients who are not senile and who have never been exposed to drugs (Fog and Pakkenberg 1970; Altrocci 1972). These movements respond to dopamine antagonists in the same way as tardive dyskinesia.

CHOREA INDUCED BY SYSTEMIC LUPUS ERYTHEMATOSUS

Chorea is an unusual manifestation of systemic lupus erythematosus. Arteritis leads to ischaemic lesions of the central nervous system; striatal pathology has been reported but the evidence is limited (Baucer *et al* 1950).

Haloperidol has been given to two patients with chorea due to systemic lupus erythematosus. As a result, the involuntary movements improved in both (Heilman *et al* 1971; Klawans 1973), suggesting the possibility of a pharmacological mechanism analogous to other choreas, characterised by a relative increase of dopaminergic function.

TORTICOLLIS

Torticollis—involuntary twisting of the head and neck—may be spasmodic or sustained. It can be an isolated finding, in which case it is unusual to establish any aetiology other than occasional genetic predisposition (Pratt 1967). Torticollis can also occur in the setting of a more generalised neurological disturbance, such as postencephalitic Parkinsonism, carbon monoxide poisoning, dystonia musculorum deformans, Huntington's chorea or drug induced dyskinesia.

The neuropathology of isolated torticollis is obscure. There has been one report of atrophy predominantly involving the caudate nucleus and putamen (Podovinský 1968).

Torticollis may prove to be pharmacologically similar to the choreas because drugs which reduce dopaminergic function, such as tetrabenazine (Swash *et al* 1972) and haloperidol (Gilbert 1972) are occasionally beneficial. Large doses of diazepam can also be useful (Duvoisin 1972).

TREMOR

Familial, senile and essential tremor form a continuum. They are characterised by regular, rhythmic and predominantly distal involuntary movements which may be prominent at rest but are usually exacerbated by action or anxiety. If there is evidence of a hereditary aetiology, this clinical picture is called familial tremor. When it starts after the age of 60 years, it is termed senile tremor. If it cannot be attributed to either genetic predisposition or old age, it is labelled essential tremor. No clinicopathological correlation has been established (Herkovits and Blackwood 1969); no pharmacological basis has been identified.

Two therapeutic approaches have proved effective. First ethanol, which is particularly useful because patients can often pursue therapy at social engagements when it is specially desirable to minimise shaking. Second, beta adrenergic blocking drugs, such as propanolol are beneficial in some but not all patients (Winkler and Young 1971; Gilligan *et al* 1972; Morgan *et al* 1973; Dupont *et al* 1973; Sweet *et al* 1974).

Beta adrenergic blockers decrease the amplitude of physiological tremor by an effect mediated at the periphery (Marsden *et al* 1967), but the site of action of these drugs is not known in familial, essential, or senile tremor. The treatment of Parkinsonian tremor is discussed in Chapter 13. Thyrotoxic tremor responds to conventional therapy directed at suppressing thyroid function (see Chapter 9). There is no satisfactory medical treatment for intention tremor, but stereotactic surgery can be helpful.

OTHER DYSKINETIC DISORDERS

METABOLIC DISTURBANCES

Metabolic disturbances commonly generate involuntary movements. The irregular flap of hepatic, renal and respiratory failure—asterixis —is sometimes accompanied by more severe involuntary movements. These motor disorders respond to treatment of the underlying biochemical abnormality (see Chapter 9).

Wilson's disease and thyrotoxic chorea have already been discussed.

The Lesch–Nyhan syndrome is caused by deficiency of hypoxanthine-guanine-phosphoribosyl-transferase. In consequence, uric acid accumulates in the tissues and the blood. Allopurinol is useful in preventing the peripheral complications of hyperuricaemia, but the cerebral manifestations do not respond to any form of treatment.

DYSLYSIS

Compulsive movement of the limbs, known as dyslysis, restless legs, or Ekbom's syndrome, is a condition of unknown origin which may benefit from phenobarbitone (Behrman 1958) or diazepam (Brain and Walton 1969). These drugs are considered in more detail in Chapters 12 and 15.

AKATHISIA

Akathisia is a state of restlessness induced in some 10% of subjects receiving major tranquillisers. It is clinically similar to dyslysis. Patients continually rock, shift their legs, tap their feet or pace up and down aimlessly. This clinical picture is often mistakenly attributed to anxiety, an error which may lead to an exacerbation of the problem if the dose of the causal neuroleptic drug is increased! Akathisia clears on stopping the therapy responsible (Chase 1972).

PAROXYSMAL KINESOGENIC CHOREOATHETOSIS

Paroxysmal kinesogenic choreoathetosis (striatal epilepsy, extrapyramidal epilepsy) is a benign, sometimes familial disease of children and young adults (Stevens 1966; Kertesz 1967). It responds to anticonvulsants, such as phenytoin and carbamazepine—drugs which are considered in detail in Chapter 12.

CREUTZFELDT-JAKOB DISEASE

Creutzfeldt-Jakob disease is a slow virus infection with extrapyramidal features. It has been reported to benefit from amantadine (Braham 1971; Hamoen 1973; Sanders and Dunn 1973), which is fully considered in Chapter 13.

HICCUP, TICS AND THE SYNDROME OF GILLES DE LA TOURETTE

This group of disorders is sometimes helped by haloperidol (Boris 1968; Connell *et al* 1967; Korczyn 1971).

DOSE REGIMENS AND ADVERSE REACTIONS

ANTIDOPAMINERGIC DRUGS

In discussing the treatment of choreoathetoid movements there have been frequent references to the use of antidopaminergic drugs. These agents can themselves induce extrapyramidal reactions; their long term therapeutic role has not been defined because of the difficulty in evaluating the balance between their beneficial and adverse effects. Drugs may reduce dopaminergic function by (1) blocking dopaminergic receptors (phenothiazines, butyrophenones, and diphenylbutypiperidines) or (2) by depleting concentrations of dopamine (tetrabenazine).

Haloperidol. Haloperidol is a butyrophenone. It is rapidly absorbed, reaching peak plasma concentrations in 2–6 hours. The plasma half-life is about 20 hours. Excretion takes place via both urine and faeces. Treatment may be started with 0.5 mg thrice daily increasing by 0.5 mg every third day until there is an adequate therapeutic response or adverse reactions occur. The usual dose range is 4–8 mg/day, though 16 mg/day may be given. Unwanted effects include sedation, hypotension and Parkinsonism. Serum transaminase levels may rise; there have been reports of leucopenia and rarely, agranulocytosis.

Perphenazine. Perphenazine is a phenothiazine. The usual maintenance dose is 12–32 mg/day. Unwanted effects are similar to those of thiopropazate (see below).

Pimozide. Pimozide is a diphenylbutylpiperidine. It is readily absorbed but only about 0.1% of the dose can be found in the brain—though much of this accumulates in the striatum. In spite of its limited penetration of the blood–brain barrier, the major actions of pimozide are all exerted through the central nervous system. Metabolites seem to be pharmacologically inert, the major pathway being dealkylation (Laduron 1971). The plasma-life is about 24 hours. An initial dose of 2 mg/day may be raised by 2 mg every third day until a good response is obtained or adverse reactions develop. Patients seldom tolerate more than 20 mg/day. The usual dose limiting factors are drowsiness and Parkinsonism; akathisia can also be troublesome.

Tetrabenazine. Tetrabenazine is pharmacologically similar to reserpine but it has a more selective action on the central nervous system. Its effects develop more quickly than reserpine and are of shorter duration, so it is easier to titrate dosage. A reasonable initial intake is 25 mg twice daily, building up the regimen by 25 mg every third day until an improvement occurs or difficulties are encountered; 75–100 mg/day is generally satisfactory. Tetrabenazine can induce drowsiness, depression, feelings of unreality, sweating, insomnia, hypotension, akathisia and Parkinsonism.

Thiopropazate. Thiopropazate is a phenothiazine. The dose range is 15–30 mg/day. Intake is adjusted according to the response and the emergence of adverse reactions, which include Parkinsonism, blurring of vision, dryness of the mouth, nasal congestion, constipation and hypotension.

BETA ADRENERGIC BLOCKING DRUGS

Beta adrenergic blocking drugs are employed in the treatment of essential, familial and senile tremor. They can induce bronchospasm and decrease the force of contraction of the heart so they are contraindicated in patients with a history of bronchial asthma or cardiac failure.

Oxprenolol. Oxprenolol reaches peak plasma levels 1–2 hours after ingestion. A starting dose of 40 mg daily can be built up with 40 mg increments every third day. Its unwanted effects are similar to those of propanolol, though it is reported to cause less bronchospasm.

Propanolol. Peak plasma concentrations of propanolol are reached 1–1½ hours after oral intake. A starting dose of 20 mg twice daily can be increased by 20 mg every third day until tremor is controlled or adverse reactions develop. A useful indication of pharmacological activity is the pulse rate—as dosage rises the pulse should not be allowed to fall below 60 beats/minute. In addition to bradycardia, bronchospasm, and cardiac failure, propanolol can induce hypotension, nausea, diarrhoea, lassitude, ataxia, insomnia, hallucinations and parasthaesiae.

CHELATING AGENTS

Penicillamine (D-penicillamine). Penicillamine is the most satisfactory treatment for Wilson's disease (Walshe 1970). It is readily absorbed and undergoes rapid excretion in the urine. A dose of 250 mg four times daily may be increased according to tolerance; prolonged treatment with more than 2 g/day commonly produces toxic reactions. Occasionally penicillamine causes nausea and vomiting. Optic neuropathy has been reported but this usually improves if pyridoxine (100 mg/day) is given. The skin can become pigmented and it may break down over pressure areas; rashes and fever can also occur. The most serious complications are leucopenia, systemic lupus erythematosus and nephrotic syndrome.

Triethylenetetramine dihydrochloride. Triethylenetetramine dihydrochloride is a satisfactory alternative to penicillamine. It is generally well tolerated, the usual maintenance dose is 400 mg thrice daily (Walshe 1969; 1973).

URICOSURIC AGENTS

Allopurinol. Allopurinol is used in the treatment of the Lesch–Nyhan syndrome. It inhibits the synthesis of uric acid by blocking xanthine oxidase. The dose range is 2–8 mg/kg/day, employing the serum concentration of uric acid as a guide to response. Adverse reactions are uncommon—they include nausea, diarrhoea, colic, headache, drowsiness, malaise, fever, pruritus, skin eruptions, peripheral neuropathy and leucopenia.

CHAPTER 15
SPASTICITY

Spasticity is an abnormal, increased resistance to passive movement of a limb caused by a lesion of the corticospinal (pyramidal) tract. Classically, this resistance has been described as displaying specific clinical features: increasing force applied by the examiner is matched by increasing resistance to movement until suddenly the patient's reaction appears to melt away like the closure of a clasp knife. This finding is unusual. Corticospinal lesions more frequently give rise to a sustained resistance to passive movement (Dimitrijevic and Nathan 1967) which may resemble the rigidity of extrapyramidal disease.

The term spasticity has persisted where the clinical context indicates that the cause is a corticospinal lesion—a pattern of predominant resistance in arm extensors and leg flexors with associated weakness, increased tendon reflexes, absent abdominal responses, extensor plantars and often flexor or adductor spasms.

PHYSIOLOGY AND PHARMACOLOGY

The physiological and pharmacological disturbances occurring in spasticity are not understood. One animal model, produced by ischaemic decerebration, is characterised by increased alpha motoneuron activity. Another, occurring after intercollicular section, is mediated by increased fusimotor drive. Investigations of human spasticity have employed the silent period, the H reflex, peripheral cooling and the response to vibration in an attempt to separate

222

predominant alpha motoneuron and fusimotor drive. Current results suggest that either or both motoneuron systems may show excessive activity (Asai and Hufschmidt 1958; Rushworth 1966; Dietrichson 1971 a and b; Knutsson *et al* 1973; McLellan 1973b).

It is probable that extensive changes of transmitter function occur when spasticity develops (Stavraky 1961). Noradrenaline, serotonin, acetylcholine, glycine and GABA are all transmitters in the spinal cord but no coherent neuropharmacological explanation of spasticity has emerged.

Some understanding of flexor and adductor spasms may stem from the observation that administration of levodopa to a cat with spinal transection leads to a marked increase in the flexor reflex induced by pinching the skin, associated with an intense discharge of both alpha mononeurons and fusimotor neurons (Andén *et al* 1964). Furthermore, recent studies by Maxwell and Sumpter (1974) indicate that central noradrenergic blockade decreases fusimotor activity.

TREATMENT

The cause of spasticity should always be treated if this is possible, because effective therapy—for example B_{12} in subacute combined degeneration of the spinal cord—will arrest progressive disease and may lead to improvement in both muscle tone and power.

If the underlying lesion cannot be treated, a decision must be made on whether muscle tone should be reduced by methods which may exacerbate paresis. The splinting effect of spastic muscles can help a patient with weak legs to stand and walk, so alleviation of spasticity without any improvement in power may result in further disability. When clinical evaluation indicates that a decrease in muscle tone is nervertheless desirable, treatment with a centrally acting muscle relaxant can be undertaken. Several drugs produce a definite though transient reduction in spasticity when administered intravenously; these compounds are much less effective when given by mouth because adverse reactions, in particular sedation, become prominent. No drug is capable of achieving a substantial, sustained decrease in spasticity without sedation but limited benefit can often be obtained.

In this Chapter the treatment of spasticity will be considered in the following stages: (1) Baclofen; (2) Diazepam; (3) Mephenesin; (4) Intrathecal phenol; (5) Drugs currently undergoing evaluation.

BACLOFEN

Baclofen is an analogue of GABA, a transmitter acting predominantly at inhibitory synapses. Baclofen decreases experimental spasticity produced by either ischaemic decerebration or intercollicular section (Bein 1972); it is also effective in spasticity in man. Patients with total spinal transection are reputed to benefit to the same extent as those with incomplete corticospinal lesions, suggesting that baclofen acts predominantly at spinal level. Several mechanisms of action have been proposed, varying from direct inhibition of alpha motoneurons and fusimotor neurons to reduction of posttetanic potentiation and facilitation of the Renshaw inhibitory feed-back loop. Knutsson *et al* (1973) consider that patients with a substantial increase in fusimotor neuron activity respond best to baclofen. McLellan (1973b) has suggested that baclofen selectively reduces the excitability of the monosynaptic reflex arc from dynamic spindles.

Therapeutic actions. Controlled studies have confirmed that spasticity is improved by baclofen and there is substantial alleviation of flexor spasms (Pedersen *et al* 1970; Hudgson and Weightman 1971; Hudgson *et al* 1972).

Pharmacokinetics. Baclofen is readily absorbed from the gastrointestinal tract, peak plasma concentrations being reached some 2 hours after oral administration (Faigle and Keberle 1972). The plasma half-life is about 3 hours. Metabolism is limited; some 85% of the drug is excreted in the urine unchanged. Baclofen crosses the blood–brain barrier rather slowly.

Dose regimen. An initial intake of 5 mg thrice daily may be increased by adding 5 mg every 3 or 4 days, until there is a satisfactory response or adverse reactions develop. It is undesirable to exceed 100 mg/day unless patients are under close supervision in hospital. Caution is required when treating patients who are also taking hypotensive drugs.

Adverse reactions. The commonest problems encountered with baclofen are sedation and nausea, which occur in some 10% of patients (de Pinto *et al* 1972). There have also been reports of hypotonia, increased weakness, vertigo, confusion, alteration in mood and reduction in blood pressure. Baclofen can induce a deterioration of the EEG in epileptic patients.

DIAZEPAM

Diazepam belongs to the benzodiazepine group of drugs—chlordiazepoxide, oxazepam, medazepam, nitrazepam, clonazepam—most widely employed for their tranquillising, sedative and anticonvulsant actions. Diazepam is also used for the treatment of spasticity; its therapeutic effect is reputed to be unrelated to sedation (Cook and Nathan 1967).

Benzodiazepines increase the concentration of acetylcholine in the brain (Consolo *et al* 1972); they also accelerate the turnover and inhibit the reuptake of noradrenaline and dopamine (Lidbrink *et al* 1973; Taylor and Laverty 1973). It is not known whether any of these properties is relevant to their action in spasticity. Neurophysiological effects which may contribute include:

1   Inhibition of brainstem activating systems. The spontaneous firing of brainstem neurons in the cat is decreased by administration of diazepam, as is the response elicited from these neurons by electrical stimulation of the sciatic nerve (Przybyla and Wang 1968).

2   Increase of presynaptic inhibition. Presynaptic inhibition in the cat is augmented by diazepam (Schmidt *et al* 1967; Schlosser 1971; Stratten and Barnes 1971).

3   Inhibition of polysynaptic spinal reflexes. Evidence for suppression of interneuronal pathways by a mechanism other than presynaptic inhibition has been presented by Brausch *et al* (1973).

4   Inhibition of fusimotor activity. Observations on tension–extension curves obtained by eliciting the stretch reflex in cats (Brausch *et al* 1973) suggest that diazepam reduced fusimotor firing.

Therapeutics actions. Controlled studies have demonstrated the therapeutic activity of diazepam in alleviating spasticity and flexor spasms (Wilson and McKechnie 1966; Margulies and Slade 1968; Corbett *et al* 1972). Pinelli (1973) has proposed that diazepam improves motor performance in spastic patients by reducing abnormal excitation in antagonistic muscles. Cook and Nathan (1967) have reported that patients with complete spinal transection benefit as much as those with incomplete lesions, indicating that at least part of the therapeutic action of diazepam is achieved at spinal level. In this respect diazepam resembles baclofen.

Pharmacokinetics. Peak plasma concentrations of diazepam are reached 2–4 hours after oral intake. There is extensive binding to plasma proteins (van der Kleijn 1969). The decay curve shows two main components, one with a half-life of 7–10 hours, the other of 2–6 days (Zbinden and Randall 1967). Administration of the same dose to different individuals reveals a 20 fold range of variation in plasma levels. Diazepam crosses the blood–brain barrier very readily; the concentration is higher in brain than blood one minute after intravenous injection (Marcucci *et al* 1971).

The major metabolic pathways are demethylation and hydroxylation (Schwartz *et al* 1965), transformations taking place rapidly. Some 70% of the products are excreted in the urine. Part of the therapeutic action of diazepam stems from the formation of active metabolites such as oxazepam. Diazepam does not induce any change in hepatic microsomal enzymes (Solomon *et al* 1971).

Dose regimen. The maximum tolerated intake of diazepam varies considerably between patients. A reasonable starting dose is 5 mg twice daily, increasing by 5mg every third day until spasticity is alleviated or sedation occurs. In some patients drowsiness develops at low dosage, but others can take 45 mg/day without undue sleepiness.

Adverse reactions. It is most unusual for patients to experience any adverse reaction other than sedation. Unfortunately this often develops at doses which are too low to accomplish worthwhile improvement in spasticity.

MEPHENESIN

Mephenesin reduces experimental spasticity. It inhibits polysynaptic reflexes but its detailed neuropharmacological actions have not been identified. Mephenesin is readily absorbed and rapidly metabolised; useful therapeutic results are seldom obtained because adverse reactions tend to mask any benefit.

The dose range for mephenesin carbamate is 1–3 g repeated three to five times a day according to response and tolerance. Nausea, confusion, diplopia, generalised weakness and syncope can all limit intake. A cerebellar syndrome may also be induced with nystagmus, incoordination and ataxia. Occasionally depigmentation of the hair can occur (Spillane 1963).

INTRATHECAL PHENOL

Intrathecal phenol was introduced to treat spasticity for reasons which subsequently proved to be incorrect—a familiar occurrence in the history of neurological therapuetics. Since certain forms of spasticity were attributed to increased fusimotor neuron activity, it was considered desirable to destroy the fusimotor axons while still allowing alpha motoneurons to operate. Early claims that phenol selectively damaged small nerve fibres led to an investigation of its action in patients with spastic paraplegia. Intrathecal injection gave encouraging results (Kelly and Gautier-Smith 1959; Nathan 1965), but further studies indicated that the lesion produced by phenol was not related to the diameter of nerve fibres (Nathan *et al* 1965). A new explanation had to be found for the clinical observations—it was concluded that phenol decreased input to the spinal cord by indiscriminate damage of posterior root fibres, the consequent incomplete deafferentation resulting in reduced motoneuron activity.

Intrathecal phenol alleviates sustained adductor spasm, allowing incontinent patients to be kept clean. This, in turn, reduces the incidence of intercurrent infections. Painful muscle spasms can be expected to decrease, but treatment with phenol should only be undertaken when all other therapeutic approaches have proved unsuccessful. Patients who may improve spontaneously should not be treated. No benefit can be achieved where contractures have developed. Other factors determining the selection of patients include the risk of impairing sensation or disturbing sphincter control.

The technique for administration involves lumbar puncture with the patient in the flexed lateral position; if necessary, the location of the needle tip can be confirmed radiologically. A solution of 10% phenol is made up in either iophendylate or glycerol, both of which are heavier than CSF. The patient is postured so that the phenol will collect at the posterior roots under attack—corresponding to the muscles most severely involved. This position is achieved by elevating the head so that the spine is at a suitable angle for the phenol to collect at the appropriate roots with the back rotated to a plane at 70° to the bed. The bevel of the needle is adjusted to face towards the floor and an initial 0.2 ml is injected. The patient is examined 15 minutes later for any neurological changes; if necessary, further injections of 0.2 ml are given every 15 minutes up to a total of 1 ml, evaluating the result after each dose.

DRUGS CURRENTLY UNDERGOING EVALUATION

A number of drugs are currently undergoing evaluation as potential therapeutic agents for spasticity.

Dantrolene. Dantrolene is a hydantoin which impairs excitation–contraction coupling in skeletal muscle (Ellis and Bryant 1972). Its precise mechanism of action is not known. In a recent study of patients with multiple sclerosis, substantial improvement in spasticity has been reported but unfortunately this was confined to a minority (Gelenberg and Poskanzer 1973). An initial dose of 25–50 mg twice daily can be increased at intervals of 3–4 days until a response is obtained or adverse reactions occur. An intake of 800 mg/day should not be exceeded. The commonest dose limiting problem is weakness. Other unwanted effects include light headedness and diarrhoea.

Dimethothiazine. Dimethothiazine is a phenothiazine which alleviates decerebrate rigidity and inhibits both dynamic and static fusimotor neurons (Keary and Maxwell 1967; Maxwell and Rhodes 1970). It has recently been reported to have a therapeutic action in spasticity (Matthews *et al* 1972; Crawley *et al* 1973). An initial dose of 200 mg on waking and 100 mg at noon may be increased to 500 mg daily if tolerated. Adverse reactions include exacerbation of flexor spasms, drowsiness, photosensitivity and obesity.

Orciprenaline. Drugs which activate beta adrenergic receptors increase the rate of relaxation of muscle and reduce the extent of fusion in response to rapidly repetitive electrical stimulation (Marsden and Meadows 1970). Such pharmacological properties may be of therapeutic value in spasticity and preliminary reports have been encouraging. It has been claimed that orciprenaline, 10 mg four times daily, can reduce spasticity and lead to increased freedom of movement (Zaimis 1973). Clonus may be exacerbated and patients sometimes complain of tremor. Orciprenaline, like other beta adrenergic agonists, can induce palpitations and cardiac arrhythmias.

CHAPTER 16
URINARY INCONTINENCE

Normal control of micturition involves a cycle of filling, development of a desire to void, postponement, initiation of bladder contraction with sphincter relaxation, and maintenance of coordinated motor function until the bladder is empty (Yeates 1973). Disturbances of micturition are common in neurological practice, for example some 80% of patients with multiple sclerosis experience urinary symptoms at some time and in about 50% these persist (Miller *et al* 1965).

In this Chapter urinary incontinence will be considered in the following stages: (1) Innervation and physiology of the bladder; (2) Pharmacology of micturition; (3) Treatment of incontinence; (4) Dose regimens and adverse reactions.

INNERVATION AND PHYSIOLOGY OF THE BLADDER

Micturition is a spinal reflex subject to supraspinal control by descending facilitation or inhibition. Parasympathetic fibres from sacral segments 2–4 supply the entire musculature, which also receives sympathetic innervation via the hypogastric plexus. Afferent fibres accompany the efferents of both these systems. Ascending and descending pathways run in the lateral columns of the spinal cord. An hierarchy of supraspinal driving, restraining and coordinating mechanisms are also involved in normal micturition. There is an area in the pons concerned with facilitation of the voiding reflex, an inhibitory region in the midbrain, and a controlling area has been identified in the superior frontal gyrus (Andrew and Nathan 1964).

The bladder muscle displays plasticity so that when stretched, tension is not sustained. If the bladder is filled from a urethral catheter there is minimal change in vesical pressure until a critical volume around 400 ml is reached. The micturition reflex is then triggered—a steep rise in vesical pressure occurs and urine is passed.

The denervated bladder can undergo autonomous waves of contraction, but intact innervation from the spinal cord is necessary for adequate emptying. Patients with chronic spinal lesions are capable of reflex micturition; it is probable that autonomous waves of contraction usually provide the final stimulus for reflex voiding (Plum 1962) though brief abdominal compression is often a useful artificial way of initiating micturition. One important area of obscurity is the failure to find any cystometric correlation with the sensation of fullness of the bladder (Denny-Brown and Robertson 1933). Another difficult problem is the analysis of the complex mechanisms concerned with postponing a desire to void until the circumstances are appropriate.

The main neurological causes of urinary symptoms are:

1 Deafferentation; this leads to distension of the bladder without the sensation of fullness. It usually results in overflow incontinence with a chronically enlarged bladder. An analogy may be drawn to hypotonia in the limbs.

2 Lower motoneuron lesions; again there is dilatation, but it is initially painful, with a sensation of fullness. Ultimately dribbling incontinence develops and the areflexic bladder commonly shrinks, though the reason for this loss of volume is not known; this phenomenon may perhaps be comparable to the formation of contractures in the denervated limb.

3 Upper motoneuron lesions; these result in facilitation of the micturition reflex, analogous to augmentation of the tendon reflexes. Repetitive reflex voiding occurs, which is often incomplete. The hyperreflexic bladder tends to have a small volume and is often termed spastic because of a supposed similarity to upper motoneuron lesions of the limbs.

PHARMACOLOGY OF MICTURITION

The traditional concept of the mechanism of micturition envisaged a detrusor muscle under cholinergic parasympathetic control and a sphincter innervated by the noradrenergic sympathetic system. Parasympathetic drive was thought to be involved in emptying the bladder while sympathetic input held it closed; an example of the classical cholinergic–noradrenergic antagonism operating throughout the autonomic nervous system and exemplified by comparison with the mechanisms responsible for constricting and dilating the pupil of the eye.

Unfortunately, this scheme is not in accord with current observations (Woodburne 1961). The neuropharmacology of micturition is not understood— it is easy to delineate large areas of ignorance and difficult to identify the few small points of knowledge. In a critical review on this topic, Plum (1962) states that the sympathetic efferent innervation in man is 'without known function in micturition'. It may be inferred that noradrenergic peripheral pathways are concerned with other roles such as those involved in sexual activity.

Considering now the cholinergic systems, it has been reported that voluntary control of urine persists after curarisation (Lapsides *et al* 1957) which blocks the cholinergic nicotinic junction between motor nerve endings and striated muscle. This leaves, as the only pathway which has not been rendered redundant, the cholinergic muscarinic (parasympathetic) innervation of smooth muscle.

TREATMENT OF INCONTINENCE

Clinical observations are consonant with the view that the peripheral synapses most directly involved in the control of micturition in man belong to the parasympathetic system. It is common neurological experience that administration of muscarinic blocking drugs, employed in the treatment of Parkinsonism, can lead to difficulty in passing urine. Correspondingly, in patients with postoperative retention, micturition can be induced by administration of cholinomimetic agents.

Incontinence associated with a bladder which is not distended should be treated with anticholinergic (muscarinic blocking) agents such as atropine, propantheline, methantheline, imipramine and emepronium. Conversely, when retention of urine leads to vesical dilatation with overflow, control of micturition may be improved by restoring the size of the bladder to normal with drugs which induce contraction by increasing cholinergic activity, such as bethanechol, carbachol, neostigmine or distigmine.

Alleviation of involuntary micturition is desirable for medical aesthetic and social reasons. In the paraplegic patient, correction of bladder function is mandatory to prevent pressure sores, urinary tract infections and hydronephrosis. If drugs fail to achieve adequate control, collecting appliances, catheterisation, stimulation via implanted electrodes or surgical diversion of urine should be undertaken (Crosbie Ross 1970).

The best safeguards against ascending urinary infection are a high fluid intake, free bladder drainage and the avoidance of prolonged recumbency. Prophylactic use of antimicrobial therapy is controversial—while occasionally advocated, it is more common to reserve treatment for acute episodes of urinary infection (Crosbie Ross *et al* 1964; Hunt and Hader 1966).

DOSE REGIMENS AND ADVERSE REACTIONS

ANTICHOLINERGIC DRUGS

Atropine. Atropine is rapidly absorbed; some 50% becomes bound to plasma proteins. Most of the drug is excreted in the urine within 24 hours, a major fraction as a glucuronide conjugate (Kalser and McLain 1970). The usual dose range of atropine (administered as the sulphate) is 0.25–1 mg by mouth, 3–4 times daily according to response and tolerance. The most frequently encountered adverse reactions are constipation, dryness of the mouth and skin, mydriasis, photophobia, defective ocular accommodation and tachycardia.

Emepronium. Emepronium is another antimuscarinic drug commonly employed in the treatment of urinary incontinence. The dose is built up from an initial intake of 50 mg twice daily, or 100 mg at night if nocturnal symptoms are prominent. Some patients tolerate as much as 600 mg/day. Overdosage leads to the same reactions as an excessive intake of atropine.

Imipramine. Imipramine may occasionally be helpful in nocturnal incontinence. The adult dose is 50 mg at night. For children of 4–10 years, 25 mg is usually adequate. This drug is discussed in more detail in Chapter 20.

Methantheline. Methantheline is similar in structure to propantheline but has more blocking action on autonomic ganglia (this antinicotinic effect is not prominent with other antimuscarinic agents). The dose range is 50–100 mg, up to 4 times daily.

Propantheline. Only a small fraction of propantheline is absorbed from the gastrointestinal tract—less than 50% (Beermann *et al* 1972). It may take 4 days to be cleared from the body. A multiple peak pattern of excretion suggests enterohepatic recirculation (Pfeffer *et al* 1968). The usual dose range is 30–75 mg daily; for nocturnal incontinence 30 mg is generally administered at night.

CHOLINERGIC DRUGS

Bethanechol. Bethanechol is reputed to have more selective muscarinic actions than carbachol. The oral dose range is 10–100 mg which may be repeated up to 4 times a day (Ursillo 1967). The usual toxic reactions are colic, flushing of the skin and sweating.

Carbachol. The oral dose range of carbachol is 0.2–0.8 mg, 2–3 times daily. Adverse reactions are similar to those of bethanechol.

Distigmine. Distigmine is an anticholinesterase agent, so muscarinic and nicotinic effects are equal. The usual oral dose for incontinence is 5 mg/day; its actions generally persist for 24 hours.

CHAPTER 17
MYASTHENIA AND MYOTONIA

Myasthenia is characterised by failure to sustain adequate muscle contraction; conversely, in myotonia symptoms stem from excessive contraction. There is no evidence to suggest that myasthenia and myotonia arise from reciprocal neurophysiological abnormalities but they do represent opposite ends of a neuropharmacological spectrum. Anticholinesterase agents such as neostigmine improve myasthenia and exacerbate myotonia while drugs such as procainamide alleviate myotonia and increase myasthenia (Drachman and Skom 1965).

Myasthenia

Myasthenia is a descriptive term for increased fatiguability of striated muscle; it is a clinical feature rather than a disease or syndrome. While weak muscles usually tire more quickly than normal, the association of good initial power with rapid fatigue is a notable finding in myasthenia gravis, the Lambert–Eaton syndrome, drug induced myasthenia, polymyositis, dermatomyositis and systemic lupus erythematosus (Walton 1969). The last three conditions are discussed in Chapter 7 so attention will here be confined to myasthenia gravis, the Lambert–Eaton syndrome and drug induced myasthenia.

MYASTHENIA GRAVIS

The majority of deaths attributable to myasthenia gravis occur within 5 years of the onset of symptoms; the disease usually stops progressing after about 10 years. Some 10–20% of patients have a thymic tumour. Other associated conditions include thyrotoxicosis, Raynaud's syndrome and pernicious anaemia (Simpson 1969). Antibodies to muscle (Strauss *et al* 1960; Feltkamp *et al* 1974) and thymus (Van der Geld *et al* 1964) occur in the serum of many patients with myasthenia gravis. An immunological aetiology has been proposed by Simpson (1960)—the possibility of a therapeutic role for immunosuppressive drugs is implicit in this suggestion.

Myasthenia gravis will be considered in the following stages: (1) Physiology; (2) Pharmacology; (3) Treatment; (4) Crises in myasthenia gravis; (5) Unstable myasthenics; (6) Medical management of thymectomy; (7) Infantile myasthenia.

PHYSIOLOGY

In normal subjects, rapidly repetitive electrical stimulation of a motor nerve results in a succession of muscle action potentials of uniform size. In myasthenia gravis there is a progressive fall in the amplitude of muscle responses (and an analogous reduction in amplitude of the recruitment pattern after sustained voluntary contraction). The antidromically propagated nerve action potentials are quite normal, so the disturbance in the amplitude of muscle action potentials must be produced at or distal to the motor nerve ending. In vitro studies on intercostal nerve-muscle preparations from patients undergoing thymectomy have shown that in myasthenia gravis the miniature end-plate potentials are of lower amplitude than normal (Elmqvist *et al* 1964).

PHARMACOLOGY

The pharmacological lesion in myasthenia gravis has persistently eluded precise identification. Attention has been focused on the neuromuscular junction following the demonstration of a therapeutic response to anticholinesterase drugs (Walker 1934) and the finding that acetylcholine is released by the arrival of impulses at motor nerve endings (Dale *et al* 1936). Many hypotheses have been put forward: (1) impaired synthesis, storage or release of acetylcholine, (2) increased breakdown or reuptake of acetylcholine, (3) the presence of a cholinergic antagonist, (4) reduced postsynaptic receptor sensitivity to acetylcholine.

Current views are controversial; while some advocate a predominantly presynaptic disorder (Elmqvist *et al* 1964; Desmedt 1966) others consider a postsynaptic lesion more likely (Grob 1971). Recent biochemical observations suggest that the synthesis of acetylcholine is impaired in myasthenia gravis (Rosenberg *et al* 1971). It has also been proposed that the thymus releases a circulating polypeptide which blocks neuromuscular conduction (Goldstein and Manganaro 1971) but the evidence for this view is limited. Because of the extensive morphological disturbances of the neuromuscular junction, Simpson (1971) argues that both presynaptic and postsynaptic mechanisms are abnormal in myasthenia gravis.

TREATMENT OF MYASTHENIA GRAVIS

It is not possible to make any simple generalisations on the most satisfactory course of management for myasthenia gravis. Three powerful but potentially hazardous approaches to treatment are available—anticholinesterase agents, corticosteroids and thymectomy. The choice of therapy will be determined by such factors as the age of the patient, the severity and duration of symptoms, the response to previous treatment, the presence of a thymoma, and the possible coexistence of other diseases.

ANTICHOLINESTERASE DRUGS

Anticholinesterase agents potentiate the action of acetylcholine by competing for acetylcholinesterase at all cholinergic synapses to which they have access. The rate of hydrolysis of anticholinesterase drugs is about a million times slower than acetylcholine. They are often termed *reversible* to distinguish them from the *irreversible* highly toxic organophosphorus insecticides and nerve gases, but the differences are quantitative rather than qualitative (Koelle 1970). The earliest anticholinesterase drug to be used in myasthenia gravis was physostigmine (eserine), an alkaloid derived from the Calabar bean, which was traditionally used as an ordeal poison in West African witchcraft. In 1934, Mary Walker wrote a letter to the *Lancet* reporting that 'the abnormal fatiguability in myasthenia gravis has been thought to be due to curare-like poisoning of the motor nerve-endings or of the "myoneural junction" in the affected muscles. It occurred to me recently that it might be worthwhile to try the effect of physostigmine, a partial antagonist to curare, on a case of myasthenia gravis.' After describing the gratifying therapeutic result, she mentioned that 'it might be significant that physostigmine inhibits the action of the esterase which destroys acetylcholine'.

Physostigmine has the disadvantage of producing adverse reactions in the central nervous system; it has been succeeded by neostigmine, which does not readily penetrate the blood–brain barrier.

Anticholinesterase agents such as neostigmine and pyridostigmine are the most satisfactory drugs for the routine treatment of myasthenia gravis. However, in rats long term administration of anticholinesterase drugs has been found to result in decreased miniature end-plate potentials and atrophy of the neuromuscular junction (Lytle and Wellband 1970; Engel *et al* 1972). It is possible that prolonged use of anticholinesterase agents may lead to a deterioration of neuromuscular transmission in patients with myasthenia gravis; this could account for the weak and wasted muscles often encountered in 'burnt out' myasthenics after many years of treatment.

Anticholinesterase drugs produce miosis by increasing acetylcholine concentrations at the parasympathetic nerve endings of the constrictor pupili muscle. The diameter of the pupil can be employed as a guide for monitoring cholinergic activity in order to maintain patients on optimum dosage—in normal lighting conditions a diameter of less than 2 mm suggests overdosage. This index of cholinergic stimulation is rendered redundant if muscarinic receptors are blocked by concomitant administration of atropine (see below).

Neostigmine. Parenteral administration of some 0.5–2 mg is equivalent to over 30 mg by mouth. One factor contributing to the difference between oral and injected dosage is extensive inactivation in the gastrointestinal tract. Subcutaneous neostigmine has a relatively short action, lasting only about 2 hours; when given orally, slow absorption results in prolongation of its effects. Neostigmine is hydrolysed at the ester linkage and also excreted unchanged in the urine.

A reasonable initial oral dose is 15 mg thrice daily; this is subsequently raised according to response and tolerance, increasing the frequency of administration before augmenting the size of each dose. Most patients take their neostigmine every 4 hours, but improved control is sometimes achieved on 3 or even 2 hourly regimens. The average daily dose is about 150 mg. Parenteral therapy is discussed when considering myasthenic crises (see below).

While miosis can be exploited as a useful peripheral effect of anticholinesterase agents, a number of adverse reactions may be produced at other synapses of the autonomic nervous system. These include abdominal colic, increased salivation, augmented bronchial secretion, bronchospasm, belching, nausea, vomiting, diarrhoea, sweating, lachrymation and hypotension. Grossly excessive intake can induce cardiac arrhythmias and, if significant quantities of neostigmine cross the blood–brain barrier, agitation, confusion or even coma.

Important adverse effects can also occur at the neuromuscular junction. Overdosage with anticholinesterase drugs leads to blockade of transmission by excessive depolarisation—so called cholinergic crisis (see below). As already mentioned, long term administration of anticholinesterase agents over many years may damage the neuromuscular junction to result in the late myopathic syndrome which often develops as a major problem refractory to all forms of treatment.

Some of the difficulties encountered with anticholinesterase agents can be controlled without loss of therapeutic response, by selective blockade of cholinergic muscarinic receptors with atropine. Nicotinic cholinergic receptors remain unaffected, so facilitation of neuromuscular transmission still occurs. For an initial dose, 0.6 mg of atropine can be taken by mouth twice daily, increasing if necessary.

Chapter 17

Pyridostigmine. Pyridostigmine has a more prolonged effect than neostigmine. After oral administration activity persists for 3 to 8 hours, so less frequent doses are necessary; 3–4 times daily is adequate. Combined administration of pyridostigmine with neostigmine is often useful because this elicits a response which is both rapid in onset and sustained in duration. An oral dose of 60 mg of pyridostigmine corresponds to 15 mg of neostigmine; parenteral administration of 1 mg pyridostigmine is approximately equivalent to 0.5 mg neostigmine.

Ambenonium. Ambenonium has a slightly longer action than pyridostigmine. It has been claimed to produce fewer peripheral muscarinic effects but it causes more toxicity in the central nervous system (Simpson 1969). An oral dose of 25 mg of ambenonium is equivalent to 15 mg of neostigmine.

Distigmine. Distigmine has the most protracted action of all the anticholinesterase drugs in current use; its effects persist for some 24 hours. The usual oral dose range is 5–20 mg/day. While it is occasionally employed in treating myasthenia gravis, its prolonged activity leads to difficulty in titrating intake. A cholinergic crisis induced by distigmine can be particularly dangerous owing to its gradual onset and the slow rate at which this drug is inactivated.

Edrophonium. Edrophonium has an extremely short action; it is therefore employed as a diagnostic tool—10 mg is administered by intravenous injection. In untreated myasthenia gravis this results in alleviation of weakness within a few seconds, which usually lasts 3–5 minutes.

The edrophonium test is also useful in distinguishing between myasthenic and cholinergic crises (see below), but when undertaken for this purpose the dose should be limited to 5 mg. Furthermore, facilities must be available for intubation and artificial ventilation; although the effect of edrophonium is of brief duration, significant deterioration can be precipitated in patients in cholinergic crisis (McLellan 1973c).

The action of edrophonium is too evanescent to have any therapeutic, as opposed to diagnostic, value.

CORTICOSTEROIDS

Following Simpson's (1960) suggestion that myasthenia gravis might be an autoimmune disease, an effort was made to treat patients with corticosteroids. Initial results were disappointing and corticosteroids fell into disrepute because an exacerbation of weakness was often precipitated when therapy was started. However, it gradually became evident that after the early deterioration, substantial improvement commonly occurred.

Warmolts and Engel (1972) have recently reported sustained therapeutic results without initial transient deterioration. They employed a regimen of high single dose oral prednisone (100 mg) on alternate days. This schedule produces less pituitary-adrenal suppression than an equivalent dose administered daily (Cope 1972). Patients were weaned off anticholinesterase drugs at the start of corticosteroid therapy. They were given antacids, potassium supplements (6 g/day KCl) and a diet low in sodium (not more than 4 g/day NaCl).

Jenkins (1972) has also obtained good therapeutic results with prednisone. His management differed from that of Warmolts and Engel in two respects. He kept patients on anticholinesterase drugs (though the dosage was often reduced as improvement occurred) and he used lower maintenance doses of prednisone in patients who responded well—50–70 mg on alternate days. A few of his patients experienced transient deterioration in muscle power at the start of treatment. Lower initial doses of prednisone (25 mg on alternate days) may reduce the incidence of early exacerbation (Seybold and Drachman 1974).

Corticosteroid therapy usually leads to improvement within 2 months (Cornelio *et al* 1973); the results appear to be unrelated to the duration of disease or previous thymectomy (Engel and Warmolts 1973). After some 3 months, remissions can frequently be maintained with doses as small as 20–40 mg of prednisone on alternate days (Humphrey 1973; Pinelli *et al* 1973).

There is no evidence on whether the lower mineralocorticoid activity of dexamethasone confers any worthwhile advantage over prednisone in the management of myasthenia gravis.

The pharmacokinetics and adverse effects of corticosteroids are discussed in Chapter 7. In view of the reports that patients occasionally experience initial transient exacerbation of myasthenia gravis, it is desirable to have facilities available for respiratory support over the first three weeks of treatment.

OTHER DRUGS

Corticotrophin. The use of corticotrophin in myasthenia gravis was first suggested 30 years ago (Torda and Wolff 1944), when it was found to increase the synthesis of acetylcholine. There has been a resurgence of interest in corticotrophin over the last decade (Grob and Namba 1966; Osserman and Genkins 1966; von Reiss *et al* 1966; Cape and Utterback 1969; Gibberd *et al* 1971).

Reporting their own experience together with a review of published accounts of 251 courses of corticotrophin in myasthenia gravis, Namba *et al* (1971) have concluded that optimum results can be obtained with short regimens employing high dosage. They advocate 100 units/day of corticotrophin administered over 8 hours in an intravenous infusion for 10 days. Daily administration of 160 units of corticotrophin gel by intramuscular injection has been suggested as an alternative to intravenous therapy (Grob *et al* 1973).

Treatment should always be administered in an intensive care unit because there is often a transient but profound deterioration in the first few days of therapy. Improvement emerges either during or shortly after the course of corticotrophin and lasts 1–6 months. Anticholinesterase drugs are usually continued, though dosage may require adjustment. Potassium supplements (6 g/day KCl), a low salt diet (not more than 4 g/day NaCl) and antacids can be added to the regimen if adverse reactions occur. The pharmacokinetics and toxicity of corticotrophin are discussed in Chapter 7.

Tetracosactrin. The synthetic congener of corticotrophin, tetracosactrin, is also effective (Ferro Milone and Nordera 1973) and carries a lower risk of hypersensitivity. Plain tetracosactrin has a very brief action so the sustained release preparation should be used, 1 mg corresponding to 100 units of corticotrophin.

The main advantage of corticotrophin and tetracosactrin over corticosteroids is the reduction of pituitary-adrenal suppression. The major disadvantages are the higher risk of fluid retention and the inconvenience of parenteral administration.

Antimetabolites and alkylating agents. Following the suggestion that myasthenia gravis may be an autoimmune disease, the possible therapeutic value of a number of powerful immunosuppressive drugs has been investigated. Rowland (1971) has recently reviewed the published accounts of 46 patients treated with mercaptopurine, cyclophosphamide, azathioprine, methotrexate, melphalan and busulphan. The results were difficult to evaluate because many other drugs were administered concomitantly. He considered current experience was too limited to permit any reliable conclusions to be drawn.

Germine esters. Early studies with germine diacetate revealed a therapeutic action in myasthenia gravis (Flacke *et al* 1966) but it was subsequently shown that this ester undergoes rapid hydrolysis to the monoacetate which is pharmacologically more potent. Germine monoacetate probably improves muscle power in myasthenia gravis by increasing sodium conductance after depolarisation of excitable membranes—like the veratrum alkaloids. The germine acetates produce less hypotension, bradycardia and emesis than the veratrum alkaloids. Initial clinical observations with germine monoacetate have been encouraging (Flacke *et al* 1973) but it has not undergone adequate evaluation.

Oxtriphylline. Oxtriphylline, a choline salt of theophylline, has been found to alleviate myasthenia gravis. It is thought to facilitate neuromuscular transmission by inhibiting phosphodiesterase, hence preventing the breakdown of cyclic adenosine monophosphate. In addition to having an action of its own, it is reputed to potentiate anticholinesterase agents and reduce the exacerbations often encountered when starting treatment with corticotrophin (Brumlik *et al* 1973). The dose range is 1.2–2.4 g/day. Experience is too limited to allow any firm appraisal of its therapeutic value.

Ephedrine. Ephedrine was reported to be beneficial in myasthenia gravis before the advent of anticholinesterase drugs (Edgeworth 1930). There have been no adequately controlled studies to confirm or refute this claim. If ephedrine has a therapeutic action, this is probably mediated through the alpha and beta noradrenergic receptors in the region of the neuromuscular junction (Bowman and Raper 1967).

Calcium gluconate. Intravenous injections of calcium gluconate improve motor performance in some patients with myasthenia gravis (Kornfeld *et al* 1969). This effect is presumably related to the important role of calcium in neuromuscular transmission (Katz 1966), but no precise mechanism of action has been established. The usual intravenous dose of calcium gluconate is 20 ml of a 10% solution administered over 5 minutes.

CRISES IN MYASTHENIA GRAVIS

Patients with myasthenia gravis may experience profound and often rapid deterioration in motor performance. These exacerbations of weakness may result from a deficiency (myasthenic crisis) or an excess (cholinergic crisis) of acetylcholine at the neuromuscular junction. Distinction between these two situations is of paramount importance because the treatment of myasthenic crisis is an increase of anticholinesterase agents whereas cholinergic crisis is managed by stopping these drugs.

The clinical setting may allow a firm diagnosis to be made, for example where a patient has exhausted his supply of tablets with consequent omission of therapy. However, the diagnosis is often more difficult; in these circumstances the edrophonium test (5 mg intravenously) is invaluable. In myasthenic crisis intravenous administration of edrophonium produces a rapid improvement, but in cholinergic crisis the change, if any, is one of deterioration. In evaluating the response to edrophonium, attention must be focused on essential bulbar and respiratory movement rather than ocular or limb muscles; a flow meter is usually employed to measure changes in respiration. Weakness in some muscle groups may be consequent upon inadequate acetylcholine while simultaneous paralysis elsewhere can be due to an excess (Simpson 1969)—myasthenic and cholinergic crises may both occur in the same patient at the same time.

MYASTHENIC CRISES

Myasthenic crises can develop spontaneously but they are commonly associated with thyrotoxicosis, infection, trauma, surgery or childbirth. They may also be precipitated by drugs which (1) have neuromuscular blocking properties, such as neomycin, (2) reduce membrane excitability, such as quinine, (3) depress respiration, such as morphine. Emotional stress, physical exertion and menstruation have also been suggested to be provocative factors.

Myasthenic crisis is a medical emergency; artificial ventilation should be readily available. Any contributing condition should be treated where possible. Anticholinesterase therapy must be increased, titrating the intake with frequent edrophonium tests to ensure that overdosage does not induce cholinergic weakness. Neostigmine 0.5 mg is given by subcutaneous or intramuscular injection, repeating the dose every 20–30 minutes according to the response. Atropine should be administered parenterally to control unwanted muscarinic effects. The rate and extent of gastrointestinal absorption is variable during myasthenic crisis so parenteral treatment may have to be continued for several days. With stabilisation of anticholinesterase requirements, a more sustained response can be achieved by substituting subcutaneous or intramuscular pyridostigmine for part or all of the neostigmine regimen.

When the patient's clinical state improves a gradual conversion can be attempted to oral anticholinesterase and antimuscarinic therapy.

CHOLINERGIC CRISIS

Weakness caused by excessive anticholinesterase intake is as much an emergency as myasthenic crisis. Once the diagnosis has been made, treatment with anticholinesterase drugs should be stopped. Muscarinic overactivity can be alleviated with atropine.

Cholinesterase reactivators have been developed as antidotes for poisoning by nerve gases and organophosphorus insecticides. The value of these reactivators in cholinergic crisis is controversial. Pralidoxime may be given by slow intravenous injection; a dose of

1–2 g can be repeated after 20 minutes if necessary. The efficacy of such treatment has been queried by Osserman and Genkins (1963) and Simpson (1969), who consider that it is preferable to allow anticholinesterase drugs to be removed by normal physiological mechanisms.

Facilities for intubation and artificial ventilation must be available for patients in cholinergic crisis. Progress can be assessed by intravenous administration of 5 mg of edrophonium. Anticholinesterase therapy may gradually be re-introduced when two successive edrophonium tests have produced a myasthenic type of response.

UNSTABLE ('BRITTLE') MYASTHENIA GRAVIS

Patients can display paradoxical reactions to treatment. Insensitivity to anticholinesterase drugs may develop at any time and there can be wide spontaneous fluctuations in the dose required. This type of problem is particularly common after thymectomy and in fulminating cases of myasthenia gravis with prominent bulbar and respiratory involvement. Sometimes patients respond to edrophonium with increased muscle power but fail to improve when given longer acting anticholinesterase agents. Occasionally there is an inexorable deterioration leading to respiratory insufficiency which cannot be attributed to either myasthenic or cholinergic crisis; corticotrophin or corticosteroid therapy can be helpful in these circumstances. Such patients may also be treated by curarisation and artificial ventilation, withholding all anticholinesterase drugs; resting the end-plates in this way often leads to a resumption of responsiveness to anticholinesterase agents after 3–10 days (Glaser 1966).

MEDICAL MANAGEMENT OF THYMECTOMY

It is now clear that thymectomy is beneficial in myasthenia gravis (Simpson 1958; Papatestas *et al* 1971; Mulder *et al* 1972), particularly if it is performed within the first 5 years of the disease. Sustained remission develops gradually, with a progressive increase in power emerging over several months. The most striking improvement occurs in patients who do not have a thymoma. Surgery is not usually undertaken in patients with weakness confined to the ocular muscles.

Thymectomy for myasthenia gravis was initially associated with a high mortality, but this has fallen over the last decade from some 20% to 5% or less. Improved artificial ventilation is one factor responsible for this change; another is the recognition that there can be rapid spontaneous variation in postoperative anticholinesterase requirements (Head 1964).

Anticholinesterase treatment does not need to be altered before operation. Opiates should be avoided in premedication and anaesthesia is maintained with minimal use of muscle relaxants.

After surgery all patients require artificial positive pressure ventilation; a tracheostomy is often necessary. Anticholinesterase drugs should be withheld for 18–24 hours postoperatively to avoid confusion between myasthenic and cholinergic crises (Genkins *et al* 1960). When re-introducing anticholinesterase therapy, neostigmine is administered by intramuscular or subcutaneous injection with frequent edrophonium tests to assess response. Dosage should be adjusted as described above in the management of myasthenic crises, using parenteral pyridostigmine if more sustained anticholinesterase activity is required. Atropine is given to prevent excessive muscarinic stimulation.

Injections can be replaced by oral treatment as the patient's clinical state improves, but this manoeuvre must be undertaken gradually because gastrointestinal absorption is variable over the postoperative period.

INFANTILE MYASTHENIA

One out of seven infants born to myasthenic mothers displays defective sucking, impaired swallowing and weak respiratory movements. Intravenous injection of edrophonium, 1 mg, improves motor performance; a more sustained response can be achieved with oral neostigmine, 1–4 mg, or pyridostigmine, 4–20 mg. Untreated babies may die, though the condition usually improves spontaneously after a few days or weeks. Very rarely a similar but persistent syndrome occurs in babies born to healthy mothers.

LAMBERT–EATON SYNDROME

For two decades it has been recognised that there exists an unusual myasthenic syndrome distinct from myasthenia gravis, which has been termed atypical myasthenia gravis, pseudomyasthenia, my-asthenic–myopathic syndrome or the Lambert–Eaton syndrome. It is characterised by (1) frequent association with bronchial carcinoma, (2) fatiguability predominantly involving proximal limb muscles, (3) relative sparing of cranial nerve territory, (4) reduced tendon reflexes, (5) characteristic electromyographic findings, (6) limited improvement with anticholinesterase drugs, (7) a good therapeutic response to guanidine.

NEUROMUSCULAR TRANSMISSION IN THE LAMBERT–EATON SYNDROME

In the Lambert–Eaton syndrome, application of a rapidly repetitive volley of electrical stimuli to a motor nerve leads to a progressive increase in the amplitude of the action potentials in successive muscle responses (Lambert and Rooke 1965). In myasthenia gravis, as already mentioned, the opposite occurs (the size of the evoked muscle action potentials does not alter in normal subjects).

The abnormalities in the Lambert–Eaton syndrome are similar to those found in experimental neuromuscular blockade produced with botulinum toxin, neomycin or magnesium, which are known to decrease the number of quanta of acetylcholine released by each nerve impulse (Lambert 1966). Minature end-plate potentials, each representing the electrical response to a quantum of acetylcholine, are of normal amplitude (Lambert and Elmqvist 1971). These observations indicate that both the quantal content of acetylcholine and muscle receptor sensitivity are normal in the Lambert–Eaton syndrome—the major functional disturbance is simply a reduction in the number of quanta.

TREATMENT OF THE LAMBERT–EATON SYNDROME

Guanidine. Guanidine is the most satisfactory treatment for the Lambert–Eaton syndrome. This drug has been known to influence neuromuscular transmission for many years; it was even prescribed for myasthenia gravis (Minot *et al* 1939) until the superiority of anticholinesterase agents was established. Guanidine appears to act by increasing the number of quanta of acetylcholine released by the arrival of each action potential at the motor nerve endings (Lambert and Elmqvist 1971).

A suitable starting dose is 250 mg thrice daily, increasing according to response and tolerance. Reasonable control can usually be achieved with 1.5–2.5 g/day. Improvement may take several days to develop and is correspondingly slow to disappear on stopping treatment. Adverse reactions include paraesthesiae, anorexia, vomiting, colic, diarrhoea, sialorrhoea, anxiety and tremor. Skin eruptions and fever may also occur.

DRUG INDUCED MYASTHENIA

Some drugs, such as neomycin, produce defects of neuromuscular transmission similar to those found in the Lambert–Eaton syndrome. Others, such as colistin, cause depolarisation blockade resembling overdosage with anticholinesterase agents (D'Arcy and Griffin 1972). Further drugs which can induce myasthenia include busulphan, dihydrostreptomycin, kanamycin, phenytoin, polymixin B, procainamide, quinine, streptomycin, trimethadione, and viomycin.

Toxic impairment of neuromuscular conduction clears on stopping the agent responsible.

Myotonia

Myotonia is 'continued active contraction of a muscle which persists after the cessation of voluntary effort or stimulation' (Brain and Walton 1969). The commonest causes are dystrophia myotonica (myotonia atrophica) and myotonia congenita (Thomsen's disease). The myotonic contraction is accompanied by electrical activity detectable on the electromyogram; it is still present after blockade of the neuromuscular junction (Denny-Brown and Nevin 1941) so it must be due to an abnormality of the muscle fibre. The typical myotonic discharge is a brief volley of impulses in which both the frequency and the amplitude of successive muscle action potentials progressively decay to produce the characteristic 'dive bomber' phenomenon on the electromyograph audiomonitor. This activity occurs both during and immediately after muscle contraction. One essential feature of myotonia seems to be abnormal excitation induced by mechanical displacement of muscle fibres; it can be precipitated by percussion of the muscle or even by small movements of the recording needle electrode.

Quinine was the first effective treatment to be found for myotonia (Wolf 1936). Subsequently phenytoin and procainamide were reported to be more satisfactory (Geschwind and Simpson 1955; Leyburn and Walton 1959). These drugs all appear to act by stabilising the sensitivity of the myotonic muscle fibre membrane; they are also useful in the treatment of muscle cramps (Layzer and Rowlands 1971).

Phenytoin (diphenylhydantoin). Details of the pharmacokinetics and toxicity of phenytoin are reviewed in Chapter 12. The usual intake is 200–400 mg/day in divided doses. Phenytoin is probably the most satisfactory drug for the treatment of myotonia because it achieves improvement comparable to procainamide with fewer adverse effects (Munsat 1967).

Procainamide. Procainamide has properties which are qualitatively similar to procaine, but its systemic actions are more prolonged and it has fewer effects on the central nervous system. It is readily absorbed from the gastrointestinal tract, reaching peak plasma concentrations in about an hour. Some 15% is bound to plasma proteins and about 60% is excreted unchanged in the urine; the remainder is slowly hydrolysed by plasma esterases. The plasma half-life is approximately 5 hours.

A satisfactory initial dose is 250 mg thrice daily, which can be increased according to therapeutic response and toxicity. Unwanted effects are commonly encountered with doses over 2–3 g/day. The commonest adverse reactions are anorexia, nausea and vomiting. Patients occasionally complain of experiencing an abnormal bitter taste. Diarrhoea, hypotension, flushing, lassitude, depression and hallucinations occur. More serious problems include blood dyscrasias, skin eruptions, fever, cardiac arrhythmias and systemic lupus erythematosus. There may be cross reactions with procaine.

Quinine. Quinine is well absorbed from the gastrointestinal tract; maximum plasma concentrations are attained in 1–3 hours. Some 70% becomes bound to plasma proteins. Inactivation is mainly achieved by hepatic degradation. The usual range of intake is 200–400 mg/day in divided doses, which generally alleviates muscle cramps and myotonia. If cramps only occur at night, 300 mg should be taken each evening. Adverse effects include tinnitus, headache, nausea, abdominal pain, skin eruptions and optic atrophy.

CHAPTER 18

PAIN

Pain is the commonest symptom in medicine and probably the least understood. It is a source of complaint in 90% of patients (Douglas-Wilson 1944) and although effective treatment has been available for centuries, the mode of action of analgesic drugs is shrouded in obscurity.

Analgesia will be considered in the following stages: (1) Psychology of pain; (2) Physiology of pain; (3) Pharmacology of pain; (4) Non-narcotic analgesics; (5) Narcotic analgesics; (6) Migraine; (7) Trigeminal neuralgia; (8) Post-herpetic neuralgia; (9) Headache due to raised intracranial pressure; (10) Special techniques for treating pain.

PSYCHOLOGY OF PAIN

The psychological context in which pain occurs is of profound importance in determining its effect. A stimulus which would normally produce considerable pain may go unnoticed if attention is distracted. Conversely, in a setting where attention is focused on the stimulus, there may be a heightened sensation and exaggerated behavioural response, out of all proportion to the extent of tissue damage. In addition to the modulation of response by circumstances, different individuals react in diverse ways to the same stimulus applied in a standardised situation.

While it is not easy to categorise the psychological factors which exacerbate pain, they are broadly covered by the concept of anxiety.

252

This has therapeutic implications because it provides a rational basis for the use of drugs which alleviate anxiety—these are often as effective as analgesics in the management of pain and in certain circumstances they may be even more important (Merskey 1973). The treatment of anxiety is considered in Chapter 20.

PHYSIOLOGY OF PAIN

Most painful stimuli, such as trauma, ischaemia and inflammation, are associated with tissue damage. This commonly results in the release of certain chemical agents, such as histamine, bradykinin and prostaglandin E, which may play a part in exciting peripheral nerve endings. It is also probable that mechanical distortion of free nerve terminals, for example by increased tension in the wall of a viscus, can generate a painful sensation (Sinclair 1973).

There are three major neurophysiological concepts of pain:

1 The *specific modality* theory—that there exist specialised nerve terminals and peripheral fibres carrying impulses to specific spinal tracts which ascend to localised pain centres in the brain.

2 The *pattern* theory—that the same afferent pathways are employed to carry impulse traffic for all forms of sensation; the different qualities, such as pain, derive from a central analysis of the spatio-temporal patterns of activity.

3 A synthesis between the above two views—that there is some degree of receptor and pathway specificity but interpretation is ultimately determined by central scanning of impulse patterns (Melzack and Wall 1962). This has been developed into a more precise hypothesis proposing that afferent impulses which mediate the sensation of pain are controlled by a gate mechanism operated by the balance between excitation in large and small peripheral nerve fibres. A preponderance of impulses in large nerve fibres closes the gate, while a relative increase of traffic in small nerve fibres opens it. The gate is also under the influence of descending pathways so that afferent activity can be modulated by central events (Melzack and Wall 1965).

There remain a number of observations which cannot be explained by the gate theory (Schmidt 1972; Iggo 1972), but the concept formulated by Melzack and Wall reconciles many of the conflicts which have arisen from evidence relating to the *specific modality* and *pattern* theories.

PHARMACOLOGY OF PAIN

The mode of action of drugs which alleviate pain is obscure, though recent studies are beginning to shed light in this area (Bonica 1974). With this background it is somewhat surprising that such a wide range of potent analgesic agents have been available for many years; there are two reasons for the paradox of effective therapy without a rational basis. First, for several centuries traditional social customs have established and repeatedly confirmed the value of opium as an analgesic. Second, extremely simple tests are available for screening potential therapeutic agents—a standard painful stimulus applied to an animal elicits a behavioural response which can readily be quantified, enabling the analgesic action of different drugs to be compared quickly and cheaply.

Analgesics fall into two major categories: narcotics (drugs which resemble morphine) and others (often referred to as non-narcotics, these are derivatives of salicylic acid and aniline). Over the last decade evidence has been accumulating which suggests that while narcotics act upon the central nervous system, non-narcotics have a predominantly peripheral effect (Melmon and Morelli 1972). These conclusions are based on the results of cross perfusion experiments (Lim *et al* 1964; Guzman and Lim 1968).

The peripheral action of non-narcotic analgesics is likely to stem from an effect at nerve endings because these drugs do not impair axonal transmission of impulses (Keele 1969). Interference with chemical mediators has been suggested (Collier 1969)—certain non-narcotic analgesics block the sensitisation of afferent nerve endings which normally results from the release of endogenous prostaglandins (Vane 1971; Ferreira 1972; Ferreira *et al* 1973).

The actions of narcotics on synaptic transmission are complex and poorly understood. Morphine inhibits the release of acetylcholine (Lees *et al* 1972) and increases the synthesis of noradrenaline and dopamine (Smith and Sheldon 1972). There have been conflicting accounts of the effect of morphine or serotonergic systems; Calcutt *et al* (1972) have suggested that narcotic dependence is associated with a disturbance in the balance between cerebral noradrenaline and serotonin.

Certain drugs which are structurally similar to morphine antagonise its actions but still have their own analgesic properties—an example is nalorphine. It is not known whether morphine agonists and antagonists act upon the same receptors (Martin and Jasinski 1972).

The lack of any coherent picture of the mechanism of action of morphine was recently spelt out by Vogt (1972): 'We measure those things of which we are aware, and for which we have assay methods, and just hope that they are going to tell us something relevant.' This hope has not yet been realised.

In the use of analgesics, a number of therapeutic principles apply:

1 Dosage should be the minimum required to reduce pain to tolerable levels of intensity.

2 The interval between doses should be the maximum that affords sustained relief from pain.

3 The severity of adverse effects considered acceptable will depend upon the clinical setting, exemplified by the contrast between a young patient with sciatica and a debilitated patient with terminally raised intracranial pressure.

4 Whenever possible, specific therapy should be undertaken—for example ergotamine for migraine, carbamazepine for trigeminal neuralgia.

5 Because narcotics and non-narcotics act at different sites, they can potentiate each other—the combination of aspirin (non-narcotic) with codeine (narcotic) is logical and effective.

NON-NARCOTIC ANALGESICS

Aspirin and paracetamol are the most widely employed non-narcotic analgesics. Phenacetin is no longer prescribed, owing to the nephropathy with which it has become associated. Amidopyrine should not be used, since it carries a relatively high risk of agranulocytosis. Because of their chemical structure, codeine, dextropropoxyphene and pentazocine are classified as narcotics although they are often given as alternatives to aspirin and paracetamol.

Large quantities of non-narcotic analgesics are consumed to alleviate pain of mild to moderate intensity. Severe pain, which has proved refactory to other therapeutic approaches, may respond to non-narcotic analgesics when these are administered in combination with tranquillisers, antidepressants and if necessary, sedatives (Merskey and Hester 1972). For example pericyazine, amitriptyline and promethazine have together been found effective in conditions such as post-herpetic neuralgia (Merskey 1973).

Aspirin. Aspirin was introduced into medicine in 1899. Over 2,000 tons are consumed each year in the United Kingdom. While aspirin is usually employed as an analgesic, it also suppresses inflammation, inhibits platelet aggregation and possesses antipyretic properties.

Aspirin is readily absorbed, reaching peak plasma levels about 2 hours after ingestion; relatively low concentrations are found in the brain. Hydrolysis to salicylic acid is rapid, salicylate metabolites having therapeutic activity. Some 50–80% of plasma salicylate is protein bound. Salicylates have a plasma half-life averaging around 4 hours. The main urinary metabolites are conjugates of glucuronic acid and glycine; the excretion of free salicylate depends on urinary pH—in alkaline urine it can amount to 85% of the ingested drug.

The usual dose of aspirin ranges from 300–900 mg, three to four times daily. The commonest adverse reactions are epigastric pain and vomiting, related to haemorrhagic shedding of gastric mucosal epithelium. Occult bleeding from the stomach occurs in at least 50% of patients and occasionally there is frank haematemesis. Overdosage can lead to hypoprothrombinaemia. The possibility of a teratogenic action has recently been raised (Richards 1969).

In spite of these toxic properties, serious adverse reactions to aspirin are very uncommon. A number of different formulations are available. Soluble aspirin is suitable for pain needing intermittent treatment where a rapid response is required. Enteric coated aspirin is useful when administration is repeated at regular intervals for persistent pain; it causes less gastric irritation but it is absorbed more slowly.

Paracetamol (acetaminophen). Paracetamol is absorbed very quickly, reaching peak plasma concentrations after $\frac{1}{2}$–1 hour; the plasma half-life is 2 hours. Some 25 % is bound to plasma protein. Conjugation occurs in the liver, predominantly with glucuronic acid; only a small fraction of free paracetamol is excreted in the urine—around 3%.

The usual dose is 0.5–1 g, repeated every 3–4 hours if necessary. Toxic reactions are very uncommon. Occasionally methaemoglobin is formed, leading to cyanosis. Hepatic and renal damage have also been reported.

NARCOTIC ANALGESICS

Extracts of poppy capsules have been used medicinally for well over two thousand years. Paracelsus compounded laudanum in the sixteenth century and morphine was isolated in 1803. The other analgesic alkaloid in opium, codeine, was identified in 1832; many congeners have since been synthesised. The basic structure of the narcotics is a phenylpiperidine ring.

The most widely used drugs in this group are codeine, dextropropoxyphene, pentazocine, pethidine and morphine. Codeine and dextropropoxyphene are prescribed for mild pain in the same way as non-narcotics; their analgesic potency is similar to aspirin or paracetamol and the risk of developing drug dependence is very low. Pentazocine is a more powerful therapeutic agent with a higher incidence of abuse. Pethidine and morphine are reserved for treatment of pain where other measures have failed or are known to be inadequate.

Codeine. Codeine is well absorbed. It is metabolised, in the liver, to morphine and norcodeine which appear in the urine with codeine, mainly as glucuronide conjugates. Some 90% of an administered dose is excreted in 24 hours. The usual intake is 30–60 mg, three to four times daily. The commonest adverse reaction is constipation; nausea, vomiting, dizziness and drowsiness can also occur.

Dextropropoxyphene. Dextropropoxyphene produces less constipation than codeine, but it is a less potent analgesic. It is readily absorbed and undergoes incomplete demethylation in the liver. The free drug is excreted over about 6 hours. The dose is 32–64 mg, three to four times daily. Occasionally dextropropoxyphene produces headache, dizziness, drowsiness or excitation.

Pentazocine. Pentazocine combines high analgesic potency with a low risk of establishing drug dependence. It is absorbed quite rapidly, reaching peak plasma concentrations in 1–3 hours. The plasma half-life is about 2 hours. Some 30% undergoes hepatic conjugation to glucuronides and excretion is completed in 24 hours. The oral dose range is 25–100 mg every 3–4 hours; the corresponding intramuscular or subcutaneous dose range is 20–60 mg, repeated at similar intervals. The main adverse reactions to pentazocine are sweating, sedation, nausea, vomiting and sometimes excitation.

Pethidine (meperidine). Pethidine occupies an intermediate position between pentazocine and morphine in both its efficacy as an analgesic and its propensity to induce dependence. It is well absorbed, reaching peak plasma concentrations 1–2 hours after oral intake. Some 40% is bound to plasma proteins. Hydrolysis, demethylation and conjugation take place in the liver; about 5% is excreted unchanged in the urine.

The dose range is 50–200 mg orally or 50–150 mg by intramuscular injection. Analgesia usually lasts 3–4 hours. Pethidine often produces euphoria. Adverse reactions include dizziness, sweating, nausea and vomiting; antimuscarinic effects can occur, such as dryness of the mouth, defective ocular accommodation and urinary retention.

Morphine. Morphine is the most potent analgesic available and, together with diamorphine (heroin), carries the highest risk of abuse. In addition to relieving pain, it produces sedation, emotional detachment and alterations of mood which can be either pleasant or distressing. Absorption of morphine is unpredictable, so it is usually administered parenterally. Metabolism occurs in the liver, mainly to form glucuronide conjugates which are excreted in the urine. Some 90% of an administered dose is removed in 24 hours.

An initial subcutaneous or intramuscular injection of 10 mg affords relief of pain in the majority of patients. Subsequent dosage is adjusted according to requirements. Adverse reactions are depression of respiration, suppression of the cough reflex, vomiting, constipation and spasm of the biliary tract. Undesirable interactions may occur with phenothiazines, tricyclic antidepressants and monoamine oxidase inhibitors. These may lead to hypotension, increased sedation and further depression of respiration. Miosis can cause difficulty in evaluating the neurological status of a patient.

MIGRAINE

Migrainous headache is attributed to recurrent dilatation of cranial arteries (Graham and Wolff 1938). The pain usually has a throbbing quality and is generally associated with nausea. Migraine is the commonest of all neurological disorders—estimates of prevalence range from 4 to 30% of the population, the ratio of women to men being approximately 2 to 1 (Blumenthal 1968; Waters 1974). A family history can be elicited in some 70% of patients (Goodell *et al* 1953). Environmental factors can often be related to the onset of attacks and occasionally migraine is precipitated by structural lesions such as aneurysms or angiomata.

The classification of different types of migraine is controversial; many of the difficulties are semantic. Five major categories have been recognised by the *ad hoc* committee of the National Institute of Neurological Diseases and Blindness (*Archives of Neurology*, 1962, **6,** 173).

1   *Classic migraine.* Predominantly unilateral with transient sensory (especially visual), motor or dysphasic prodromes.
2   *Common migraine.* Frequently bilateral, with less clearly defined prodromes.
3   *Cluster headache* (Horton's headache, migrainous neuralgia, histaminic headache). Unilateral attacks grouped together, usually accompanied by peripheral vasodilatation, sweating, rhinorrhoea and increased lachrymation.
4   *Hemiplegic and ophthalmoplegic migraine.* Neurological deficit persisting after the headache.
5   *Others.* This is an ill-defined group including *lower half headache,* some forms of *atypical facial pain* and certain cranial neuralgias

(sphenopalatine and Vidian) which may produce a migrainous type of syndrome.

PATHOPHYSIOLOGY OF MIGRAINE

The traditional concept of the pathophysiology of migraine attributes the prodrome to intracranial vasoconstriction and the headache to extracranial vasodilatation. This hypothesis has certain important therapeutic implications—that the prodrome should be improved by intracranial vasodilators (such as carbon dioxide), while the headache should respond to vasoconstrictors.

Current views on the vascular basis of the prodrome are controversial. Marshall (1973b) and Skinhoj (1973) have recently reported falls in cerebral blood flow during prodromal symptoms. In contrast, Bruyn (1968b) has reviewed angiographic studies on over 110 patients and concludes 'that the evidence in by far the majority is equivocal, contradictory and certainly not clinching the case for the customary and traditional theory of spasm of major cerebral vessels'. These divergent opinions may perhaps be resolved by postulating vasoconstriction in vessels which are too small to be seen in carotid angiograms.

There is less conflict over the relationship between the headache and vasodilatation. Nevertheless, there are important discrepancies—for example heat, histamine and acetylcholine can all produce dilatation of cranial vessels without pain (Ostfeld 1962).

PHARMACOLOGY OF MIGRAINE

The pharmacology of migraine is poorly understood. There have been many observations and even more speculations but it is not possible to unite them into any coherent hypothesis. The difficulties are increased by failure to confirm some of the findings originally reported.

Serotonin. The concentration of serotonin in the plasma has been found to fall during a migrainous headache, while the urinary excretion of its major metabolite, 5-hydroxyindoleacetic acid, has been claimed to rise (Sicuteri *et al* 1961; Curran *et al* 1965; Anthony *et al* 1967). Reserpine, which reduces tissue levels of serotonin, can precipitate headaches in migrainous patients (Kimball *et al* 1960).

These observations have led to the suggestion that migraine may be produced by a circulating agent which releases and subsequently depletes serotonin (Lance 1969). According to this view, serotonin normally mediates a tonic vasoconstrictor action on cranial blood vessels. Against this hypothesis, administration of serotonin or its immediate precursor, 5-hydroxytryptophan, fails to produce any consistent effect in migrainous patients (Friedman 1968).

Tyramine. Some patients notice that their migraine is precipitated by the intake of cheese or red wine, which contain tyramine. It has been reported that in this type of migraine, oral administration of tyramine provokes the same attacks (Hanington 1967). One possible interpretation is that reduction in the activity of intestinal monoamine oxidase may allow dietary tyramine to be absorbed.

Sandler (1972) has developed this concept further by suggesting that tyramine produces migraine by triggering the release of prostaglandins, injection of which is known to cause headache (Carlson 1967).

Endocrine changes. Attacks of headache are related to menstruation in 60% of migrainous women and in such cases improvement can often be achieved by giving a short course of a diuretic, at the time of each period (see below).

The majority of patients notice an improvement in their attacks during pregnancy, but occasionally migraine first appears at this time (Lance 1969). The confusion over causal relationships is increased by the fact that while oral contraceptives commonly exacerbate migraine, these drugs have also been claimed to possess therapeutic activity (Lundberg 1962).

Other active agents. Wolff (1963) has suggested that in addition to arterial dilatation, a local sterile inflammatory reaction occurs at the site of migrainous pain. Noradrenaline, acetylcholine, histamine, bradykinin and neurokinin have all been proposed as possible links in the causal chain of events leading to vasodilatation and inflammation, but there is no firm evidence to substantiate any of these claims.

TREATMENT OF MIGRAINE

The difficulties which may be encountered in treating migraine are reflected by the number of drugs that have been advocated. At the beginning of the nineteenth century, Heberden suggested 'valerian, fetid gums, myrrh, musk, camphor, opium, extract of hemlock, sneezing powders' (Sacks 1970). Less than 20 years ago recommended treatment included injections of milk, horse serum, placental hormones and peptones, or oral administration of bile salts, thyroid extract, strychnine and magnesium sulphate (Wilson 1955).

The prodrome

In view of the widespread opinion that prodromes result from vasospasm of cerebral vessels, a number of vasodilators have been employed as potential therapeutic agents—for example carbon dioxide, amylnitrite, nicotinic acid, nicotinyl alcohol and tolazoline. These are seldom helpful and often exacerbate the subsequent headache (Taverner 1968).

The headache

Mild headaches can be controlled with paracetamol, aspirin or codeine. If these prove inadequate, the best treatment is ergotamine. Occasionally pentazocine or pethidine prove necessary. Severe, prolonged, intractable headache (status migrainosus) has been reported to respond to intravenous hydrocortisone (100 mg) or oral prednisone (40–60 mg/day for 2 days) which presumably act by suppressing localised inflammatory changes occurring around dilated blood vessels (Sicuteri *et al* 1967; Edmeads 1973).

Ergotamine. Ergotamine is the most widely prescribed drug in the management of migraine. Although ergot was first advocated by

Eulenberg in 1878, its therapeutic effects were not firmly established until the studies of Graham and Wolf (1938).

Ergotamine has complex actions, the most important of which is direct stimulation of smooth muscle. In some tissues this appears to be achieved through alpha noradrenergic receptors. Ergotamine also blocks alpha noradrenergic receptors, so it may operate as a partial agonist (see Chapter 4). In addition, serotonergic receptors are blocked by ergotamine. The extent to which these pharmacological properties contribute to the therapeutic action of ergotamine is not known.

Ergotamine should be given at the earliest sign of onset of an attack. A number of alternative routes are available for administration. Oral preparations are often combined with caffeine (100 mg) or an antiemetic agent such as cyclizine (50 mg). The following regimens are useful:

1 Sublingual. Initially 1–2 mg is given, followed by 1 mg hourly if required, not exceeding 6 mg in one day or 12 mg in one week.
2 Aerosol inhalation. Inhalers usually deliver 0.36 mg at each application. Up to 5 doses may be administered at 15 minute intervals in one day; no more than 15 inhalations should be taken in one week. This route is particularly prone to result in overdosage.
3 Suppositories. A satisfactory starting dose is 2 mg, repeating hourly if necessary but not exceeding 6 mg in one day or 12 mg in one week.
4 Subcutaneous or intramuscular injection. Initially 0.25–0.5 mg is administered, repeating hourly if required, but not normally giving more than 1.5 mg in one day or 4 mg in one week. Cluster headaches present a special problem of frequent attacks in rapid succession followed by a relatively long interval free of symptoms. In this situation 0.25 mg can be injected thrice daily every day for two weeks over the cluster period, though treatment should be stopped if any adverse reactions develop.

Toxicological experience of ergotamine derives from centuries of poisoning from the original source, the grain fungus *Claviceps purpurea*. The classical features arise from vasoconstriction—the limbs become cold, pale and numb with muscle pain on exertion and ultimately gangrene—a syndrome known through the middle ages as St. Anthony's Fire. Other toxic problems mimic many of the

symptoms of migraine such as headache, nausea, vomiting, diarrhoea
and dizziness. Weakness, pruritus, miosis, confusion, drowsiness
and convulsions can occur. Patients with occlusive arterial disease
or abnormal liver function are particularly vulnerable to adverse
reactions; ergotamine is contraindicated in pregnancy. Ergotism is
managed by withdrawing the drug and if necessary administering
vasodilators and antiemetics.

Migraine prophylaxis

Diuretics. Migraine related to menstruation usually improves if a
diuretic such as hydrochlorothiazide 50 mg is administered daily for
5 days, starting 3 days before each period. For details of pharmacokinetics and toxicity see Chapter 12.

Minor tranquillisers. Since emotional factors often play a major role
in precipitating migraine, substantial benefit can often be achieved
by continuous administration of diazepam or prochlorperazine.
These drugs are discussed more fully in Chapters 15 and 19.

Antidepressants. Low doses of antidepressants can reduce the
frequency of migrainous headaches. Amitriptyline, 25–50 mg taken
at night, is often effective (Gomersall and Stuart 1973). For further
details see Chapter 20.

Dihydroergotamine. Ergot derivative may be useful in the prophylaxis
of migraine. It is usual to use dihydroergotamine rather than
ergotamine, because the former is less likely to produce ischaemic
toxic reactions. The dose is 1–2 mg thrice daily by mouth, which
is commonly administered in preparations also containing caffeine.

Propranolol. It has recently been claimed that propranolol is
effective in the prophylactic treatment of migraine (Weber and
Reinmuth 1972). This drug is discussed in more detail in Chapter 14.

Clonidine. Clonidine has been advocated for the prevention of
migraine (Sjaastad and Stensrud 1971; Shafar *et al* 1972), though

there is no general agreement on its efficacy (Shaw and Saunders 1972). Its pharmacological properties are complex; they include activity as a noradrenergic agonist. The dose employed for migraine is 0.025 to 0.075 mg twice daily, which is considerably lower than that prescribed for hypertension. Adverse reactions include drowsiness (usually transient), depression, dryness of the mouth, constipation, pruritus, and hypotension.

Cyproheptidine. Cyproheptidine is a serotonin antagonist which also has a prominent antihistamine action. It is reputed to reduce the incidence and severity of migrainous headaches. A low dose, 2 mg thrice daily, can be increased gradually to 12–24 mg/day. Intake is commonly limited by sedation.

Methysergide. Methysergide, a serotonergic blocking agent, was used extensively for migraine prophylaxis until it became recognised that fibrosis was occasionally induced in retroperitoneal and thoracic tissues (including the heart). This serious toxic reaction led many physicians to stop prescribing methysergide, but Lance (1969) considers that 2–6 mg daily is a safe dose provided patients are kept under close medical supervision.

Pizotifen. Pizotifen is another serotonin antagonist. It has recently undergone a number of studies in migraine, which indicate that it may be therapeutically useful (Lance and Anthony 1970; Speight and Avery 1972; Andersson 1973). A dose of 3 mg/day achieves results similar to 15 mg/day of prochlorperazine (Hubbe 1973).

TRIGEMINAL NEURALGIA

Trigeminal neuralgia (tic douloureux) produces paroxysms of severe pain in the distribution of a division of the trigeminal nerve. Trigeminal neuralgia usually develops in the second half of life; when it presents in younger patients it is often associated with multiple sclerosis. The pathology and aetiology remain unknown. Similar neuralgias can involve other cranial nerves, in particular the glosso-pharyngeal.

The treatment of choice for trigeminal neuralgia is carbamazepine (Penman 1968); phenytoin can also be useful (Chinitz *et al* 1966). These drugs may, in addition, be effective in other cranial neuralgias and in paroxysmal pain elsewhere—for example in Fabry's disease or tabes dorsalis.

The dose regimens and adverse reactions of carbamazepine and phenytoin have already been described in Chapter 12. Their action in trigeminal neuralgia is presumably related to the properties discussed when considering them as anticonvulsants.

Patients who fail to respond to carbamazepine or phenytoin can be treated effectively by ganglionic injection of alcohol (Penman 1968).

POST-HERPETIC NEURALGIA

The results of treating post-herpetic neuralgia are seldom satisfactory. Recent evidence suggests that patients who receive amantadine (see Chapter 13) during their episode of shingles are less likely to develop persistent pain (Galbraith 1973). It has been reported that a 3 week course of corticosteroids can be helpful in the management of early post-herpetic neuralgia (Juel-Jensen and MacCallum 1972).

Sometimes improvement can be achieved by vibration (for 20 minutes thrice daily) or repeated cooling (with ethylchloride spray) of the involved area of skin. Such measures often have to be maintained for several weeks or even months. The therapeutic task in post-herpetic neuralgia is provision of a long term regimen to alleviate the burden of persistent discomfort which may otherwise drive patients to suicide. In this setting an optimal response is usually obtained by combining antidepressant therapy with a tranquilliser and a mild analgesic. Amitriptyline or imipramine are suitable antidepressants; chlorpromazine or pericyazine are satisfactory tranquillisers. Paracetamol, aspirin or dextropropoxyphene can be employed to provide analgesia. Apart from pericyazine, these drugs are all considered elsewhere (amitriptyline, imipramine and chlor-promazine in Chapter 20; paracetamol, aspirin and dextropro-poxyphene earlier in this Chapter).

Pericyazine. Pericyazine is a phenothiazine which has been claimed to be particularly useful in the management of pain (Merskey 1973). Pharmacokinetics and toxicity are similar to chlorpromazine. An initial dose of 2.5 mg twice daily can be increased slowly until a reasonable balance is obtained between therapeutic effects and adverse reactions. Sedation is the commonest dose limiting problem, so maximum benefit can usually be achieved by giving an evening dose twice as large as the morning dose, thereby ensuring that the drowsiness induced by pericyazine is usefully employed to prevent insomnia. With this regimen a daily intake of 60–90 mg can often be maintained. Caution is necessary with the higher doses; elderly patients seldom tolerate more than 30 mg/day.

HEADACHE DUE TO RAISED INTRACRANIAL PRESSURE

Mechanical distortion of pain sensitive structures (such as the venous sinuses and the proximal portions of major intracranial arteries) is probably responsible for the headache of raised intracranial pressure (Pallis and Rice Edwards 1974).

Localised brain swelling is a common complication of intracranial lesions. More generalised cerebral oedema is found in encephalitis, malignant hypertension, hypercapnia, hepatic encephalopathy, lead encephalopathy, cerebral ischaemia and the syndrome of benign intracranial hypertension. Where possible, treatment is directed at the cause but additional palliative therapy is also beneficial.

The relationship between cerebral oedema and intracranial pressure is not direct—an increase of 2.5% in brain water can result in a fourfold rise in CSF pressure (Rosomoff and Zugibe 1963).

EXPERIMENTAL CEREBRAL OEDEMA

In experimental studies of cerebral oedema, lesions are usually induced on one side of the brain. Oedema can then be measured by determining the ratio of wet weight to dry weight in affected tissue and comparing the result with homologous portions of the contralateral hemisphere. Although there is considerable overlap, cerebral swelling may be subdivided into types which display predominantly extracellular, intracellular or intramyelin oedema.

Extracellular oedema. Focal necrotic damage produced by freezing of localised brain regions results in some 50% of swelling in sub-cortical white matter but only 5% in grey matter; it appears that the interstitial spaces of white matter are more distensible than those of grey matter. Oedema fluid resembles plasma exudate, suggesting that disruption of the blood–brain barrier leads to extracellular spread of fluid along the paths of least resistance (Tower 1972).

Intracellular oedema. Circulatory inadequacy leads to intracellular oedema amounting to about 20%, which mainly involves the cerebral cortex. When this has occurred it is difficult to re-establish adequate cerebral perfusion because the capillary lumen is compressed by swollen endothelial cells and perivascular glia; the problem is exacerbated by the associated local rise in blood viscosity (Ames *et al* 1968; Chiang *et al* 1968; Brierley *et al* 1973).

Intramyelin oedema. Certain toxic agents produce cerebral oedema by splitting the myelin lamellae to generate vacuoles (Aleu *et al* 1963). This can lead to enlargement of subcortical white matter by more than 30%.

SPACE OCCUPYING LESIONS AND OBSTRUCTIVE HYDROCEPHALUS

Space occupying lesions and obstructive hydrocephalus displace brain tissue to result in herniation, ischaemia and localised oedema. Space occupation usually causes interstitial swelling (Tower 1972) which predominantly involves white matter (Stewart-Wallace 1939).

ENCEPHALITIS

Diffuse inflammatory involvement of the brain can lead to wide-spread cerebral oedema. From a therapeutic viewpoint, it is important to establish whether raised intracranial pressure is making a significant contribution to the clinical features of a patient with encephalitis (see Chapter 5).

CEREBRAL ISCHAEMIA

As already mentioned, experimental studies suggest that brain oedema is one important factor determining the extent of cerebral perfusion that can become re-established after an episode of ischaemia. Treatment of oedema should, therefore, be undertaken in patients who survive a period of inadequate cerebral blood flow following cerebral infarction, subarachnoid haemorrhage (which is commonly associated with arterial spasm), or cardiac arrest.

BENIGN INTRACRANIAL HYPERTENSION

In benign intracranial hypertension (otitic hydrocephalus, pseudo-tumour cerebri) there is raised intracranial pressure without any identifiable causal lesion. The salient features are headache, papilloedema and vomiting; the main danger is irreversible visual failure consequent upon the papilloedema. Benign intracranial hypertension usually clears over a matter of months, seldom persisting over a year. Since there are no localised pressure differences within the intracranial cavity, there is no risk of herniation of brain.

Benign intracranial hypertension has been reported associated with otitis media, hypocalcaemia and certain endocrinological changes such as occur at the menarche, in pregnancy, with secondary amenorrhoea, or in Addison's disease. It can also be induced by administration of tetracycline, nalidixic acid, oral contraceptives or vitamin A. The commonest precipitating factor is probably withdrawal of long term corticosteroid therapy (Neville and Wilson 1970).

The functional disturbance in benign intracranial hypertension has not been identified. Absorption of intrathecally injected radioactive iodinated human serum albumin is decreased, suggesting a defect in the removal of CSF at the arachnoid villi (Bercaw and Greer 1970). Support for this hypothesis derives from observations on an animal model of benign intracranial hypertension produced by cessation of prolonged corticosteroid therapy (Johnston 1973).

TREATMENT OF RAISED INTRACRANIAL PRESSURE

Dexamethasone. Dexamethasone inhibits the extravasation of dye-protein complexes from plasma after cold injury to the brain. Microscopic studies indicate that it decreases astrocytic swelling and reduces the extracellular space of the white matter (Long *et al* 1972). Glucocorticoids also inhibit the enlargement and vacuolation of astrocytes cultured in media of low osmolarity (Sano *et al* 1972).

Early proposals suggested that corticosteroids interefere with the accumulation of sodium (Fox 1964) and water (Taylor *et al* 1965) in pathological brain. Sato (1967) has argued that they inhibit the production of CSF.

Dexamethasone is the most widely used glucocorticoid for the treatment of brain swelling (Patten *et al* 1972). It is particularly effective in the management of cerebral oedema due to tumours (Maxwell *et al* 1972; Weinstein *et al* 1973), infarction (Patten *et al* 1972), subarachnoid haemorrhage and benign intracranial hypertension (Hooshmand 1972b).

Dexamethasone is similar to other glucocoticorids (see Chapter 7) in its general pharmacological properties, though it binds less to plasma proteins, causes less salt retention and has a relatively long plasma half-life, around 3 hours.

For the acute treatment of raised intracranial pressure, 8–10 mg may be given intravenously, followed by intramuscular injection of 4 mg every 6 hours. The dose for tumours should be titrated according to requirements and side effects; it is often possible to maintain patients for prolonged periods on 0.5–1.0 mg/day orally. In cerebral infarction, subarachnoid haemorrhage or cardiac arrest, an intramuscular injection of 4 mg every 6 hours is usually maintained for 10 days; the dose can then be tailed off over 7 days (see Chapter 6). For benign intracranial hypertension 4 mg thrice daily should be adequate, reducing the dose after 10 days.

Adverse reactions to dexamethasone are similar to those discussed when considering other glucocorticoids.

Acetazolamide. Acetazolamide reduces the rate of formation of CSF (Tschirgi *et al* 1954). The active transport of solute still takes place at the choroid plexus, but there is inhibition of the flow of water which would normally follow the establishment of an osmotic gradient across the epithelium (Davson 1970).

The decrease in CSF formation induced by acetazolamide has been reported to be of therapeutic value in benign intracranial hypertension (Davidoff 1956), though this conclusion is controversial (Greer 1968). For details of the dose regimen see Chapter 12.

Dehydrating agents. Dehydrating agents relieve increased intracranial pressure by shrinking the brain; their action is much less sustained that that of dexamethasone, but they produce their effect more rapidly.

Diuretics such as frusemide (40 mg intravenously) can be employed for this purpose. Intravenous mannitol (2 g/kg as a 25% solution infused over 30 minutes) is effective for a few hours. More prolonged reduction of intracranial tension can be achieved with oral glycerol (1 g/kg, thrice daily). Intravenous glycerol is also useful, particularly in ischaemic strokes (see Chapter 6). Unfortunately the amelioration of cerebral oedema achieved with hypertonic solutions may be followed by a rise in intracranial pressure; this does not occur with dexamethasone (Hooshmand *et al* 1969).

SPECIAL TECHNIQUES FOR TREATING PAIN

A variety of surgical procedures are employed in the treatment of pain—section of a peripheral nerve or root, spinothalamic tractotomy and stereotactic thalamotomy (Illingworth 1973). Peripheral nerve blockade with a local anaesthetic can sometimes induce prolonged alleviation of pain (Powell 1955). Causalgia often responds to sympathectomy (Bonney 1973). Other procedures which have been claimed to help pain include repeated withdrawal and re-injection of CSF (Lipton 1973) and intrathecal administration of phenol, hypertonic saline or cold saline (Hitchcock and Prandini 1973).

The technique currently attracting most attention is electrical stimulation of peripheral nerves (Wall and Sweet 1967) or spinal cord (Nashold and Friedman 1972). The rationale is that suitably adjusted electric shocks should be capable of selectively stimulating large nerve fibres to result in closure of the gate mechanism proposed by Melzack and Wall (1965). Activation of large nerve fibres may also be responsible for the alleviation of pain sometimes achieved by superficial mechanical vibration, for example in the treatment of post-herpetic neuralgia.

CHAPTER 19
NAUSEA AND VERTIGO

Nausea and vertigo often occur together and they are frequently alleviated by the same drugs. However, each may be experienced alone, so it is convenient to consider them separately, dealing with pharmacology first, and then treatment.

Nausea

PHARMACOLOGY

Nausea is a sensation of sickness which is felt in the epigastrium and usually precedes vomiting. It tends to fluctuate, in waves which are accompanied by pallor, sweating, tachycardia and salivation; there is loss of tone in the stomach and reverse peristalsis.

Peripheral causes include disturbances in the thorax or abdomen (e.g. myocardial infarction or peptic ulceration) and abnormal vestibular stimulation (e.g. motion sickness or Ménière's syndrome).

Central mechanisms mediating nausea and vomiting are complex. It is teleologically appropriate that chemoreceptors are located in the brainstem near the area postrema, where the blood–brain barrier is relatively ineffective and therefore substances circulating in blood have ready access. The chemoreceptors monitor the levels of circulating toxic materials, including drugs, so that if excessive concentrations build up, nausea and vomiting occur. This constitutes a homeostatic control system which provides continuous surveillance

of dietary intake and elimination of any unwanted materials from
the gastrointestinal tract. In addition to the emesis induced by
certain foods and drugs, central vomiting can result from raised
intracranial pressure, emotional crises, or accumulation of toxic
metabolites, as occurs in renal and hepatic failure.

There is pharmacological evidence for the existence of two closely
associated controlling areas in the brainstem—a *chemoreceptor
trigger zone* responsible for detecting circulating toxic materials,
which projects to an *emetic centre* that also receives inputs from the
viscera, the labyrinth and the cerebral cortex (Fig. 43). The detailed
pharmacology of vomiting has not been elucidated, but a few components have been dissected away from the major body of ignorance.

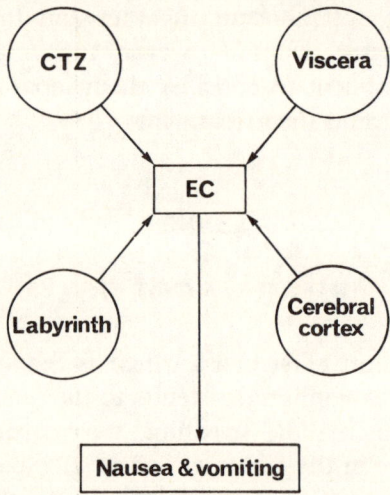

Fig. 43. Diagrammatic summary of the pathways concerned with the
control of emesis. CTZ is the chemoreceptor trigger zone. EC is the
emetic centre.

DOPAMINERGIC SYSTEMS

A number of observations suggest that a dopaminergic pathway is
concerned with the induction of emesis.

1 Precursors of dopamine, such as levodopa, cause nausea and
vomiting; in animals, this response can still be elicited after gastrointestinal deafferentation.

2 Relatively specific dopaminergic agonists, such as apomorphine and piribedil, are also potent emetic agents.
3 Dopaminergic blocking drugs, such as the butyrophenones and phenothiazines, are effective antiemetic drugs.

CHOLINERGIC (MUSCARINIC) SYSTEMS

The evidence for involvement of cholinergic synapses is more limited. It derives largely from the observation that muscarinic blocking drugs alleviate motion sickness.

HISTAMINERGIC SYSTEMS

The mode of action of antihistaminic agents has not been established. These drugs all possess cholinergic (muscarinic) blocking properties which could be responsible for their antiemetic effect; there is no compelling evidence for the existence of a histaminergic mechanism.

TREATMENT

Before attempting to alleviate nausea, it is important to establish that treatment is necessary. If nausea is produced by ingestion of a gastric irritant (e.g. methylalcohol) or overdosage with a drug (e.g. digoxin) the most satisfactory outcome is expulsion of the toxic material from the gastrointestinal tract by vomiting. Similarly, nausea may be an essential clue for the early diagnosis of a disease (e.g. infective hepatitis), so therapy should not be started before a cause has been found.

A large number of drugs are available for the treatment of nausea and vomiting:

DOPAMINERGIC BLOCKING DRUGS

Chlorpromazine. The pharmacokinetics, dosage and toxicity of chlorpromazine are discussed in Chapter 20.

Prochlorperazine. Prochlorperazine is readily absorbed from the gastrointestinal tract. The usual dose is 10–30 mg/day by mouth,

12.5–25 mg/day by intramuscular injection, or 25–50 mg/day by suppository. Divided doses are employed for all routes. Adverse effects are similar to those of chlorpromazine; in particular dryness of the mouth, orthostatic hypotension, drowsiness and extrapyramidal reactions. There have been occasional reports of marrow depression and cholestatic jaundice.

Haloperidol. The pharmacokinetics, dosage and toxicity of halo-periodol are discussed in Chapter 14. In the treatment of nausea, about 5 mg are equivalent to 50 mg of chlorpromazine (Dyrberg 1962).

ANTICHOLINERGIC DRUGS

Hyoscine. Hyoscine has many properties similar to atropine (see Chapter 17) but displays sedative rather than stimulant actions on the central nervous system. It is readily absorbed from the gastrointestinal tract and much becomes bound to plasma proteins. The usual dose is 0.6 mg orally or by subcutaneous injection. Hyoscine is particularly effective in motion sickness; doses as low as 0.1 mg are often therapeutic (Brand *et al* 1967).

ANTIHISTAMINES

Antihistamines are used extensively to control nausea. They have antimuscarinic actions leading to adverse effects similar to atropine (see Chapter 16); they also tend to induce sedation.

Meclozine. Meclozine is widely employed for sustained prophylaxis of nausea because of its long duration of action, which may extend to 24 hours. The usual oral dose is 25 mg twice daily; it takes at least an hour for an antiemetic response to develop.

Cyclizine. Cyclizine is an antihistamine with a rapid onset of action— within some 20 minutes of oral intake. The usual dose is 50 mg by mouth thrice daily. Injections of 50 mg or suppositories of 100 mg are given when there is vomiting.

OTHER DRUGS

Metoclopramide. Metoclopramide, a derivative of procainamide, has recently become widely used as an antiemetic. It hastens gastric emptying by increasing peristalsis—a property which may contribute to the control of vomiting. The oral dose is 10 mg thrice daily. Intramuscular or intravenous injections of 10 mg can be given if the patient is vomiting. Adverse reactions include extrapyramidal disorders, drowsiness and constipation.

Vertigo

PHARMACOLOGY

Vertigo is a hallucination of movement. Information concerning the position of the body reaches the central nervous system from a number of different pathways, including vision and a wide range of sensory receptors in the skin, joints and muscles. The vestibular system is concerned with detecting and transmitting acceleration. The semicircular canals are sensitive to angular acceleration while the otolith organ responds to linear acceleration, including gravitational forces. Vertigo is produced by diseases affecting the vestibular apparatus or its central connections.

The current state of profound obscurity concerning the pharmacology of vertigo is illustrated by its absence from the the index of such authoritative works as Goodman and Gilman's *Pharmacological basis of therapeutics* (1970). In the words of Laurence (1973) 'There is not yet enough knowledge of the physiology of the symptoms for drug therapy to be on a scientific basis'. Approaches which have been advocated include such contradictory measures as histaminic stimulants, histaminic blockers, vasoconstrictors, vasodilators, central nervous stimulants and central nervous depressants. In the absence of any adequate pharmacological information, the treatment of vertigo is pragmatic.

TREATMENT

Frequent attacks of vertigo are treated by regular administration of agents which suppress vestibular function. Cinnarizine and prochlorprazine are probably the most satisfactory drugs (Dix and Morales-Garcia 1972; Hinchcliffe 1972). Hydrochlorothiazide has been reported to have a worthwhile prophylactic action in Ménière's syndrome, possibly by alleviating endolymphatic hydrops (Klockhoff and Lindblom 1966). If attacks of vertigo are prolonged, it may be useful to give intramuscular chlorpromazine or rectal prochlorperazine.

Cinnarizine. Cinnarizine is an antihistamine with a prominent depressive action on vestibular function. Philipszoon (1962) has measured the reaction to vestibular stimulation in a double-blind setting; his results indicate that cinnarizine reduces the responses to both angular and linear acceleration. Patients with peripheral causes of vertigo obtained the greatest benefit.

The usual dose of cinnarizine is 15–30 mg thrice daily but when patients feel an attack of vertigo developing they can immediately take double their usual dose. The duration of action of cinnarizine is about 4 hours. Sedation may be encountered.

Prochlorperazine. Suppositories of 25–50 mg prochlorperazine are useful if vertiginous episodes are prolonged. As a prophylactic agent 5 mg may be administered orally three times a day. Prochlorperazine is discussed further earlier in this Chapter.

Chlorpromazine. Intramuscular chlorpromazine can be given for acute attacks of vertigo; the usual dose is 50 mg. This drug is considered in more detail in Chapter 20.

Hydrochlorothiazide. Hydrochlorothiazide is reputed to alleviate vertigo in Ménière's syndrome and may also help deafness. The dose is 50 mg/day; pharmacokinetics and adverse reactions are described in Chapter 12.

CHAPTER 20
ANXIETY, DEPRESSION AND INSOMNIA

Anxiety

A bewildering range of drugs is available for the treatment of anxiety, depression and insomnia. Each new product is launched amid claims for its superiority over previous therapy, but the cogency of these assertions usually reflects expertise in marketing rather than adequately documented facts. In this Chapter attention is confined to drugs which have proved to be satisfactory over several years of use and no attempt will be made to evaluate the somewhat dubious advantages that may have been attributed to their numerous congeners, many of which have failed to withstand the test of time.

MAJOR TRANQUILLISERS

Phenothiazines and butyrophenones are usually employed in the treatment of severe anxiety such as that encountered in psychosis or exceptional environmental stress. These drugs block noradrenergic and dopaminergic receptors in the central nervous system. In addition, their prolonged administration leads to a fall in the concentrations of noradrenaline and dopamine in the brain (Sourkes 1972). Rauwolfia alkaloids, such as reserpine, are also major tranquillisers and they too reduce central catecholamine function—though they have now been abandoned because of relatively prominent adverse reactions.

The pharmacological basis of anxiety and its alleviation are not understood, but as the major tranquillisers share similar properties

279

in relation to catecholamines, it is likely that effects upon nor-adrenergic or dopaminergic synapses are concerned with their therapeutic action. The most widely used phenothiazine is chlorpromazine and the most extensively prescribed butyrophenone is haloperidol.

Chlorpromazine. Chlorpromazine is rapidly absorbed and undergoes enterohepatic recirculation. It is quickly distributed, the brain concentration being higher than plasma but lower than many other organs, such as lung and liver. The metabolic pathway involves hydroxylation with subsequent conjugation to form glucuronides. Excretion of metabolites is equal in urine and faeces. Chlorpromazine and its metabolites remain in the body for a prolonged period, which may extend to 18 months.

Treatment can be started with 25 mg thrice daily, increasing until adverse reactions occur or a satisfactory response is obtained. An average dose is 100–200 mg/day. Exceptionally, doses of 2–5 g/day have been employed in the treatment of severe, disabling psychosis.

Unwanted effects include sedation, lassitude, palpitations, orthostatic hypotension, nasal congestion, a dry mouth, constipation, impotence, galactorrhoea, weight gain, photosensitivity and seizures. Jaundice is a rare but important manifestation of hypersensitivity. Blood dyscrasias are occasionally encountered. High doses may lead to the formation of opacities in the cornea and lens. Extrapyramidal reactions are discussed in Chapters 13 and 14. Elderly debilitated patients are particularly sensitive to intramuscular chlorpromazine; an injection of 100 mg can be equivalent to 400–500 mg by mouth—such doses may induce profound sedation and hypotension (Nemetz 1969). Widespread muscle rigidity and hypothermia can also occur following overdosage.

Haloperidol. For details of pharmacokinetics, dose regimens and toxicity of haloperidol see Chapter 14.

MINOR TRANQUILLISERS

One of the commonest symptoms in neurology is mild anxiety, which may be related to organic disease, social problems or genetic predisposition. Traditional remedies for anxiety include alcohol, tobacco, cannabis and opiates. In clinical practice drugs are employed that are less likely to be abused, though dependence upon prescribed minor tranquillisers certainly does occur.

The most satisfactory drugs for anxiety are the benzodiazepines (e.g. diazepam), meprobamate and the barbiturates (e.g. phenobarbitone). Out of the many neuropharmacological actions of all these drugs, it is not clear which is responsible for alleviating anxiety though it may be relevant that they all have anticonvulsant properties and excessive doses produce sedation.

Diazepam. For details of pharmacokinetics, dose regimens and toxicity of diazepam see Chapter 15.

Meprobamate. Meprobamate was initially developed as a muscle relaxant with a more prolonged action than mephenesin. It is readily absorbed, reaching peak plasma concentration in 1–2 hours. Like the barbiturates, meprobamate induces increased activity of hepatic microsomal enzymes. It is oxidised and conjugated, the products being excreted in the urine. The usual dose is 200 mg taken 2–6 times a day. The commonest adverse effect is sedation. Anorexia, nausea and vomiting occur, and hypotension can be troublesome; skin eruptions and blood dyscrasias have also been reported. The overall toxicity of meprobamate is comparable to that of phenobarbitone.

Phenobarbitone. For details of pharmacokinetics, dose regimens and toxicity of phenobarbitone see Chapter 12.

Depression

The neuropharmacology of depression is not understood, but as in the case of anxiety, a number of strands of indirect evidence implicate the catecholamines. Whereas catecholamine antagonists alleviate anxiety the opposite applies to depression—drugs which facilitate catecholamine transmission elevate mood.

Monoamine oxidase inhibitors are the most obvious example of antidepressant agents which augment central catecholamines. While these were once widely used to treat depression they have now been virtually abandoned because of the potentially dangerous consequences of interactions with certain foods (containing tyramine) and drugs.

The tricyclic anti-depressants—amitriptyline, imipramine and their congeners—are currently considered to exert their therapeutic effect by blocking catecholamine reuptake, which results in an increased quantity of transmitter in the synaptic cleft. These actions are in accord with the view that cerebral amines play an important part in the control of mood. Indirect evidence consonant with this hypothesis derives from the finding that lithium, which is used to treat mania, decreases catecholamine transmission. Furthermore reserpine depletes brain monoamines and precipitates depression.

Some 30% of patients do not respond to treatment with tricyclic agents (Davis and Janowsky 1974). Failure can sometimes be attributed to pharmacokinetic factors—different patients taking the same dose of tricyclic drugs display a wide variety of plasma concentrations.

Amitriptyline. Amitriptyline is well absorbed and up to 50% is excreted in 24 hours. An initial dose of 25 mg thrice daily may be increased gradually according to tolerance up to 200 or even 300 mg/day. Two or three weeks elapse before the full therapeutic effect is manifest. Amitriptyline often causes sedation; other toxic reactions are similar to those of imipramine, but usually less severe.

Imipramine. Imipramine is rapidly absorbed and up to 90% becomes bound to plasma protein. It undergoes demethylation, hydroxylation and conjugation; some 40% is excreted in the urine over 24 hours. The usual starting dose is 25 mg thrice daily, increasing by 25 mg every 2 days until unwanted effects are encountered. The maintenance dose range is 100–300 mg/day. It generally takes 2–3 weeks for depression to improve. The commonest adverse reactions resemble those of atropine—dryness of the mouth, defective ocular accomodation, constipation, urinary retention and tachycardia. Other problems which may be encountered include orthostatic hypotension, lassitude, headache, sweating, oedema, paraesthesiae, tremor, excitement, hallucinations, delusions, convulsions, skin eruptions, jaundice and galactorrhoea.

Insomnia

Normally two distinct patterns of sleep can be recognised—'rapid eye movement sleep' (dreaming and fast electroencephalographic activity) and 'orthodox sleep' (slow electroencephalographic activity).

At the start of the night there is a phase of orthodox sleep for about an hour; this is followed by periods of rapid eye movement sleep that last approximately 20 minutes, alternating with cycles of orthodox sleep which are each sustained for some 90 minutes. Hypnotic drugs disrupt this sequence by reducing the proportion of rapid eye movement sleep.

It has been estimated that in the United Kingdom 10% of the population use drugs to induce sleep (Dunlop 1970). Long term administration of hypnotics is generally regarded as undesirable; sensitive tests of performance reveal impaired reaction time extending well into the following day. In clinical practice these problems have to be balanced against the obvious distress caused by repeated nights of insomnia.

The mode of action of hypnotics is not understood. Different drugs may produce their effects in dissimilar ways, such as modifying synaptic transmission or altering membrane stability.

There are four main groups of hypnotics—benzodiazepines, barbiturates, chloral derivatives and antihistamines.

BENZODIAZEPINES

Nitrazepam. Oral administration leads to peak plasma concentrations in about 2 hours; some 85% is bound to plasma protein (Rieder and Wendt 1973). The plasma half-life is 7–10 hours (Mattson 1972).

Nitrazepam is one of the most frequently prescribed hypnotics. The usual dose is 5–10 mg. Adverse effects are very uncommon; drowsiness may persist into the following day and elderly patients can become confused.

BARBITURATES

The traditional classification of barbiturates into short, medium and long acting categories does not receive support from clinical experience and may now be regarded as redundant (Laurence 1973). The most satisfactory barbiturate hypnotics are probably pento-barbitone and quinalbarbitone.

Pentobarbitone (pentobarbital). Some 50% of pentobarbitone in the plasma is bound to proteins; about 80% is inactivated by hepatic hydroxylation. Pharmacokinetic and adverse reactions are similar to those described for phenobarbitone (see Chapter 12). The usual hypnotic dose is 100–200 mg.

Quinalbarbitone (secobarbital). This drug is similar in all respects to pentobarbitone. The dose is 100–200 mg.

CHLORAL DERIVATIVES

The pharmacological action of a number of hypnotic drugs, such as chloral hydrate and triclofos, is largely dependent upon formation of an active metabolite—trichloroethanol.

Chloral hydrate. Chloral hydrate is rapidly absorbed and quickly metabolised to trichloroethanol. The usual dose is 0.3–2 g for adults and 50 mg/kg for children. It is commonly prescribed for the very young and the very old because it carries a relatively low risk of inducing excitation or confusion. Chloral hydrate has a pungent, bitter taste and it is a gastric irritant.

Triclofos. Triclofos is hydrolysed in the stomach to trichloroethanol, which is readily absorbed. The usual dose is 0.5–2 g. Occasionally triclofos produces headache or nausea.

ANTIHISTAMINES

Promethazine. Promethazine is a phenothiazine which impairs transmission at cholinergic, noradrenergic and serotonergic synapses; it is also a local anaesthetic agent. Promethazine has a prominent sedative action and it is sometimes prescribed as a hypnotic. The usual dose is 25–50 mg. Because of its protean pharmacological effects a number of dose dependent adverse reactions may be encountered. The commonest problem is dryness of the mouth; occasionally hypersensitive and idiosyncratic reactions occur, such as jaundice, blood dyscrasias and photosensitivity. In infants promethazine can cause excitement, pyrexia and convulsions.

CHAPTER 21
THE USE OF PLACEBO

Administration of placebo plays an essential part in the design of many double-blind studies undertaken to evaluate the efficacy and toxicity of new drugs. In these circumstances it is ethically desirable to warn patients that more than one form of treatment will be given. Placebos often produce a limited improvement in symptoms, so there is no deception in the conduct of an investigation of this type.

Inactive preparations are more commonly used in another context—the management of disorders for which no effective curative or even palliative therapy is available. In many terminal diseases loss of insight softens reality for the patient but often the intellect is well preserved. When the patient recognises his relentless deterioration, it has been traditional practice to prescribe placebos in an effort to sustain hope and so improve the quality of life. This approach is widely employed in conditions which run a relatively short downhill course such as motoneuron disease, but placebos are less useful when there is a protracted accumulation of neurological deficits over many years as, for example, in multiple sclerosis.

Investigations have been undertaken to compare the effect of different colours, tastes, smells and routes of administration of placebos, but few would take these exercises very seriously.

A distinction is sometimes drawn between *pure* placebos which are pharmacologically inert and *impure* placebos that have actions remotely relevant to the disease process. It has been suggested that the latter are unsatisfactory because they may deceive the physician as much as his patient. Of more importance is the need to avoid specific pitfalls in the choice of placebo, such as vitamin preparations containing folic acid (which can precipitate subacute combined degeneration of the spinal cord in patients with B_{12} deficiency) or pyridoxine (which blocks the therapeutic action of levodopa).

Placebos should never be employed where a diagnosis is in doubt because they can delay the recognition of a disease by modifying symptoms; in this way they may impede the introduction of effective therapy.

Placebos are no substitute for supportive medical consultations. Patients with unremitting diseases need frequent opportunities to ventilate their problems. In addition to the major limitations imposed by their illness, discussion usually reveals many small difficulties that can be overcome by simple, practical advice which eases the burden of coping with routine daily activities.

In deciding whether to prescribe a placebo, much depends on the patient's personality and attitudes. Someone who is well adjusted to his circumstances may prefer to face reality by being confronted with the facts by his physician. However, most patients expect medical science to arrest their deterioration or at least slow down the inexorable progress of their disease. Placebos can postpone the realisation that these hopes are unattainable. Provided inactive preparations are introduced without extravagant claims early therapeutic failure does not lead to immediate despair, although persistently declining neurological function generates recurring requests for something new to be done.

One placebo can be replaced by another in an attempt to give continuing encouragement until after a series of disappointments, the position becomes clear to the patient. At this stage, frustration and apprehension are appropriate reactions, but drugs are available for alleviating this predicament. Tranquillisers (see Chapter 20) are widely used to treat anxiety arising in a psychiatric setting; these agents are also capable of blunting many of the normal responses to intractable disease. Benzodiazepines and phenothiazines can improve the mental state without unduly impairing the intellect or inducing excessive sedation. In addition, antidepressants may be helpful.

Over the last few weeks of life awareness is usually clouded by toxic confusional states resulting from infection, metabolic disturbances or analgesic overdosage, but occasionally there is grim lucidity. When patients are troubled by the fearful uncertainties of terminal illness, opiates can often achieve a state of emotional adjustment which allows death to be accepted with peaceful detachment.

REFERENCES

AARLI J.A. (1973) *Acta neurol. scand.* **49,** Suppl. 53, 11.

ACHESON J., DANTA G. and HUTCHINSON E.C. (1969) *Brit. med. J.* **1,** 614.

ACHESON J. and HUTCHINSON E.C. (1964) *Lancet* **2,** 871.

ACHESON J. and HUTCHINSON E.C. (1971) *Quart. J. Med.* **40,** 15.

ACKERMAN G.L. (1970) *Ann. intern. Med.* **72,** 511.

ADAMS R.D. (1968). In *Handbook of Clinical Neurology*, Vol. 6. Ed. Vinken P.J. and Bruyn G.W. North Holland Publishing Co, Amsterdam.

ADOUR K.K., WINGERD J., BELL D.N., MANNING J.J. and HURLEY J.P. (1972) *New Engl. J. Med.* **287,** 1268.

ALBERTI K.G.M.M., DARLEY J.H., EMERSON P.M. and HOCKADAY T.D.R. (1972) *Lancet* **2,** 391.

ALEU F.P., KATZMAN R. and TERRY R.D. (1963) *J. Neuropath. exp. Neurol.* **22,** 403.

ALEXANDERSON B. and BORGA O. (1972) *Europ. J. clin. Pharmacol.* **4,** 196.

ALLING C., VANIER M.T. and SVENNERHOLM L. (1971) *Brain Res.* **35,** 325.

ALTROCCI P.H. (1972) *Arch. Neurol. (Chic.)* **26,** 506.

AMES A., WRIGHT R.L., KOWADA M., THURSTON J.M. and MAJNO G. (1968) *Amer. J. Path.* **52,** 437.

ANDÉN N.E., BUTCHER S.G., CORRODI H., FUXE K. and UNGERSTEDT U. (1970a) *Europ. J. Pharmacol.* **11,** 303.

ANDÉN N.E., CARLSSON A., KERSTELL J., MAGNUSSON T., OLSSON R., ROOS B.E., STEEN B., STEG G., SVANBORG A., THIEME G. and WERDINIUS B. (1970b) *Acta. med. scand.* **187,** 247.

ANDÉN N.E., DAHLSTRÖM A., FUXE K., LARSSON K., OLSON L. and UNGERSTEDT U. (1966) *Acta physiol. scand.* **67,** 313.

ANDÉN N.E., FUXE K., HAMBERGER B. and HÖKFELT T. (1966) *Acta physiol. scand.* **67,** 306.

ANDÉN N.E., JUKES M.G.M., LUNDBERG A. and VYKLICKY L. (1964) *Nature (Lond.)* **202,** 1344.

ANDERSSON P.G. (1973) *Excerpta med. Int. Congr. Ser.* **296,** 27.

ANDREW J. and NATHAN P.W. (1964) *Brain* **87,** 233.

ANDEWS C.J. and BURKE D. (1973) *J. Neurol. Neurosurg. Psychiat.* **36,** 321.

ANGEL R.W., HOFMANN W.W. and EPPLER W. (1966) *Neurology (Minneap.)* **16,** 529.

ANGLE C.R. and McINTIRE M.S. (1968) *J. Pediat* **73**, 124.

ANTHONY J.J. (1970) *Arch. Neurol. (Chic.)* **22**, 450.

ANTHONY M., HINTERBERGER H. and LANCE J.W. (1967) *Arch. Neurol. (Chic.)* **16**, 544.

APLEY J., CLARKE S.K.R., ROOME A.P.C.H., SANDRY S.A., SAYGI G., SILK B. and WARHURST D.C. (1970) *Brit. med. J.* **1**, 596.

ARMITAGE P. (1960). In *Controlled clinical trials*. Ed. Hill A.B. Blackwell, Oxford.

ARVIDSSON J., ROOS B.E. and STEG G. (1966) *Acta physiol. scand.* **67**, 398.

ASAI K. and HUFSCHMIDT H.J. (1958) *Dtsch. Z. Nervenheilk* **178**, 289.

AUR R.J.A., SIMONE J., HUSTU H.O., WALTERS T., BORELLA L., PRATT C. and PINKEL D. (1971) *Blood* **37**, 272.

AUSTIN J.H. (1958) *Brain* **81**, 157.

AVERY G.S., DAVIES E.F. and BROGDEN R.N. (1972) *Drugs* **4**, 7.

AXELROD J., MUELLER R.A. and THEONEN H. (1970) In *New Aspects of Storage and Release Mechanisms of Catecholamines*. Ed. Schümann H.J. and Kroneberg G. Springer, Berlin.

AYD J. (1961) *J. Amer. med. Ass.* **175**, 1054.

BACK E.H. (1969) *Lancet* **2**, 1005.

BAGSHAWE K.D., MACGRATH I.T. and GOLDING P.R. (1969) *Lancet* **2**, 1258.

BAK I.J., CHOI W.B., HASSLER R., USUNOFF K.G. and WAGNER A. (1974). In *Dopaminergic Mechanisms*. Ed. Calne D.B., Chase T.N. and Barbeau A. Raven Press, New York.

BAKER R.W.R., THOMPSON R.H.S. and ZILKHA K.J. (1964) *J. Neurol. Neurosurg. Psychiat.* **27**, 408.

BALAGTAS R.C., LEVIN S., NELSON K.E. and GOTOFF S.P. (1970) *J. Pediat.* **77**, 957.

BALDESSARINI R.J. and LIPINSKI J.F. (1973) *New Engl. J. Med.* **289**, 427.

BALDESSARINI R.J., LIPINSKI J.F. and CHACE K.V. (1972) *Biochem. Pharmacol.* **21**, 77.

BARBEAU A. (1961) *Excerpta med. Int. Congr. Ser.* **38**, 152.

BARBEAU A. (1972). In *Proceedings of the 4th International Symposium on Parkinson's Disease*. Ed. Siegfried J. Huber, Bern.

BARBEAU A. (1974). In *Second Canadian–American Conference on Parkinson's Disease*. Ed. McDowell F.H. and Barbeau A. Raven Press, New York.

BARBEAU A., CHASE T.N. and PAULSON G.W. (1973). *Huntington's chorea, 1872–1972*. Raven Press, New York.

BARBEAU A. and FRIESEN H. (1970) *Lancet* **1**, 1180.

BARBEAU A. and McDOWELL F.H. (1970). *L-dopa and Parkinsonism*. Davis, Philadelphia.

BARONDES S.H. (1964) *Science* **146**, 779.

BARR W.H. (1968). *Amer. J. pharm. Educ.* **32**, 958.

BARTHOLINI G., BURKARD W.F., PLETSCHER A. and BATES H.M. (1967) *Nature (Lond.)* **215**, 852.

BAUER F.K., RILEY W.C. and COHEN F.B. (1950) *Ann. intern. Med.* **33**, 1042.

BAUMGARTEN H.G., BJÖRKLUND A., LACHENMAYER L., NOBIN A. and STENEVI U. (1971) *Acta physiol. scand.* Suppl. **373**, 1.

BEATTIE A.D. and GOLDBERG A. (1972) *Medicine (London)* No. 12, 774.

BEATTIE A.D., MOORE M.R., GOLDBERG A. and WARD R.L. (1973) *Brit. Med. J.* **3**, 257.

BEERMAN B., HELLSTRÖM K. and ROSÉN A. (1972) *Clin. Pharmacol. Ther.* **13**, 212.

BEESON P.B. and McDERMOTT W. (1971). *Cecil-Loeb Textbook of Medicine.* Saunders, Philadelphia.

BEEVERS D.G., FAIRMAN M.J., HAMILTON M. and HARPUR J.E. (1973) *Lancet* **1**, 1407.

BEHRMAN S. (1958) *Brit. med J.* **1**, 1454.

BEIN H.J. (1972). In *Moderne aspekte der muskelverkrampfung*, International Symposium, Wien, 1971. Ciba-Geigy, Basel.

BELLER A.J., SAHAR A. and PRAISS I. (1973) *J. Neurol. Neurosurg. Psychiat.* **36**, 757.

BELSEY M.A. and TARDO C. (1967) *Ann. N.Y. Acad. Sci.* **145**, 482.

BENNETT R., HUGHES G.R.V., BYWATERS E.G.L. and HOLT P.J.L. (1972) *Brit. med. J.* **4**, 342.

BERCAW B.L. and GREER M. (1970) *Neurology (Minneap.)* **20**, 787.

BERNHEIMER H., BIRKMAYER W. and HORNYKIEWICZ O. (1961) *Klin. Wschr.* **41**, 465.

BIRCHER J., MÜLLER J., GUGGENHEIM P. and HAEMMERLI U.P. (1966) *Lancet* **1**, 890.

BIRD E.D., MACKAY A.V.P., RAYNER C.N. and IVERSEN L.L. (1973) *Lancet* **1**, 1090.

BIRDWOOD G.F.B., GILDER S.S.B. and WINK C.A.S. (1971). *Parkinson's Disease. A new approach to treatment.* Academic Press, London.

BIRKET-SMITH E., LUND M., MIKKELSEN B., VESTERMARK S., OLSEN P.Z. and HOLM P. (1973) *Acta neurol. scand.* **49**, Supp. 53, 18.

BIRKET-SMITH E. and MIKKELSEN B. (1972) *Acta neurol. scand.* **48**, 385.

BIRKMAYER W. (1969) *Wien. klin. Wschr.* **81**, 10.

BIRKMAYER W. and HORNYKIEWICZ O. (1961) *Wien. klin. Wschr.* **73**, 787.

BIRKS R.I. and MACINTOSH F.C. (1961) *Canad. J. Biochem. Physiol.* **39**, 787.

BLACK P., GRAYBILL J.R. and CHARACHE P. (1973) *J. Neurosurg.* **38**, 705.

BLADIN P.F. (1973) *Med. J. Aust.* **1**, 683.

BLASCHKO H. (1973) *Brit. med. Bull.* **29**, 105.

BLEIDNER W.E., HARMON J.B., HEWES W.E., LYNES T.E. and HERMANN E.C. (1965) *J. Pharmacol. exp. Ther.* **150**, 484.

BLOOM F.E., ALGERI S., GROPETTI A., REVUELTA A. and COSTA E. (1969) *Science* **166**, 1284.

BLOOM F.E., COSTA E. and SALMOIRAGHI G.C. (1965) *J. Pharmacol. exp. Ther.* **150**, 244.

BLUMENTHAL L.S. (1968). In *Handbook of Clinical Neurology*, Vol. 5. Ed. Vinken P.J. and Bruyn G.W. North Holland Publishing Co, Amsterdam.

BOCHNER F., HOOPER W.D., TYRER J.H. and EADIE M.J. (1972) *J. Neurol. Neurosurg. Psychiat.* **35**, 873.

BOLLETTI M. and BERTAGGIA A. (1971) *Gazz. med. Ital.* **130**, 171.

BONICA J.J. (1974) *International Symposium on Pain.* Raven Press, New York.

BONNEY G.L.W. (1973) *Brit. J. Hosp. Med.* **9**, 593.

BOOKER H.E. (1972). In *Antiepileptic drugs.* Ed. Woodbury D.M., Penry J.K. and Schmidt R.P. Raven Press, New York.

BORIS M. (1968) *J. Amer. med. Ass.* **205**, 648.

BOWMAN W.C. and RAND M.J. (1961) *Brit. J. Pharmacol.* **17**, 176.

BOWMAN W.C. and RAPER C. (1967) *Ann. N.Y. Acad. Sci.* **139**, 541.

BØE J., SOLBERG C.O. and SAETER T. (1965) *Brit. med. J.* **1**, 1094.

BRADBURY M.W. and DAVSON H. (1964). In *Absorption and distribution of drugs.* Ed. Binns T.B. Livingstone, Edinburgh.

BRAHAM J. (1971) *Brit. med. J.* **4**, 212.

BRAIN R. and WALTON J.N. (1969). *Diseases of the Nervous System.* Oxford University Press, London.

BRAND J.J., COLQUHOUN W.P., GOULD A.H. and PERRY W.L.M. (1967) *Brit. J. Pharmacol.* **30**, 463.

BRAUSCH U., HENATSCH H.D., STUDENT C. and TAKANO K. (1973). In *The Benzodiazepines.* Ed. Gorattini S., Mussini E. and Randall L.O. Raven Press, New York.

BRECKENRIDGE A., ORME M.L'E., DAVIES L., THORGEIRSSON S.S. and DAVIES D.S. (1973) *Clin. Pharmacol. Ther.* **14**, 514.

BRETT E.M. (1966) *J. neurol. Sci.* **3**, 52.

BRETT E.M. (1973) *Brit. J. Hosp. Med.* **9**, 177.

BRIERLEY J.B., MELDRUM B.S. and BROWN A.W. (1973) *Arch. Neurol (Chic.)* **29**, 367.

BRODER L.E. and CARTER S.K. (1972). *Meningeal leukaemia.* Plenum Press, New York.

BRODIE B.B., KURZ H. and SCHANKER L.S. (1960) *J. Pharmacol. exp. Ther.* **130**, 20.

BROGDEN R.N., SPEIGHT T.M. and AVERY G.S. (1971) *Drugs*, **2**, 262.

BRUCK J., GERSTENBRAND F., GRUNDIG E. and PROSENZ P. (1965). *Conf. Hung. pro Therapia et Investigation in Pharmacologia*, 149–158. Kultura, Budapest.

BRUMLIK J., JACOBS R. and KARCZMAR A.G. (1973) *Clin. Pharmacol. Ther.* **14**, 380.

BRUYN G.W. (1962) *Psychiat. Neurol. Neurochir.* **65**, 430.

BRUYN G.W. (1968a). In *Handbook of Clinical Neurology*, Vol. 6. Ed. Vinken P.J. and Bruyn G.W. North Holland Publishing Co, Amsterdam.

BRUYN G.W. (1968b). In *Handbook of Clinical Neurology*, Vol. 5. Ed. Vinken P.J. and Bruyn G.W. North Holland Publishing Co, Amsterdam.

BUCHANAN R.A. (1972). In *Antiepileptic drugs*. Ed. Woodbury D.M., Penry J.K. and Schmidt R.P. Raven Press, New York.

BUCHANAN R.A., FERNANDEZ L. and KINKEL A.W. (1969) *J. clin. Pharmacol*. **9**, 393.

BUCHTHAL F. and LENNOX-BUCHTHAL M.A. (1972) In *Antiepileptic drugs*. Ed. Woodbury D.M., Penry J.K. and Schmidt R.P., Raven Press, New York.

BULL G. and HEMSWORTH B.A. (1963) *Nature (Lond.)* **199**, 487.

BURGEN A.S.V., BURKE G. and DESBORATS-SHONBAUM M. (1956) *Brit. J. Pharmacol*. **22**, 313.

BURN J.H. and RAND M.J. (1965) *Ann. Rev. Pharmacol*. **5**, 163.

BUTCHER L.L., ENGEL J. and FUXE K. (1970) *J. Pharm. Pharmacol*. **22**, 313.

BUTLER T.C. (1956) *J. Pharmacol. exp. Ther*. **116**, 326.

BUTLER T.C. (1957) *J. Pharmacol. exp. Ther*. **119**, 1.

BUTLER T.C. and WADDELL W.J. (1956) *Proc. Soc. exp. Biol. (N.Y.)* **93**, 544.

BUXTON P.H. and HAYWARD M. (1967) *J. Neurol. Neurosurg. Psychiat*. **30**, 511.

CALCUTT C.R., HANDLEY S.L., SPARKES C.G. and SPENCER P.S.J. (1972). In *Agonist and antagonist actions of narcotic analgesic drugs*. Ed. Kosterlitz H.W., Collier H.O.J. and Villareal J.E. Macmillan, London.

CALNE D.B. (1970). *Parkinsonism: physiology, pharmacology and treatment*. Edward Arnold, London.

CALNE D.B. (1971) *Brit. med. J*. **3**, 693.

CALNE D.B. (1973). *Progress in the treatment of Parkinsonism*. Raven Press, New York.

CALNE D.B., CLAVERIA L.E., TEYCHENNE P.F., HASKAYNE L. and LODGE-PATCH I. (1974) *Trans. Amer. neurol. Ass.*, in press.

CALNE D.B., REID J.L., VAKIL S.D., RAO S., PETRIE A., PALLIS C.A., GAWLER J., THOMAS P.K. and HILSON A. (1971) *Brit. med. J*. **3**, 729.

CALNE D.B., SPIERS A.S.D., STERN G.M., LAURENCE D.R. and ARMITAGE P. (1969a) *Lancet* **2**, 973.

CALNE D.B., STERN G.M., LAURENCE D.R., SHARKEY J. and ARMITAGE P. (1969b) *Lancet* **1**, 744.

CAMP W.A. and FRIERSON J.G. (1962) *Arch. Neurol. (Chic.)* **7**, 432.

CANNON W.B. (1939) *Amer. J. med. Sci*. **198**, 737.

CAPE C.A. and UTTERBACK R.A. (1969) *J. Neurol. Neurosurg. Psychiat*. **32**, 290.

CARLSON L.A. (1967). In *Prostaglandins*. Ed. Bergström S. and Samuelsson B. Interscience, New York.

CARLSSON A. (1970). In *L-dopa and Parkinsonism*. Ed. Barbeau A. and McDowell F.H. Davis, Philadelphia.

CARLSSON A. and LINDQVIST M. (1962) *Acta physiol. scand*. **54**, 87.

CARTER A.B. (1960) *Quart. J. Med*. **29**, 611.

CARTER C.H. (1971) *Clin. Med*. **78**, 33.

CAWEIN M.J. (1969) *New Engl. J. Med*. **281**, 1489.

CEREGHINO J.J., VAN METER J.C., BROCK J.T., PENRY J.K., SMITH L.D. and WHITE B.G. (1973) *Neurology (Minneap.)* **23**, 357.

CHANG T., DILL W.A. and GLAZKO A.J. (1972) In *Antiepileptic drugs*. Ed. Woodbury D.M., Penry J.K. and Schmidt R.P. Raven Press, New York.

CHASE T.N. (1972) *Res. Publ. Ass. Res. nerv. ment. Dis.* **50**, 448.

CHASE T.N. and WATANABE A.M. (1972) *Neurology (Minneap.)* **22**, 384.

CHATEAU R., FAU R., GROSLAMBERT R. and PERRET J. (1966) *Rev. Neurol.* **114**, 65.

CHIANG J., KOWADA M., AMES A., WRIGHT J.L. and MAJNO G. (1968) *Amer. J. Path.* **52**, 455.

CHINITZ A., SEELINGER D.F. and GREENHOUSE A.H. (1966) *Amer. J. med. Sci.* **252**, 62.

CHIPMAN M. and KAUL S. (1972) *Neurology (Minneap.)* **22**, 401.

CHRISTENSEN E., MOLLER J.E. and FAURBYE A. (1970) *Acta psychiat. scand.* **46**, 14.

CHRISTIANSEN C., RØDBRO P. and LUND M. (1973) *Brit. med. J.* **4**, 693.

CLAVERIA L.E., CALNE D.B. and ALLEN J.G. (1973) *Brit. med J.* **2**, 641.

CLAVERIA L.E., TEYCHENNE P., CALNE D.B., PETRIE A. and BASSENDINE M.F. (1974). In *Dopaminergic Mechanisms*. Ed. Calne D.B., Chase T.N. and Barbeau A. Raven Press, New York.

CLEMMESEN J., FUGLSANG-FREDERIKSEN V. and PLUM C.M. (1974) *Lancet* **1**, 705.

COATSWORTH J.J. (1971). *Studies on the clinical efficacy of marketed antiepileptic drugs*. National Institute of Neurological Diseases and Stroke, Monograph No. 12. U.S. Dept. Health, N.I.H., Bethesda.

COLLIER H.O.J. (1969) *Nature (Lond.)* **223**, 35.

CONNELL P.H., CORBETT J.A., HORNE D.J. and MATTHEWS A.M. (1967) *Brit. J. Psychiat.* **113**, 375.

CONSOLO S., LADINSKY H., PERI G. and GARATTINI S. (1972) *Europ. J. Pharmacol.* **18**, 251.

COOK J.B. and NATHAN P.W. (1967) *J. neurol. Sci.* **5**, 33.

COPE C.L. (1972) *Adrenal steroids and disease*. Pitman Medical, London.

CORBETT J.L., SPALDING J.M.K. and HARRIS P.J. (1973) *Brit. med. J.* **3**, 423.

CORBETT M., FRANKEL H.L. and MICHAELIS L. (1972) *Paraplegia* **10**, 19.

CORNELIO F., NEGRI S., BORRONI V. and FERRARIO L. (1973) *Excerpta med. Int. Congr. Ser.* **296**, 82.

COTZIAS G.C., PAPAVASILIOU P.S., FEHLING C., KAUFMAN B. and MENA I. (1970) *New Engl. J. Med.* **282**, 31.

COTZIAS G.C., VAN WOERT M.H. and SCHIFFER L.M. (1967) *New Engl. J. Med.* **276**, 374.

COURTICE F.C. and SIMMONDS W.J. (1951) *Aust. J. exp. Biol. med. Sci.* **29**, 255.

COYLE J.T. and SNYDER S.H. (1969) *Science* **166**, 899.

CRANE G.E. (1973a) *Science* **181**, 124.

CRANE G.E. (1973b) *Brit. J. Psychiat.* **122**, 395.

CRANE G.E. and PAULSON G. (1967) *Int. J. Neuropsychiat.* **3**, 286.

CRAWLEY F.E.H., KENNEDY P., SWASH M. (1973) *Brit. J. Pharmacol.* **47**, 613P.

CROSBIE ROSS J. (1970). In *Modern trends in urology*, Vol. 3. Ed. Riches E. Butterworths, London.

CROSBIE ROSS J., GIBBON N.O.K. and DAMANSKI M. (1964) *Lancet* **1**, 779.

CUMINGS J.N., HUGHES B.P., MORGAN-HUGHES J. and MAIR W.G.P. (1973). In *Recent advances in clinical pathology*. Ed. Dyke S.C. Churchill Livingstone, Edinburgh.

CURRAN D.A., HINTERBERGER H. and LANCE J.W. (1965) *Brain* **88**, 997.

CURRIE S. and WALTON J.N. (1971) *J. Neurol. Neurosurg. Psychiat.* **34**, 447.

CURTIS D.R., DUGGAN A.W., FELIX D. and JOHNSTON G.A.R. (1970) *Nature (Lond.)* **228**, 676.

CURTIS D.R., GAME C.J.A., JOHNSTON G.A.R., McCULLOCH R.M. and MACLACHLAN R.M. (1972) *Brain Res.* **43**, 242.

CURTIS D.R., PHILLIS J.W. and WATKINS J.C. (1961) *J. Physiol. (Lond.)* **158**, 296.

CUTLER R.W.P., PAGE L., GALICICH J. and WATTERS G.V. (1968) *Brain* **91**, 707.

DAHLBÄCK O., ELMQVIST D., JOHNS T.R., RADNER S. and THESLEFF S. (1961) *J. Physiol. (Lond.)* **156**, 336.

DAHLSTRÖM A. and FUXE K. (1964) *Acta physiol. scand.* **60**, 293.

DALBY M.A. (1969) *Brit. med. J.* **2**, 422.

DALBY M.A. (1971) *Epilepsia (Amst.)* **12**, 325.

DALE H.H., FELDBERG W. and VOGT M. (1936) *J. Physiol. (Lond.)* **86**, 353.

DAM M. (1972) *Acta neurol. scand.* **48**, Suppl. 49, 13.

DAMÁSIO A.R., CASTRO-CALDAS A. and LEVY A. (1973). In *Progress in the treatment of Parkinsonism*. Ed. Calne D.B. Raven Press, New York.

D'ARCY P.F. and GRIFFIN J.P. (1972) *Iatrogenic diseases*. Oxford University Press, London.

DAVIDOFF L.M. (1956) *Neurology (Minneap.)* **6**, 605.

DAVIES D.S. and PRICHARD B.N.C. (1973). *Biological effects of drugs in relation to their plasma concentrations*. Macmillan, London.

DAVIS J.M. and JANOWSKY D.S. (1974) *Brit. J. Hosp. Med.* **11**, 219.

DAVSON H. (1967) *The physiology of the cerebrospinal fluid*. Churchill, London.

DAVSON H. (1970) *A textbook of general physiology*, Vol. 1. Williams and Wilkins, Baltimore.

DAVSON H. (1972) *Develop. Med. Child Neurol.* **14**, Suppl. 27, 1.

DAVSON H. and BRADBURY M. (1965) *Symp. Soc. exp. Biol.* **19**, 349.

DAVSON H., KLEEMAN C.R. and LEVIN E. (1961) *J. Physiol. (Lond.)* **159**, 67P.

DAWKINS R.L. (1965) *J. Path. Bact.* **90**, 619.

DE GRACIANSKY P. and GRUPPER C. (1961) *Brit. J. vener. Dis.* **37**, 247.

DE JONG R.H. and WAGMAN I.H. (1963) *Anesthesiology* **24**, 684.

DELAY J. and DENIKER P. (1968) In *Handbook of Clinical Neurology*, Vol. 6. Ed. Vinken P.J. and Bruyn G.W. North Holland Publishing Co, Amsterdam.

DEL CASTILLO J. and KATZ B. (1954) *J. Physiol. (Lond.)* **124**, 560.

DE LEMOS R.A. and HAGGERTY R.J. (1969) *Pediatrics* **44**, 30.

DEMIS D.J., BROWN C.S. and CROSBY W.H. (1964) *Amer. J. Med.* **37**, 195.

DENGLER H.J., SPIEGEL H.E. and TITUS E.O. (1961) *Nature (Lond.)* **191**, 816.

DENNY-BROWN D. and NEVIN S. (1941) *Brain* **64**, 1.

DENNY-BROWN D. and ROBERTSON E.G. (1933) *Brain* **55**, 150.

DENT C.E., RICHENS A., ROWE D.J.F. anc STAMP T.C.B. (1970) *Brit. med. J.* **4**, 69.

DE PINTO O., POLIKAR M. and DEBONO G. (1972) *Postgrad med. J.* Suppl. 5, **48**, 18.

DESMEDT J.W. (1966) *Ann. N.Y. Acad. Sci.* **125**, 209.

DES PREZ R. (1971) In *Cecil-Loeb Textbook of Medicine*. Ed. Beeson P.B. and McDermott W. Saunders, Philadelphia.

DHASMANA K.M. and SPILKER B.A. (1973) *Brit. J. Pharmacol.* **47**, 437.

DIETRICHSON P. (1971a) *Acta neurol. scand.* **47**, 22.

DIETRICHSON P. (1971b) *Acta neurol. scand.* **47**, 163.

DILL A.W., KAZENKO A., WOLF L.M. and GLAZKO A.J. (1956) *J. Pharmacol. exp. Ther.* **118**, 270.

DIMITRIJEVIĆ M.R. and NATHAN P.W. (1967) *Brain* **90**, 1.

DIVRY P., BOBAN J., COLLARD J., PINCHARD A. and NOLS E. (1959) *Acta neurol. belg.* **59**, 337.

DIX M.R. and MORALES-GARCIA C. (1972) *Brit. J. Hosp. Med.* **7**, 623.

DLUHY R.G., LAULER D.P. and THORN G.W. (1973) *Med. Clin. N. Amer.* **57**, 115.

DOBELL A.R.C., WYANT J.D., SEAMANS K.B. and GLOOR P. (1966) *J. thorac. cardiovas. Surg.* **52**, 469.

DOLLERY C.T. and DAVIES D.S. (1970) *Brit. med. Bull.* **26**, 233.

DOLLERY C.T., GEORGE C.F. and ORME M.L'E. (1972) *Progr. Cardiol.* **1**, 31.

DOUGLAS-WILSON I. (1944) *Brit. med. J.* **1**, 413.

DRACHMAN D.A., PATERSON P.Y., BERLIN B.S. and ROGUSKA J. (1970) *Arch. Neurol. (Chic.)* **23**, 385.

DRACHMAN D.A. and SKOM J. (1965) *Arch. Neurol. (Chic.)* **13**, 316.

DRAKE C.G. and STAVRAKY G.W. (1948) *J. Neurophysiol.* **11**, 229.

DROZ B. and LEBLOND C.P. (1963) *J. comp. Neurol.* **121**, 325.

DUMERMUTH G. and KOVACS E. (1973) *Acta neurol. scand.* **49**, Suppl. 53, 26.

DUNLOP D. (1970) *Brit. med. Bull.* **26**, 236.

DUPONT E., HANSEN H.J. and DALBY M.A. (1973) *Acta neurol. scand.* **49**, 75.

DUVOISIN R. (1972) *Med. Clin. N. Amer.* **56**, 1321.

DYRBERG V. (1962) *Acta anaesth. scand.* **6**, 37.

EDGEWORTH H. (1930) *J. Amer. med. Ass.* **94**, 1136.

EDMEADS J. (1973) *Headache* **13**, 91.

EDWARDS V.E., SUTHERLAND J.M. and TYRER J.H. (1970) *J. Neurol. Neurosurg. Psychiat.* **33**, 415.

EEG-OLOFSSON O. (1973) *Acta neurol. scand.* **49**, Suppl. 53, 29.

EHRINGER H. and HORNYKIEWICZ O. (1960) *Klin. Wschr.* **38**, 1236.

ELDJARN L., TRY K., STOKKE O., MUNTHE-KAAS A.W., REFSUM S., STEINBERG D., AVIGAN J. and MIZE C. (1966) *Lancet* **1**, 691.

ELLIS F.R., KEANEY N.P., HARRIMAN D.G.F., SUMNER D.W., KYEI-MENSAH K., TYRRELL J.H., HARGREAVES J.B., PARIKH R.K. and MULROONEY P.L. (1972) *Brit. med. J.* **3**, 559.

ELLIS K.O. and BRYANT S.H. (1972) *Naunyn-Schmiedeberg's Arch. Pharmak. exp. Path.* **274**, 107.

ELMQVIST D., HOFMANN W.W., KUGELBERG J. and QUASTEL D.M.J. (1964) *J. Physiol. (Lond.)* **174**, 417.

ENERO M.A., LANGER S.Z., ROTHLIN R.P. and STEFANO F.J.E. (1972) *Brit. J. Pharmacol.* **44**, 672.

ENGEL A.G., LAMBERT E.H. and SAMTA T. (1972) *Neurology (Minneap.)* **22**, 401.

ENGEL J., CRUZ M.E. and SHAPIRO B. (1971) *Lancet* **2**, 824.

ENGEL W.K. and WARMOLTS J.R. (1973) *Excerpta med. Int. Congr. Ser.* **296**, 82.

EPSTEIN M.H. and O'CONNOR J.S. (1966) *J. Neurol Neurosurg. Psychiat.* **29**, 251.

ESIRI M.M. and TOMLINSON A.H. (1971) *J. neurol. Sci.* **15**, 35.

ESPLIN D.W. (1957) *J. Pharmacol. exp. Ther.* **120**, 301.

EULENBERG A. (1878) In *Ziemssen's Encyclopaedia of the practice of medicine*. Ed. Buck A.H. Sampson Low, London.

EVANS D.A.P. (1969) In *Selected topics in genetics*. Ed. Clarke C.A. Oxford University Press, London.

EVANS G. (1972) In *Cerebral vascular disease*. Ed. McDowell F. and Whisnant J.P. Grune and Stratton, New York.

FAERØ O., KASTRUP K.W., LYKKEGAARD NIELSEN E., MELCHIOR J.C. and THORN I. (1972) *Epilepsia* **13**, 279.

FAHN S. (1973). In *Huntington's Chorea 1872–1972*. Ed. Barbeau A., Chase T.N. and Paulson G.W. Raven Press, New York.

FAHN S. and DAVID E. (1973) *Excerpta med. Int. Congr. Ser.* **296**, 43.

FAIGLE J.W. and KEBERLE H. (1972) *Postgrad. med. J.* Suppl. 5, **48**, 9.

FALCK B., HILLARP N.Å., THIEME G. and TORP A. (1962) *J. Histochem. Cytochem.* **10**, 348.

FALCONER M.A. (1970) *J. Neurosurg.* **33**, 233.

FARNEBO L.O., FUXE K., HAMBERGER B. and LJUNGDAHL H. (1970) *J. Pharm. Pharmacol.* **22**, 733.

FARRIS W.A. and BLAW M.E. (1972) *Arch. Neurol. (Chic.)* **27**, 99.

FELDBERG W. and VOGT M. (1948) *J. Physiol. (Lond.)* **107**, 372.

FELDMAN R.G., MAYER R.M. and TAUB A. (1970) *Neurology (Minneap.)* **20**, 599.

FELTKAMP T.E.W., VAN DEN BERG-LOONEN P.M., NIJENHUIS L.E., ENGELFRIET, C.P., VAN ROSSUM A.L., VAN LOGHEM J.J. and OOSTERHUIS H.J.G.H. (1974) *Brit. med. J.* **1**, 131.

FERREIRA S.H. (1972) *Nature (Lond.)* **240**, 200.

FERREIRA S.H., MONCADA S. and VANE J.R. (1973) *Brit. J. Pharmacol.* **49**, 86.

FERRO MILONE F. and NORDERA G. (1973) *Excerpta med. Int. Congr. Ser.* **296**, 84.

FIBIGER H.C., McGEER E.G. and ATMADJA S. (1973) *J. Neurochem* **21**, 373.

298 *References*

Fibiger H.C., Pudritz R.E., McGeer P.L. and McGeer E.G. (1972) *J. Neurochem.* **19**, 1697.

Fingl E. (1972) In *Antiepileptic drugs*. Ed. Woodbury D.M., Penry J.K. and Schmidt R.P. Raven Press, New York.

Finke J. and Spiegelberg U. (1973) *Nervenarzt*. **44**, 104.

Finnerty F.A. (1968) *Amer. Heart J.* **75**, 559.

Fischer J.E. and James J.H. (1972) *Amer. J. Surg.* **123**, 222.

Flacke W.E., Blume R.P., Scott W.R., Foldes F.F. and Osserman K.E. (1971) *Ann. N.Y. Acad. Sci.* **183**, 316.

Flacke W.E., Caviness V.S. and Samaha F. (1966) *New Engl. J. Med.* **275**, 1207.

Fletcher E.A. and Redfern P.H. (1970) *J. Pharm. Pharmacol.* **22**, 957.

Fog R. and Pakkenberg H. (1970) *Acta neurol. scand.* **46**, 249.

Forgan-Smith R., Ellard G.A., Newton D. and Mitchison D.A. (1973) *Lancet* **2**, 374.

Förster C. (1972) *Münch. med. Wschr.* **114**, 399.

Fox J.L. (1964) *J. Neurosurg.* **21**, 909.

Frank G. (1971) *Stroke* **2**, 369.

Fraser R. (1974). Personal communication.

Freeman J.E., Johnston P.G.B. and Voke J.M. (1973) *Brit. med. J.* **4**, 523.

Freiman I. and Geefhuysen J. (1970) *J. Pediat.* **76**, 895.

Friedman A.P. (1968). In *Handbook of Clinical Neurology*, Vol. 5. Ed. Vinken P.J. and Bruyn G.W. North Holland Publishing Co, Amsterdam.

Fuxe K. and Hökfelt T. (1971) *Triangle (En.)* **10**, 74.

Galbraith A.W. (1973) *Brit. med. J.* **4**, 693.

Gallagher B.B. and Baumel I.P. (1972). In *Antiepileptic drugs*. Ed. Woodbury D.M., Penry J.K. and Schmidt R.P. Raven Press, New York.

Garattini S., Mussini E., Marcucci F. and Guaitani A. (1973). In *The Benzodiazepines*. Ed. Garattini S., Mussini E. and Randall L.O. Raven Press, New York.

Garfield J. (1969) *Brit. med. J.* **2**, 7.

Garrod L.P., O'Grady F. and Lambert H.P. (1973). *Antibiotic and chemotherapy*. Churchill–Livingstone, Edinburgh.

Gastaut H., Courjon J., Poiré R. and Weber M. (1971) *Epilepsia (Amst.)* **12**, 197.

Gastaut H., Naquet R., Poiré R. and Tassinari C.A. (1965) *Epilepsia (Amst.)* **6**, 167.

Gathier J.C. and Bruyn G.W. (1970). In *Handbook of Clinical Neurology*, Vol. 8. Ed. Vinken P.J. and Bruyn G.W. North Holland Publishing Co, Amsterdam.

Gelenberg A.J. and Poskanzer D.C. (1973) *Neurology (Minneap.)* **23**, 1313.

Gelfand M. (1973). In *Tropical Neurology*. Ed. Spillane J.D. Oxford University Press, London.

GENKINS G., KREEL I., JACOBSON E., OSSERMAN K.E. and BARONOFSKY I.D. (1960) *Bull N.Y. Acad. Med.* **36**, 826.

GERSTENBRAND F., PATEISKY K. and PROSENZ P. (1963) *Psychiat. et Neurol. (Basel)* **146**, 246.

GESCHWIND N.A. and SIMPSON J.A. (1955) *Brain* **78**, 81.

GIBBERD F.B., DUNNE J.F., HANDLEY A.J. and HAZLEMAN B.L. (1970) *Brit. med. J.* **1**, 147.

GIBBERD F.B., NAVAB F. and SMITH C.L. (1971) *J. Neurol. Neurosurg. Psychiat.* **34**, 11.

GIBBS C.J. and GAJDUSEK D.C. (1969) *Science* **165**, 1023.

GILBERT G.J. (1972) *Lancet* **2**, 234.

GILLES C.H.M. (1974) *Brit. J. Hosp. Med.* **11**, 8.

GILLIGAN B.S., VEALE J.L. and WODAK J. (1972) *Med. J. Aust.* **1**, 320.

GILMAN A. (1964) *Amer. J. Med.* **36**, 167.

GLASER G.H. (1966) *Ann. N.Y. Acad. Sci.* **135**, 335.

GLOWINSKI J. (1972). In *Perspectives in Neuropharmacology*. Ed. Snyder S.H. Oxford University Press, New York.

GODIN Y., HEINER L., MARK J. and MANDEL P. (1969) *J. Neurochem.* **16**, 869.

GODWIN-AUSTEN R.B. and CLARK T. (1971) *Brit. med. J.* **4**, 25.

GOLDBAUM L.R. and SMITH P.K. (1954) *J. Pharmacol. exp. Ther.* **111**, 197.

GOLDSTEIN G. (1965) *Med. J. Aust.* **1**, 715.

GOLDSTEIN G. and MANGANARO A. (1971) *Ann. N.Y. Acad. Sci.* **183**, 230.

GOMERSHALL J.D. and STUART A. (1973) *J. Neurol. Neurosurg. Psychiat.* **36**, 684.

GOMPERTZ D. (1972). In *Eighth symposium on advanced medicine*. Ed. Neale G. Pitman, London.

GOODELL H., LEWONTIN R. and WOLFF H.G. (1953) *Res. Publ. Ass. nerv. ment. Dis.* **33**, 346.

GOODMAN L.S. and GILMAN A. (1970). *The Pharmacological Basis of Therapeutics*. Macmillan, London.

GORDON A. and PARSONS M. (1972) *Brit. J. Hosp. Med.* **7**, 651.

GRAHAM J.R. and WOLFF H.G. (1938) *Arch. Neurol. Psychiat.* **39**, 737.

GRANT R.H.E. and STORES O.P.R. (1970) *Brit. med. J.* **4**, 644.

GREENFIELD J.G. (1955). In *James Parkinson 1755–1824*. Ed. Macdonald Critchley. Macmillan, London.

GREER M. (1968) *Clin. Neurosurg.* **15**, 161.

GROB D. (1971) *Ann. N.Y. Acad. Sci.* **183**, 248.

GROB D. and NAMBA T. (1966) *J. Amer. med. Ass.* **198**, 703.

GROB D., NAMBA T., BRUNNER N.G. and BERGER C.L. (1973) *Excerpta med. Int. Congr. Ser.* **296**, 83.

GUZMAN F. and LIM R.K.S. (1968) *Med. Clin. N. Amer.* **52**, 3.

HAAN D. and TILSNER V. (1966) *Med. Klin.* **61**, 1184.

HAAS D.C. (1973) *Neurology (Minneap.)* **23**, 55.

HAGBERG B. (1968) *Develop. Med. Child Neurol.* **10**, 302.

HAHN T.J., BIRGE S.J., SCHARP C.R. and AVIOLI L.V. (1972) *J. clin. Invest.* **51**, 741.

HAIRE M., FRASER K.B. and MILLAR J.H.D. (1973) *Brit. med. J.* **3**, 612.

HAMILTON C.H., SHELLEY W.M. and TUMULTY P.A. (1971) *Medicine (Baltimore)* **50**, 1.

HAMOEN A.M. (1973) *Brit. med. J.* **3**, 272.

HANINGTON E. (1967) *Brit. med. J.* **2**, 550.

HARRIS E.L. and FITZGERALD J.D. (1970). *The principles and practice of clinical trials.* Livingstone, Edinburgh.

HARRISON M.J.G., BROWNBILL D., LEWIS P.D. and ROSS RUSSELL R.W. (1973) *Arch. Neurol. (Chic.)* **28**, 389.

HARRISON M.J.G., MARSHALL J., MEADOWS J.C. and ROSS RUSSELL R.W. (1971) *Lancet* **2**, 743.

HARVEY P. (1974). Personal communication.

HEAD J.M. (1964) *Ann. Surg.* **160**, 123.

HEBB C. (1970) *Ann. Rev. Physiol.* **32**, 165.

HEBB C.O. and WAITES G.M.H. (1956) *J. Physiol. (Lond.)* **132**, 667.

HEFFRON W. and EATON R.P. (1970) *Ann. intern. Med.* **73**, 425.

HEIKKILA R.E. and COHEN G. (1972) *Europ. J. Pharmacol.* **20**, 156.

HEILMAN K.M., KOLLER W.C. and LE MASTER P.C. (1971) *Neurology (Minneap.)* **21**, 963.

HEIMANS R.L.H., RAND M.J. and FENNESSY M.R. (1972) *J. Pharm. Pharmacol.* **24**, 875.

HENNING M. and RUBENSON A. (1970) *J. Pharm. Pharmacol.* **22**, 241.

HERKOVITS E. and BLACKWOOD W. (1969) *J. Neurol. Neurosurg. Psychiat.* **32**, 509.

HERNDON J.H., STEINBERG D. and UHLENDORF B.W. (1969) *New Engl. J. Med.* **281**, 1034.

HERTTING G., AXELROD J. and WHITBY L.G. (1961) *J. Pharmacol. exp. Ther.* **134**, 146.

HINCHCLIFFE R. (1972) *Acta oto-laryng. (Stockh.)* Suppl. 305, 10.

HINTON J.M. (1963) *Brit. J. Pharmacol.* **20**, 319.

HIPPIUS v. H. and LOGEMAN G. (1970) *Arzneimittelforsch* **20**, 894.

HISHIKAWA Y., IDA H., NAKAI K. and KANEKO Z. (1966) *J. neurol. Sci.* **3**, 453.

HITCHCOCK E. and PRANDINI M.N. (1973) *Lancet* **1**, 310.

HOEHN M.M. and YAHR M.D. (1969). In *Third Symposium on Parkinson's Disease.* Ed. Gillingham F.J. and Donaldson I.M.L. Livingstone, Edinburgh.

HÖKFELT T. (1968) *Z. Zellforsch* **91**, 1.

HÖKFELT T. and FUXE K. (1972). In *Brain–Endocrine Interaction.* Ed. Knigge K.M., Scott D.E. and Weindl A. Karger, Basel.

HÖKFELT T. and LJUNGDAHL Å. (1972). In *Studies of neurotransmitters at the synaptic level.* Ed. Costa E., Iversen L.L. and Paoletti R. Raven Press, New York.

HONDA H. and GINDIN A. (1972) *J. Amer. med. Ass.* **219**, 55.

HOOSHMAND H. (1972a) *Arch. Neurol. (Chic.)* **27**, 205.

HOOSHMAND H. (1972b) *Neurology (Minneap.)* **22**, 451.

HOOSHMAND H., DOVE J., HOUFF S. and SUTER C. (1969) *Arch. Neurol. (Chic.)* **21**, 499.

HORNYKIEWICZ O. (1966) *Pharmacol. Rev.* **18**, 925.

HORTON E.W. (1973) *Brit. med. Bull.* **29**, 148.

HOUGHTON G.W. and RICHENS A. (1974) *Brit. J. clin. Pharmacol.* **1**, 155.

HOWSE P.M. and MATTHEWS W.B. (1973) *J. Neurol. Neurosurg. Psychiat.* **36**, 27.

HÜBBE P. (1973) *Acta neurol. scand.* **49**, 108.

HUDGSON P. and WEIGHTMAN D. (1971) *Brit. med. J.* **4**, 15.

HUDGSON P., WEIGHTMAN D. and CARTLIDGE N.E.F. (1972) *Postgrad. med. J.* Suppl. 5, **48**, 37.

HUGHES I.E., SMITH H. and KANE P.O. (1962) *Lancet* **1**, 616.

HUGHES R.C., POLGAR J.G., WEIGHTMAN D. and WALTON J.N. (1971) *Brit. med. J.* **2**, 487.

HUMPHREY J.G. (1973) *Excerpta med. Int. Congr. Ser.* **296**, 84.

HUNT T.E. and HADER W.J. (1966) *Med. Serv. J. Can.* **22**, 548.

HUNTER K.R. (1973). In *Progress in the treatment of Parkinsonism*. Ed. Calne D.B. Raven Press, New York.

HUNTER K.R., LAURENCE D.R., HOLLMAN A. and STERN G.M. (1971) *Lancet* **1**, 932.

HUNTER K.R., LAURENCE D.R., SHAW K.M. and STERN G.M. (1973) *Lancet* **2**, 929.

HUNTER R., BLACKWOOD W., SMITH M.C. and CUMMINGS J.N. (1968) *J. neurol. Sci.* **7**, 263.

IGGO A. (1972). In *Pain*. Ed. Janzen R., Keidel W.D., Herz A., Steichele C., Payne J.P. and Burt R.A.P. Churchill, London.

ILLINGWORTH R.D. (1973) *Brit. J. Hosp. Med.* **9**, 589.

ILLIS L.S. (1967). In *Modern trends in neurology*, Vol. 4. Ed. Williams D. Butterworths, London.

ILLIS L.S. and GOSTLING J.V.T. (1972). *Herpes simplex encephalitis*. Scientechnica, Bristol.

ILLIS L.S. and MERRY R.T.G. (1972) *J. roy. Coll. Phycns. London* **7**, 34.

INMAN T. (1862). In *A year book of medicine, surgery and allied sciences for 1862*. New Sydenham Society, London.

IVERSEN L.L. (1967) *The uptake and storage of noradrenaline in sympathetic nerves*. Cambridge University Press, Cambridge.

IVERSEN L.L. (1970) *Advanc. Biochem. Psychopharmacol.* **2**, 109.

IVERSEN L.L. (1972). In *Perspectives in Neuropharmacology*. Ed. Snyder S.H. Oxford University Press, New York.

IVERSEN L.L. (1973) *Brit. med. Bull.* **29**, 130.

302　　　　　　　　　*References*

JASPER H.H., WARD A.A. and POPE A. (1969). *Basic Mechanisms of the Epilepsies.* Little, Brown, Boston.

JEAVONS P.M. and BOWER B.D. (1964). *Infantile spasms. Clinics in developmental medicine, No. 15.* Spastics society and William Heinemann, London.

JEAVONS P.M. and CLARK J.E. (1974) *Brit. med. J.* **2,** 584.

JENKINS R.B. (1972) *Lancet* **1,** 765.

JENKINS R.B., MENDELSON S.H., LAMID S. and KLAWANS H.L. (1972) *Brit. med. J.* **3,** 512.

JENKINSON D.H. (1973) *Brit. med. Bull.* **29,** 142.

JOHNSON R.T. and RICHARDSON E.P. (1968) *Medicine (Baltimore)* **47,** 337.

JOHNSTON I. (1973) *Lancet* **2,** 418.

JUEL-JENSEN B.E. and MACCALLUM F.O. (1972). *Herpes simplex, varicella and zoster.* William Heinemann, London.

KAKULAS B.A. (1966a) *Nature (Lond.)* **210,** 1115.

KAKULAS B.A. (1966b) *J. Path. Bact.* **91,** 495.

KALBAG R.M. and WOOLF A.L. (1972). In *Handbook of Clinical Neurology,* Vol. 12. Ed. Vinken P.J. and Bruyn G.W. North Holland Publishing Co, Amsterdam.

KALSER S.C. and McLAIN P.L. (1970) *Clin. Pharmacol. Ther.* **11,** 214.

KARAT A.B.A., JEEVARATNAM A., KARAT S. and RAO P.S.S. (1970) *Brit. med. J.* **1,** 198.

KARAT A.B.A., JEEVARATNAM A., KARAT S. and RAO P.S.S. (1971) *Brit. med. J.* **4,** 514.

KATZ B. (1966). *Muscle, nerve and synapse.* McGraw-Hill, New York.

KAY H.E.M., KNAPTON P.J., O'SULLIVAN J.P., WELLS D.G., HARRIS R.F., INNES E.M., STUART J., SCHWARTZ F.C.M. and THOMPSON E.N. (1972) *Arch. Dis. Childh.* **47,** 344.

KAZAMATSURI H., CHIEN C. and COLE J.O. (1972a) *Arch. gen. Psychiat.* **27,** 95.

KAZAMATSURI H., CHIEN C. and COLE J.O. (1972b) *Arch. gen. Psychiat.* **27,** 100.

KEARY E.M. and MAXWELL D.R. (1967) *Brit. J. Pharmacol.* **30,** 400.

KEBABIAN J.W., PETZOLD G.L. and GREENGARD P. (1972) *Proc. nat. Acad. Sci. (Wash.)* **69,** 2145.

KEELE C.A. (1969) *Proc. roy. Soc. Med.* **62,** 535.

KELLY R.E. and GAUTIER-SMITH P.C. (1959) *Lancet* **2,** 1102.

KEMPER J.W., BAGGENSTOSS A.H. and SLOCUMB C.H. (1957) *Ann. intern. Med.* **46,** 831.

KERTESZ A. (1967) *Neurology (Minneap.)* **17,** 680.

KETY S.S. (1965). In *Isotopes in Experimental Pharmacology.* Ed. Roth L.J. University of Chicago Press, Chicago.

KILLAM K.F., KILLAM E.K. and NAQUET R. (1967). *Electroenceph. clin. Neurophysiol.* **22,** 497.

KIMBALL R.W., FRIEDMAN A.P. and VALLEJO E. (1960) *Neurology (Minneap.)* **10,** 107.

KING T.T. (1973) *Brit.J. Hosp. Med.* **10**, 250.

KLAUS W., LÜLLMANN H. and MUSCHOLL E. (1960) *Pflügers Arch. ges. Physiol.* **271**, 761.

KLAWANS H. (1973). *The pharmacology of extrapyramidal movement disorders.* Karger, Basel.

KLAWANS H.L., ILAHI M.M. and SHENKER D. (1970a) *Acta neurol. scand.* **46,** 409.

KLAWANS H.L. and McKENDALL R.R. (1971) *J. neurol. Sci.* **14**, 189.

KLAWANS H.L., PAULSON G.W. and BARBEAU A. (1970b) *Lancet* **2**, 1185.

KLAWANS H.L. and RUBOVITS R. (1972) *Neurology (Minneap.)* **22**, 107.

KLEIJN E. VAN DER (1968) *Arch. int. Pharmacodyn.* **179**, 225.

KLEIN J.O., HERSCHEL M., THERAKAN R.M. and INGALL D. (1971) *J. infect. Dis.* **124**, Suppl. 124, 224.

KLOCKHOFF I. and LINDBLOM U. (1966) *Acta oto-laryng. (Stockh.)* **61**, 459.

KNUDSEN E.A. and AASTRUP B. (1965) *Brit. J. vener. Dis.* **41**, 177.

KNUTSSON E., LINDBLOM U. and MARTENSSON A. (1973) *Brain* **96**, 29.

KOCEN R.S. and PARSONS M. (1970) *Quart. J. med.* **39**, 17.

KOELLE G.B. (1970). In *The pharmacological basis of therapeutics.* Ed. Goodman L.S. and Gilman A. Macmillan, London.

KOOIKER J.C. and SUMI S.M. (1974) *Neurology (Minneap.)* **24**, 68.

KOPIN I.J. (1972). In *Perspectives in Neuropharmacology.* Ed. Snyder S.H. Oxford University Press, New York.

KORCZYN A.D. (1971) *Brit. med. J.* **2**, 590.

KORCZYN A.D. (1972) *Neuropharmacology* **11**, 601.

KORCZYN A.D. and GOLDBERG G.J. (1972) *Brit. J. Psychiat.* **121**, 75.

KOREY S.R. (1951) *Proc. Soc. exp. Biol. (N.Y.)* **76**, 297.

KORNFELD P., SOMLYO A. and OSSERMAN K.E. (1969) *Arch. Neurol. (Chic.)* **21,** 466.

KORNFELD P., SAMUELS A.J., WOLF R.L. and OSSERMAN K.E. (1970) *Neurology (Minneap.)* **20**, 634.

KRAYENBÜHL H. (1967) *Clin. Neurosurg.* **14**, 1.

KRUSE R. (1968) *Mschr. Kinderheilk* **116**, 378.

KURTZKE J.F., BEEBE G.W., NAGLER B., NEFZGER M.D., AUTH T.L. and KURLAND L.T. (1970) *Arch. Neurol. (Chic.)* **22**, 215.

KUTT H. (1971) *Ann. N.Y. Acad. Sci.* **179**, 704.

KUTT H., WINTERS W., KOKENGE R. and McDOWELL F. (1964) *Arch. Neurol. (Chic.)* **11**, 642.

LADER M. (1970) *J. roy. Coll. Phycns. Lond.* **5**, 87.

LADURON P. (1971) *Clin. Trials J.* **8**, Suppl. 2, 19.

LAMBERT E.H. (1966) *Ann. N.Y. Acad. Sci.* **135**, 367.

LAMBERT E.H. and ELMQVIST D. (1971) *Ann. N.Y. Acad. Sci.* **183**, 183.

LAMBERT E.H. and ROOKE E.D. (1965). In *Remote effects of cancer on the nervous system.* Ed. Lord Brain and Norris F.H. Grune and Stratton, New York.

LAMBERT H.P. (1974) *Brit. J. Hosp. Med.* **11**, 268.

LANCE J.W. (1969). *The mechanism and management of headache*. Butterworths, London.

LANCE J.W. and ANTHONY M. (1970) *Brit. med. J.* **2**, 327.

LANGER S.Z. and TRENDELENBURG U. (1968) *J. Pharmacol. exp. Ther.* **163**, 290.

LAPIDES J., SWEET R.B. and LEWIS L.W. (1957) *J. Urol.* **77**, 247.

LAURENCE D.R. (1973). *Clinical Pharmacology*. Churchill, London.

LAVERTY R. (1973) *Brit. med. Bull.* **29**, 152.

LAXENAIRE M., TRIDON P. and POIRE P. (1966) *Acta psychiat. scand.* **42**, Suppl. 192, 137.

LAYZER R.B. and ROWLAND L.P. (1971) *New Engl. J. Med.* **285**, 31.

LEES G.M., KOSTERLITZ H.W. and WATERFIELD A.A. (1972). In *Agonist and antagonist actions of narcotic analgesic drugs*. Ed. Kosterlitz H.W., Collier H.O.J. and Villareal J.E. Macmillan, London.

LEIBOWITZ U., KAHANA E. and ALTER M. (1969) *Brain* **92**, 115.

LENNOX W.J. (1945) *J. Amer. med. Ass.* **129**, 1069.

LEPPER M.H. and DOWLING H.F. (1951) *Arch. intern. Med.* **88**, 489.

LE QUESNE P.M. (1970) In *Handbook of Clinical Neurology*, Vol. 7. Ed. Vinken P.J. and Bruyn G.W. North Holland Publishing Co, Amsterdam.

LE QUESNE P.M. (1974). In *Peripheral Neuropathy*. Ed. Dyck P.J., Thomas P.K. and Lambert E.H. Saunders, Philadelphia.

LEVY L.L. and FENICHEL G.M. (1965) *Neurology (Minneap.)* **15**, 716.

LEWIS P.D. and HARRISON M.J.G. (1969) *Brit. med. J.* **4**, 404.

LEYBURN P. and WALTON J.N. (1959) *Brain* **82**, 81.

LICHTENSTEIGER W., MUTZNER V. and LANGEMAN N. (1967) *J. Neurochem.* **14**, 489.

LIDBRINK P., CORRODI H., FUXE K. and OLSON L. (1973). In *The Benzodiazepines*. Ed. Garattini S., Mussini E. and Randall L.O. Raven Press, New York.

LIM R.K.S., GUZMAN F., RODGERS D.W., GOTO K., BRAUN C., DICKERSON G.D. and ENGLE R.J. (1964) *Arch. int. Pharmacodyn.* **152**, 25.

LIPTON S. (1973) *Brit. J. Hosp. Med.* **9**, 583.

LITHANDER A. (1966). *Antimicrobial agents and chemotherapy—1965*, 435.

LIVETT B.G. (1973) *Brit. med. Bull.* **29**, 93.

LLOYD K.G., DAVIDSON L. and HORNYKIEWICZ O. (1973). In *Progress in the treatment of Parkinsonism*. Ed. Calne D.B. Raven Press, New York.

LOCOCK C. (1857) *Lancet* **1**, 528.

LØMO T. and ROSENTHAL J. (1971) *J. Physiol. (Lond.)* **216**, 52D.

LONG D.M., MAXWELL R.E. and FRENCH L.A. (1972). In *Steroids and brain edema*. Ed. Reulen H.J. and Schürmann K. Springer-Verlag, Berlin.

LORENTZ I.T. (1966) *Bull. post-grad. Comm. Med. Univ. Sydney* **22**, 31.

LORENTZ DE HAAS A.M. and KUILMAN M. (1964) *Epilepsia* **5**, 90.

LOUGHNAN P.M., GOLD H. and VANCE J.C. (1973) *Lancet* **1**, 70.

LOUS P. (1954) *Acta pharmacol. (Kbh)* **10**, 147.

LOVELACE R.E. and HOROWITZ S.K. (1968) *Arch. Neurol. (Chic.)* **18**, 69.

LUND M. and TROLLE E. (1973) *Acta neurol. scand.* **49**, Suppl. 53, 82.

LUNDBERG P.O. (1962) *Acta endocr.* (*Kbh.*) **40**, Suppl. 68, 5.

LUNDE P.K.M., RANE A., YAFFE S.J., LUND S.J. and SJOQVIST F. (1970) *Clin. Pharmacol. Ther.* **11**, 846.

LYON R.L. (1962) *Brit. med. J.* **1**, 1308.

LYTLE R.B. and WELLBAND W.A. (1970) *Anat. Rec.* **166**, 339.

MACCOLLUM W.A.G. (1970) *Brit. med. J.* **1**, 760.

MACFADYEN D.J., REEVE C.E., BRATTY P.J.A. and THOMAS J.W. (1973) *Neurology* (*Minneap.*) **23**, 592.

MALAVIYA A.N., MANY A. and SCHWARTZ R.S. (1968) *Lancet* **2**, 485.

MANGI R.J., KUNDARGI R.S., QUINTILIANI R. and ANDRIOLE V.T. (1973) *Ann. intern. Med.* **78**, 347.

MARCUCCI F., GUAITANI A., FANELLI R., MUSSINI E. and GARATTINI S. (1971) *Europ. J. Pharmacol.* **20**, 1711.

MARGULIES M.E. and SLADE W.R. (1968) *Clin. Med.* **75**, 47.

MARSDEN C.D. (1973) *Proc. roy. Soc. Med.* **66**, 871.

MARSDEN C.D., FOLEY T.H., OWEN D.A.L. and McALLISTER R.G. (1967) *Clin. Sci.* **33**, 53.

MARSDEN C.D. and MEADOWS J.C. (1970) *J. Physiol.* (*Lond.*) **207**, 429.

MARSDEN C.D., REYNOLDS E.H., PARSONS V., HARRIS R. and DUCHEN L. (1973) *Brit. med. J.* **4**, 526.

MARSHALL J. (1968). *The management of cerebrovascular disease.* Churchill, London.

MARSHALL J. (1972). In *Handbook of Clinical Neurology*, Vol. 12. Ed. Vinken P.J. and Bruyn G.W. North Holland Publishing Co, Amsterdam.

MARSHALL J. (1973a) *Brit. J. Hosp. Med.* **10**, 240.

MARSHALL J. (1973b) *Excerpta med. Int. Congr. Ser.* **296**, 27.

MARTIN J.B. (1973) *New Engl. J. Med.* **288**, 1384.

MARTIN W.R. and JASINSKI D.R. (1972). In *Pain.* Ed. Janzen R., Keidel W.D., Herz A., Steichele C., Payne J.P. and Burt R.A.P. Churchill, London.

MARTINDALE W. (1973). *The Extra Pharmacopoeia.* The Pharmaceutical Press, London.

MATHEW N.T. and CHANDY J. (1970) *J. neurol. Sci.* **11**, 243.

MATHEW N.T., MEYER J.S., RIVERA V.M., CHARNEY J.Z. and HARTMAN A. (1972) *Lancet* **2**, 1327.

MATTHEW H. (1972). Medicine (London). No. 4, 273.

MATTHEWS F.P. (1958) *Amer. J. Psychiat.* **114**, 1034.

MATTHEWS P.B.C. and RUSHWORTH G. (1957) *J. Physiol.* (*Lond.*) **135**, 263.

MATTHEWS W.B. (1958) *Brain* **81**, 193.

MATTHEWS W.B. (1965) *J. Neurol. Neurosurg. Psychiat.* **28**, 23.

MATTHEWS W.B., RUSHWORTH G. and WAKEFIELD G.S. (1972) *Acta neurol. scand.* **48**, 635.

MATTSON R.H. (1972). In *Antiepileptic Drugs.* Ed. Woodbury D.M., Penry J.K. Schmidt R.P. Raven Press, New York.

MAXWELL D.R. and RHODES K.F. (1970) *Brit. J. Pharmacol.* **39**, 520.

MAXWELL D.R. and SUMPTER E.A. (1974) *Brit. J. Pharmacol.* **50**, 355.

MAXWELL R.E., Long D.M. and FRENCH L.A. (1972). In *Steroids and brain edema*. Ed. Reulen H.J. and Schürmann K. Springer-Verlag, Berlin.

MAYNERT E.W. (1969) *Epilepsia (Amst.)* **10**, 145.

MAYNERT E.W. (1972). In *Antiepileptic drugs*. Ed. Woodbury D.M., Penry J.K. and Schmidt R.P. Raven Press, New York.

MAYNERT E.W. and VAN DYKE H.B. (1949) *Pharmacol. Rev.* **1**, 217.

MCAFEE D.A. and GREENGARD P. (1972) *Science* **178**, 310.

MCALPINE D., LUMSDEN C.E. and ACHESON D. (1965). *Multiple Sclerosis: a reappraisal*. Livingstone, Edinburgh.

MCARDLE B. (1969). In *Disorders of voluntary muscle*. Ed. Walton J.N. Churchill, London.

MCCULLOCH M.W., RAND M.J. and STOREY D.F. (1973) *Brit. J. Pharmacol.* **49**, 141P.

MCDOWELL F.H. (1971). In *Cecil-Loeb Textbook of Medicine*. Ed. Beeson P.B. and McDermott W. Saunders, Philadelphia.

MCDOWELL F.H. and BARBEAU A. (1974) *Second Canadian–American Conference on Parkininson's Disease*. Raven Press, New York.

MCDOWELL F.H. and MARKHAM C.H. (1971). *Recent advances in Parkinson's disease*. Blackwell, Oxford.

MCLELLAN D.L. (1973a) *J. Neurol. Neurosurg. Psychiat.* **36**, 342.

MCLELLAN D.L. (1973b) *J. Neurol. Neurosurg. Psychiat.* **36**, 555.

MCLELLAN D.L. (1973c) *Brit. med. J.* **3**, 634.

MCLELLAN D.L., CHALMERS R.J. and JOHNSON J.H. (1974) *Lancet* **1**, 104.

MCLENNAN H. and YORK D.H. (1967) *J. Physiol. (Lond.)* **189**, 393.

MEINARDI H. (1972). In *Antiepileptic drugs*. Ed. Woodbury D.M., Penry, J.K. and Schmidt R.P. Raven Press, New York.

MELDRUM B.S., BALZAMO E., WADA J.A. and VUILLON-CACCIUTTOLO G. (1972) *Physiol. Behav.* **9**, 615.

MELDRUM B.S. and BRIERLEY J.B. (1973) *Arch. Neurol. (Chic.)* **28**, 10.

MELMON K.L. and MORELLI H.F. (1972). *Clinical Pharmacology*. Macmillan, N.Y.

MELZACK R. and Wall P.D. (1962) *Brain* **85**, 331.

MELZACK R. and WALL P.D. (1965) *Science* **150**, 971.

MERRILL J.P. (1970). In *Harrison's principles of internal medicine*. Ed. Wintrobe M.M., Thorn G.W., Adams R.D., Bennett I. L., Braunwald E., Isselbacher K.J. and Petersdorf R.G. McGraw-Hill, New York.

MERRITT H.H. and PUTNAM T.J. (1938) *J. Amer. med. Ass.* **111**, 1068.

MERSKEY H. (1973) *Brit. J. Hosp. Med.* **9**, 574.

MERSKEY H. and HESTER R.N. (1972) *Postgrad. med. J.* **48**, 594.

MERTIN J., SHENTON B.K. and FIELD E.J. (1973) *Brit. med. J.* **2**, 777.

MEYER J.S., GILROY J., BARNHART M.E. and JOHNSON J.F. (1965). In *Cerebral Vascular Diseases*. Ed. Millikan C. H., Sickert R. G. and Whisnant J.P. Grune and Stratton, New York.

MEYLER L. and PECK H.M. (1972). *Drug Induced Diseases.* Vol. 4. Excerpta Medica, Amsterdam.

MIKKELSEN B. and BIRKET-SMITH, E. (1973) *Acta neurol. scand.* **49,** Suppl. 53,91.

MILEDI R. (1960) *J. Physiol. (Lond.)* **151,** 1.

MILEDI R. and POTTER L.T. (1971) *Nature (Lond.)* **233,** 599.

MILLAR J.H.D., VAS C.J., NORONHA M.J., LIVERSEDGE L.A. and RAWSON M.D. (1967) *Lancet* **2,** 429.

MILLAR J.H.D., ZILKHA K.J., LANGMAN M.J.S., PAYLING WRIGHT H., SMITH A.D., BELIN J. and THOMPSON R.H.S. (1973) *Brit. med. J.* **1,** 765.

MILLER E., WIENER L. and BLOOMFIELD D. (1973) *Arch. Neurol. (Chic.)* **29,** 99.

MILLER H., NEWELL D.J. and RIDLEY A. (1961) *Lancet* **2,** 1120.

MILLER H., SIMPSON C.A. and YEATES W.K. (1965) *Brit. med. J.* **1,** 1265.

MILLER FISHER C., MOHR J.P. and ADAMS R.D. (1970). In *Harrison's principles of internal medicine.* Ed. Wintrobe M.M., Thorn G.W., Adams R.D., Bennett I.L., Braunwald E., Isselbacher K.J. and Petersdorf R.G. McGraw-Hill, New York.

MILLIKAN C.H. (1971) *Stroke* **2,** 201.

MINOT A.S., DODD K. and RIVEN S.S. (1939) *J. Amer. med. Ass.* **113,** 553.

MITCHELL J.R., ARIAS L. and OATES J.A. (1967) *J. Amer. med. Ass.* **202,** 973.

MONES R.J. (1973) *J. Neurol. Neurosurg. Psychiat.* **36,** 362.

MORGAN M.H., HEWER R.L. and COOPER R. (1973) *J. Neurol. Neurosurg. Psychiat.* **36,** 618.

MORELL F., BRADLEY W. and PTASHNE M. (1958) *Neurology (Minneap.)* **8,** 140.

MORRISON A.B. and WEBSTER R.A. (1973) *Neuropharmacology* **12,** 715.

MORSELLI P.L., CASSANO G.B., PLACIDI G.F., MUSCETTOLA G.B. and RIZZO M. (1973). In *The Benzodiazepines.* Ed. Garattini S., Mussini E. and Randall L.O., Raven Press, New York.

MORSELLI P.L., RIZZO M. and GARATTINI S. (1971) *Ann. N.Y. Acad. Sci.* **179,** 88.

MORZARIA R.N., WALTON I.G. and PICKERING D. (1969) *Brit. med. J.* **2,** 511.

MULDER D.G., BRAITMAN H., LI W. and HERRMANN C. (1972) *J. thorac. cardiovasc. Surg.* **63,** 105.

MUNSAT T.L. (1967) *Neurology (Minneap.)* **17,** 359.

MUNTHE-KAAS A.W. and STRANDJORD, R.E. (1973) *Acta neurol. scand.* **49,** Suppl. 53, 97.

MUSACCHIO J.M., KOPIN I.J. and WEISE V.K. (1965) *J. Pharmacol. exp. Ther.* **148,** 22.

MUSCHOLL E. and MAITRE L. (1963) *Experientia (Basel)* **19,** 658.

NAESTOFT J., LUND M., LARSEN N.E. and HVIDBERG E. (1973) *Acta neurol. scand.* **49,** Suppl. 53, 103.

NAKAE K., YAMAMOTO S., SHIGEMATSU I. and KONO R. (1973) *Lancet* **1,** 171.

NAMBA T., BRUNNER N.G., SHAPIRO M.J. and GROB D. (1971) *Neurology (Minneap.)* **21,** 1008.

NASHOLD B.S. and FRIEDMAN H. (1972) *J. Neurosurg.* **36,** 590.

NATHAN P.W. (1965) *Brit. med. J.* **1,** 1096.

NATHAN P.W. and SEARS T.A. (1963) *Anaesthesia* **18,** 467.

NATHAN P.W., SEARS T A. and SMITH M.C. (1965) *J. neurol. Sci.* **2,** 7.

NEARY D., THURSTON H. and POHL J.E.F. (1973) *Brit. med. J.* **3,** 474.

NEMETZ P.S. (1969) *Brit. med. J.* **1,** 186.

NEVILLE B.G.R. and WILSON J. (1970) *Brit. med. J.* **3,** 554.

NEWMAN R.L. and HOLT R.J. (1971) *J. infect. Dis.* **124,** Suppl. 124, 254.

NG K.Y., COLBURN R.W. and KOPIN I.J. (1971) *Nature (Lond.)* **230,** 331.

NICHOLLS J.G. (1956) *J. Physiol. (Lond.)* **131,** 1.

NICK J. and NICOLLE M.H. (1964) *Bull. Soc. méd. Hôp., Paris* **115,** 275.

NOACH E.L., WOODBURY D.M. and GOODMAN L.S. (1958) *J. Pharmacol. exp. Ther.* **122,** 301.

NORRELL H., WILSON C.B., SLAGEL D.E. and CLARK D.B. (1974) *Cancer (Philad.)* **33,** 923.

NYBACK H., SEDVALL G. and KOPIN I.J. (1967) *Life Sci.* **6,** 2307.

NYHAN W.L. (1972) *Arch. intern. Med.* **130,** 186.

OHYE C., BOUCHARD R., BOUCHER R. and POIRIER L.J. (1970) *J. Pharmacol. exp. Ther.* **195,** 700.

OLDENDORF W.H. (1971) *Trans. Amer. neurol. Ass.* **96,** 46.

OLDENDORF W.H. (1973a) *Amer. J. Physiol.* **224,** 967.

OLDENDORF W.H. (1973b) *Amer. J. Physiol.* **224,** 1450.

OLSON M.E., CHERNICK N.L. & POSNER J.B. (1974) *Arch. Neruol. (Chic.)* **30,** 122.

ORME M.L'E. (1972) *Medicine (London)* No. 4, 302.

ORTH D.N., ALMEIDA H., WALSH F.B. and HONDA M. (1967). *J. Amer. med. Ass.* **201,** 485.

OSBORNE R.H. and BRADFORD H.F. (1973) *Nature (Lond.)* **244,** 157.

OSSERMAN K.E. and GENKINS G. (1963) *J. Amer. med. Ass.* **183,** 97.

OSSERMAN K.E. and GENKINS G. (1966) *J. Amer. med. Ass.* **198,** 699.

OSTFELD A.M. (1962). *The common headache syndromes: Biochemistry, pathophysiology, therapy.* Thomas, Springfield.

OXBURY J.M. (1974) Personal communication.

PAKKENBERG H. (1968) *Acta neurol. scand.* **44,** 391.

PALLIS C.A. and LEWIS P.D. (1974) *The Neurology of Gastrointestinal Disease.* Saunders, London.

PALLIS C. and RICE-EDWARDS M. (1974) Raised Intracranial Pressure. In *Modern Radiotherapy.* Ed. Deeley T.J. Butterworth, London.

PALMER K.N.V. (1965) *Lancet* **1,** 733.

PAPATESTAS A.E., ALPERT L.I., OSSERMAN K.E., OSSERMAN R.S. and KARK A.E. (1971) *Amer. J. Med.* **50,** 465.

PAPPAS G.D. and WAXMAN S.G. (1972) In *Structure and function of synapses.* Ed. Pappas G.D. and Purpura D.P. Raven Press, New York.

PARKES J.D., SHARPSTONE P. and WILLIAMS R. (1970) *Lancet* **2**, 1341.

PARKS L.C., WATANABE A.M. and KOPIN I.J. (1970) *Lancet* **2**, 1014.

PARSONAGE M. (1972) In *Tegretol in Epilepsy*. Ed. Wink C.A.S. Nicholls, Manchester.

PARSONAGE M. (1973) *Brit. J. Hosp. Med.* **9**, 613.

PARSONAGE M.J. and NORRIS J.W. (1967) *Brit. med. J.* **3**, 85.

PATERSON J. (1972) *Medicine (London)* No. 4, 294.

PATERSON R., DE PASQUALE N. and MANN S. (1961) *Medicine (Baltimore)* **40**, 95.

PATTEN J., MENDALL B., BRUUN B., CURTIN W. and CARTER S..(1972) In *Steroids and brain edema*. Ed. Reulen, H.J. and Schürmann K. Springer-Verlag, Berlin.

PEARCE J. (1972) *Psychiat. et Neurol. (Basel)* **3**, 3.

PEARSON C.M. (1969) In *Disorders of voluntary muscle*, Ed. Walton J.N. Churchill, London.

PEDERSEN E., ARLIEN-SOBERG P., GRYNDERUP V. and HENRIKSEN O. (1970) *Acta neurol. scand.* **46**, 257.

PENMAN J. (1968) In *Handbook of Clinical Neurology*, Vol. 5. Ed. Vinken P.J. and Bruyn G.W. North Holland Publishing Co, Amsterdam.

PERRY T.L., HANSEN S. and KLOSTER M. (1973) *New Engl. J. Med.* **288**, 337.

PFEFFER M., SCHOR J.M., BOLTON S. and JACOBSEN R. (1968) *J. pharm. Sci.* **58**, 1375.

PHILIPSZOON A.J. (1962) *Clin. Pharmacol. Ther.* **3**, 184.

PHILLIS J.W. (1970) *The Pharmacology of Synapses*. Pergamon, Oxford.

PHILLIS J.W. and YORK D.H. (1968) *Brain Res.* **10**, 297.

PINCUS J.H., REYNOLDS E.H. and GLASER G.H. (1972) *J. Amer. med. Ass.* **221**, 496.

PINELLI P. (1973) In *The Benzodiazepines*. Ed. Garattini S., Mussini E. and Randall L.O. Raven Press, New York.

PINELLI P., TONALI P. and SCOPPETTA C. (1973) *Excerpta med. Int. Congr. Ser.* **296**, 85.

PLETSCHER A. (1969) In *Psychotropic drugs and dysfunction of the basal ganglia*. Ed. Crane G.E. and Gardner R. National Institute of Mental Health, Bethesda.

PLUM F. (1962) In *Modern trends in Neurology*, Vol. 3. Ed. Williams D. Butterworths, London.

PLUM F., ALVORD E.C. and POSNER J.B. (1963) *Arch. Neurol. (Chic.)* **9**, 571.

PLUM F. and POSNER J.B. (1966) *Diagnosis of stupor and coma*. Davis, Philadelphia.

PODIVINSKÝ F. (1968) In *Handbook of Clinical Neurology*. Vol. 6. Ed. Vinken P.J. and Bruyn G.W. North Holland Publishing Co, Amsterdam.

POIRIER L.J., LANGELIER P., ROBERGE A., BOUCHER R. and KITSIKIS A. (1972) *J. neurol. Sci.* **16**, 401.

POIRIER L.J., SINGH P., SOURKES T.L. and BOUCHER R. (1967) *Brain Res.* **6**, 654.

PONCE P.L. (1972) In *Antiepileptic drugs*. Ed. Woodbury D.M. Penry J.K., Schmidt R.P. Raven Press, New York.

POSER C.M. (1972) *Med. Clin. N. Amer.* **56**, 1343.

POSKANZER D.C. and KERR D.N.S. (1961) *Amer. J. med.* **31**, 328.

POTTER L.T. (1970) *J. Physiol. (Lond.)* **206**, 145.

POTTER L.T. (1973). In *Drug Receptors*. Ed. Rang H.P. Macmillan, London.

POTTER L.T. and MOLINOFF P.B. (1972) In *Perspectives in Neuropharmacology*. Ed. Snyder S.H. Oxford University Press, New York.

POWELL H.D.W. (1955) *Brit. med. J.* **2**, 829.

PRANGE A.J., MEEK J.L. and LIPTON M.A. (1970) *Life Sci.* **9**, 901.

PRATT R.T.C. (1967) *The genetics of Neurological disorders*. Oxford University Press, London.

PRICHARD B.N.C. and GILLAM P.M.S. (1969) *Brit. med. J.* **1**, 7.

PRINEAS J.W., MASON A.S. and HENSON R.A. (1965) *Brit. med. J.* **1**, 1034.

PRYSE-PHILLIPS W. (1969) *Epilepsy*. Wright, Bristol.

PRZYBYLA A.C. and WANG S.C. (1968) *J. Pharmacol. exp. Ther.* **163**, 439.

PUTKONEN T., SALO O.P. and MUSTAKALLIO K.K. (1966) *Brit. J. vener. Dis.* **40**, 273.

QUINLAN C.D. and MARTIN E.A. (1970) *J. Neurol. Neurosurg. Psychiat.* **33**, 817.

RADÓ J.P. (1973) *Brit. med. J.* **3**, 479.

RALL D.P. (1971) In *Fundamentals of Drug Metabolism and Drug Disposition*. Ed. La Du B.N., Mandel, H.G. and Way E.L. Williams and Wilkins, Baltimore.

RALSTON A.J., SNAITH R.P. and HINLEY J.P. (1970) *Lancet* **1**, 867.

REES R.J.W., PEARSON J.M.H. and WATERS M.F.R. (1970) *Brit. med. J.* **1**, 89.

REESE T.S. and KARNOVSKY M.J. (1967) *J. Cell Biol.* **34**, 207.

REID J.L., CALNE D.B., GEORGE C.F. and VAKIL S.D. (1972a). *Clin. Sci.* **43**, 851.

REID J.L., CALNE D.B., VAKIL S.D., ALLEN J.G. and DAVIES C.A. (1972b) *J. neurol. Sci.* **17**, 45.

REIVICH M., JEHLE J., SOKOLOFF L. and KETY S.S. (1969) *J. appl. Physiol.* **27**, 296.

REYNOLDS E.H. (1967) *Lancet* **1**, 1086.

REYNOLDS E.H. (1970) In *Modern trends in neurology*. Ed. Williams D. Butterworths, London.

REYNOLDS E.H., ROTHFELD P. and PINCUS J.H. (1973) *Brit. med. J.* **2**, 398.

RICHARDS I.D.G. (1969) *Brit. J. prev. soc. Med.* **23**, 218.

RICHENS A. and ROWE D.J.F. (1970) *Brit. med. J.* **4**, 73.

RIDLEY A. (1969) *Quart. J. Med.* **38**, 307.

RIEDER J. and WENDT G. (1973) In *The Benzodiazepines*. Ed. Garattini S., Mussini E. and Randall L.O. Raven Press, New York.

RINNE U.K., SONNINEN V. and HYPPÄ M. (1971) *Life Sci.* **10**, 549.

RITCHIE J.M., COHEN P.J. and DRIPPS R.D. (1970) In *The pharmacological basis of therapeutics*. Ed. Goodman L.S. and Gilman A. Macmillan, London.

ROSE A.S., KUZMA J.W., KURTZKE J.F., NAMEROW N.S., SIBLEY W.A. and TOURTELLOTTE W. (1970) *Neurology (Minneap.)* **20,** (Part 2), 1.

ROSEMAN E. (1961) *Neurology (Minneap.)* **11,** 912.

ROSENBERG R.N., DALESSIO D.J., TREMBLAY J. and WOODMAN D. (1971) *Science* **173,** 644.

ROSNER F., LEE S.L., KAGEN M. and MORRISON A.N. (1970) *Lancet* **1,** 250.

ROSOMOFF H.L. and ZUGIBE F.T. (1963) *Arch. Neurol. (Chic.)* **9,** 26.

ROSS RUSSELL R.W. and HARRISON J.G. (1973) *Brit. J. Hosp. Med.* **10,** 244.

ROSSI G.F., DI ROCCO C., MAIRA G. and MEGLIO M. (1973) In *The Benzodiazepines*. Ed. Garattini S., Mussini E. and Randall L.O. Raven Press, New York.

ROWLAND L.P. (1971) *Ann. N.Y. Acad. Sci.* **183,** 351.

ROWLAND M. (1972) In *Clinical pharmacology*. Ed. Melmon K.L. and Morelli H.F. Macmillan, New York.

ROXBURGH P.A. (1970) *Brit. J. Psychiat.* **116,** 277.

RUBIN R.C., HENDERSON E.S., OMMAYA A.K., WALKER M.D. and RALL D.P. (1966) *J. Neurosurg.* **25,** 430.

RUBENSTEIN M.K. (1965) *J. nerv. ment. Dis.* **141,** 291.

RUSHWORTH G.W. (1966) *Paraplegia* **4,** 130.

SACKS O. (1970) *Migraine, the evolution of a common disorder*. Faber and Faber, London.

SANDERS W.L. and DUNN T.L. (1973) *J. Neurol. Neurosurg. Psychiat.* **36,** 581.

SANDLER M. (1972) *Lancet* **1,** 618.

SANO K., HATANAKA H. and KAMANO S. (1972) In *Steroids and brain edema*. Ed. Reulen H.J. and Schürmann K. Springer-Verlag, Berlin.

SARUBBI F.A., SPARLING P.F. and GLEZEN W.P. (1973) *Arch. Neurol. (Chic.)* **29,** 268.

SATO O. (1967) *Brain Nerve (Tokyo)* **19,** 485.

SATOYOSHI E. (1973) *Excerpta med. Int. Congr. Ser.* **296,** 38.

SCADDING J.G. (1967) *Sarcoidosis*. Eyre and Spottiswoode, London.

SCATTON B., CHERAMY A., BESSON M.J. and GLOWINSKI J. (1970) *Europ. J. Pharmacol.* **13,** 131.

SCHADÉ J.P. and FORD D.H. (1973) *Basic Neurology*. Elsevier, Amsterdam.

SCHANKER L.S. (1966) *Antimicrobial agents and chemotherapy*—1965, 1044.

SCHAPIRA K., McCLELLAND H.A., GRIFFITHS N.R. and NEWELL D.J. (1970) *Brit. med. J.* **2,** 437.

SCHLOSSER W. (1971) *Arch. int. Pharmacodyn.* **194,** 93.

SCHMIDT R.F. (1972) In *Pain*. Ed. Janzen R., Keidel W.D., Herz A., Steichele C., Payne J.P. and Burt R.A.P. Churchill, London.

SCHMIDT R.F., VOGEL M.E. and ZIMMERMAN M. (1967) *Naunyn-Schmiedebergs Arch. Pharmak. exp. Path.* **258,** 69.

SCHMIDT R.P. and WILDER B.J. (1968) *Epilepsy.* Blackwell, Oxford.

SCHNECK S.A. and PENN I. (1971) *Lancet* **1,** 983.

SCHOTT B., COTTE M.R. and REVAL M. (1960) *J. Méd., Lyon* **41,** 1037.

SCHUMACHER G.A. (1971) National Multiple Sclerosis Society, 25th Anniversary Conference, Los Angeles.

SCHWAB R.S., ENGLAND A.C., POSKANZER D.C. and YOUNG R.R. (1969) *J. Amer. med. Ass.* **208,** 1168.

SCHWARTZ M.A., KOECHLIN B.A., POSTMA E., PALMER S. and KROL G. (1965) *J. Pharmacol. exp. Ther.* **149,** 413.

SCHWARTZ M.S. and SCOTT D.F. (1971) *Lancet* **2,** 1399.

SCOTT D. (1968) *Science* **161,** 80.

SCOTT R.B. (1973) *Price's textbook of the practice of medicine.* Oxford University Press, London.

SEEMAN P. (1972) *Pharmacol. Rev.* **24,** 583.

SEYBOLD M.E. and DRACHMAN D.B. (1974) *New. Eng. J. Med.* **290,** 81.

SHABO A.S. and MAXWELL D.S. (1968a) *J. Neurosurg.* **29,** 451.

SHABO A.S. and MAXWELL D.S. (1968b) *J. Neurosurg.* **29,** 464.

SHACKELFORD P.G., BOBINSKI J.E., FEIGIN R.D. and CHERRY J.D. (1972) *New Engl. J. Med.* **287,** 634.

SHAFAR J., TALLETT E.R. and KNOWLSON P.A. (1972) *Lancet* **1,** 403.

SHAPIRO W.R. (1972) *Neurology (Minneap.)* **22,** 401.

SHAPIRO W.R., CHERNICK N.L. and POSNER J.B. (1973) *Arch. Neurol. (Chic.)* **28,** 96.

SHAW D.A. and SAUNDERS M. (1972) In *The migraine headache and Dixarit, proceedings of a symposium held at Churchill College, Cambridge.* Boehringer Ingelheim, London.

SHERWIN A.L., EISEN A.A. and SOKOLOWSKI C.D. (1973) *Arch. Neurol. (Chic.)* **29,** 73.

SHERWIN A.L. and ROBB J.P. (1972) In *Antiepileptic Drugs.* Ed. Woodbury D.M., Penry J.K. and Schmidt, R.P. Raven Press, New York.

SIBLEY W.A. (1970) In *Handbook of Clinical Neurology*, Vol. 9. Ed. Vinken P.J. and Bruyn G.W. North Holland Publishing Co, Amsterdam.

SICUTERI F., FRANCHI G. and DEL BIANCO P.L. (1967) *Int. Arch. Allergy* **31,** 78.

SICUTERI F., TESTI A. and ANSELMI B. (1961) *Int. Arch. Allergy* **19,** 55.

SIEGAL B.A., STUDER R.K. and POTCHEN E.J. (1972) *Arch. Neurol. (Chic.)* **27,** 209.

SIEGENTHALER D. and REGLI F. (1966) *Schweiz med. Wschr.* **96,** 765.

SIEGFRIED J. (1972). *Proceedings of the 4th International Symposium on Parkinson's Disease.* Huber, Bern.

SILVERSTEIN A., FEUER M.M., and SILTZBACH L.E. (1965) *Arch. Neurol. (Chic.)* **12,** 1.

SIMPSON F.O. and HODGE J.V. (1967) In *Antihypertensive agents.* Ed. Schlittler E. Academic Press, New York.

SIMPSON J.A. (1958) *Brain* **81**, 112.

SIMPSON J.A. (1960) *Scot. med. J.* **5**, 419.

SIMPSON J.A. (1969) In *Diseases of voluntary muscle*. Ed. Walton J.N., Churchill, London.

SIMPSON J.A. (1971) *Ann. N.Y. Acad. Sci.* **183**, 241.

SINCLAIR D. (1973) *Brit. J. Hosp. Med.* **9**, 568.

SINGER K. and CHENG M.N. (1971) *Brit. med. J.* **4**, 22.

SIRTORI C.R., BOLME P. and AZARNOFF D.L. (1972) *New Engl. J. Med.* **287**, 729.

SJAASTAD O. and STENSRUD P. (1971) *Acta neurol. scand.* **47**, 120.

SKINHØJ E. (1973) *Arch. Neurol. (Chic.)* **29**, 95.

SMITH A.D. (1973) *Brit. med. Bull.* **29**, 123.

SMITH C.B. and SHELDON M.I. (1972) In *Agonist and antagonist actions of narcotic analgesic drugs*. Ed. Kosterlitz H.W., Collier H.O.J. and Villareal J.E. Macmillan, London.

SMITH H.V., VOLLUM R.L., TAYLOR L.M. and TAYLOR K.B. (1956) *Tubercle* **37**, 301.

SMITH R. and STERN G. (1967) *Brain* **90**, 593.

SMITH R. and STERN G. (1968) *J. neurol. Sci.* **8**, 511.

SMITH S.E. and RAWLINS M.D. (1973) *Variability in Human Drug Response*, Butterworths, London.

SOLOMON H.M., BARAKAT M.J. and ASHLEY C.J. (1971) *J. Amer. med. Ass.* **216**, 1997.

SOURKES T.L. (1972) In *Basic Neurochemistry*. Ed. Wayne Albers R., Siegal G.J., Katzman R. and Agranoff B.W. Little, Brown, Boston.

SPEIGHT T.M. and AVERY G.S. (1972) *Drugs*, **3**, 159.

SPIEDAL B.D. and MEADOW S.R. (1972) *Lancet* **2**, 839.

SPIERS A.S.D. (1974) In *Leukaemia*. Damashek W. and Gunz F.W. 3rd edition, Grune and Stratton, New York.

SPILLANE J.D. (1963) *Brit. med. J.* **1**, 997.

SPILLANE J.D. (1965) *Proc. roy. Soc. Med.* **57**, 135.

STAMP T.C.B., ROUND J.M., ROWE D.J.F. and HADDAD J.G. (1972) *Brit. med. J.* **4**, 9.

STANBURY J.B., WYNGAARDEN J.B., and FREDRICKSON D.S. (1972) *The metabolic basis of inherited diseases*. McGraw-Hill, New York.

STRAVRAKY G.W. (1961) *Supersensitivity following lesions of the nervous system*. University of Toronto Press, Toronto.

STEG G. (1964) *Acta physiol. scand.* **61**, Suppl. 225, 1.

STEVENS H. (1966) *Arch. Neurol. (Chic.)* **14**, 415.

STEWART-WALLACE A.M. (1939) *Brain* **62**, 426.

STRATTEN W.P. and BARNES C.D. (1971) *Neuropharmacology* **10**, 685.

STRAUSS A.J.L., SEEGAL B.C., HSU K.C., BURKHOLDER P.M., NASTUK W.L. and OSSERMAN K.E. (1960) *Proc. Soc. exp. Biol. (N.Y.)* **105**, 184.

SULLIVAN J.A., HARKEN D.E. and GORLIN R. (1968) *New Engl. J. Med.* **279**, 576.

SWANK R.L. (1970) *Arch. Neurol. (Chic.)* **23**, 460.

SWASH M. (1973) *Brit. J. Hosp. Med.* **8**, 269.

SWASH M., ROBERTS A.H., ZAKKO H. and HEATHFIELD K.W.G. (1972) *J. Neurol. Neurosurg. Psychiat.* **35**, 186.

SWEET R.D., BLUMBERG J., LEE J.E. and MCDOWELL F.H. (1974) *Neurology (Minneap.)* **24**, 64.

SWEET R.D., LEE J.E. and MCDOWELL F.H. (1971) *Clin. Pharmacol. Ther.* **13**, 23.

SWEET R.D., LEE J.E., SPIEGEL H.E. and MCDOWELL F. (1972) *Neurology (Minneap.)* **22**, 520.

SWINBURN W.R. and LIVERSEDGE L.A. (1973) *J. Neurol. Neurosurg. Psychiat.* **36**, 124.

TABAQCHALI S. and PALLIS C. (1970) *Gut* **11**, 1024.

TAVERAS J.M. and WOOD E.H. (1964) *Diagnostic Neuroradiology*. Williams and Wilkins, Baltimore.

TAVERNER D. (1968) In *Handbook of Clinical Neurology*, Vol. 5. Ed. Vinken P.J. and Bruyn G.W. North Holland Publishing Co, Amsterdam.

TAVERNER D., COHEN S.B. and HUTCHINSON B.C. (1971) *Brit. med. J.* **4**, 20.

TAYLOR J.M., LEVY W.A., HERZOG I., SCHEINBERG L.C. and MCCOY G. (1965) *Neurology (Minneap.)* **15**, 667.

TAYLOR K.M. and LAVERTY R. (1973) In *The Benzodiazepines*. Ed. Garattini S., Mussini E. and Randall L.O. Raven Press, New York.

TAYLOR R.E. (1959) *Amer J. Physiol.* **196**, 1071.

THIEBAUT F. (1968) In *Handbook of Clinical Neurology*, Vol. 6. Ed. Vinken P.J. and Bruyn G.W. North Holland Publishing Co, Amsterdam.

THIERRY A.M., STINUS L., BLANC G. and GLOWINSKI J. (1973) *Brain Res.* **50**, 230.

THOMAS P.K., HOLLINRAKE K., LASCELLES R.G., O'SULLIVAN D.J., BAILLOD R.A., MOORHEAD J.F. and MACKENZIE J.C. (1971) *Brain* **94**, 761.

THOMAS P.K., LASCELLES R.G., HALLPIKE J.F. and HEWER R.L. (1969) *Brain* **92**, 589.

TOMLINSON A.H. and MACCALLUM F.O. (1970) *Ann. N.Y. Acad. Sci.* **173**, 20.

TORCHIANA M.L., LOTTI V.J. and STONE C.A. (1973) *Europ. J. Pharmacol.* **21**, 343.

TORDA D. and WOLFF H.G. (1944) *Proc. Soc. exp. Biol. Med. (N.Y.)* **57**, 137.

TOURTELLOTTE W.W. and HAERER A.F. (1965) *Arch. Neurol. (Chic.)* **12**, 536.

TOWER D.B. (1972) In *Basic neurochemistry*. Ed. Wayne Albers R., Siegal G.J., Katzman R. and Agranoff B.W. Little, Brown, Boston.

TRANZER J.P. and THOENEN H. (1968) *Experientia (Basel)* **24**, 155.

TRENDELENBURG U. (1966) *Pharmacol. Rev.* **18**, 629.

TSAIRIS P., DYCK P.J. and MULDER D.W. (1972). *Arch. Neurol. (Chic.)* **27**, 109.

TSCHIRGI R.D., FROST R.W. and TAYLOR J.L. (1954) *Proc. Soc. exp. Biol. (N.Y.)* **87**, 373.

TUGWELL P. and JAMES S.L. (1972) *Postgrad. med. J.* **48**, 667.

TUMULTY P.A. (1970) In *Harrison's principles of internal medicine*. Ed. Wintrobe M.M., Thorn G.W., Adams R.D., Bennett I.L., Braunwald E., Isselbacher K.J. and Petersdorf R.G., McGraw-Hill, New York.

TURNER P. and RICHENS A. (1973) *Clinical Pharmacology.* Livingstone, Edinburgh.
TYRER J.H., EADIE M.J., SUTHERLAND J.M. and HOOPER W.D. (1970) *Brit. med. J.* **4,** 271.

UNGERSTEDT U. (1968) *Europ. J. Pharmacol.* **5,** 107.
UNGERSTEDT U. (1971) *Acta physiol. scand.* Suppl. **367,** 1.
UNGERSTEDT U. and LJUNGBERG T. (1974). In *Dopaminergic Mechanisms.* Ed. Calne D.B., Chase T.N. and Barbeau A. Raven Press, New York.
UPTON A.R.M. (1972) *Brit. med. J.* **2,** 226.
UPTON A.R.M., BARWICK D.D. and FOSTER J.B. (1971). *Lancet* **1,** 290.
URETSKY N.J. and IVERSEN L.L. (1969). *Nature (Lond.)* **221,** 557.
URSILLO R.C. (1967) In *The neurogenic bladder.* Ed. Boyarsky S. Williams and Wilkins, Baltimore.

VAJDA F., WILLIAMS F.M., DAVIDSON S., FALCONER M.A. and BRECKENRIDGE A. (1974) *Clin. Pharmacol. Ther.* **15,** 597.
VAKIL S.D., CALNE D.B. and REID J.L. (1973) In *Progress in the treatment of Parkinsonism.* Ed. Calne D.B., Raven Press, New York.
VAN DER GELD H.W.R., FELTKAMP T.E.W. and OOSTERHUIS H.J.G.H. (1964) *Proc. Soc. exp. Biol. (N.Y.)* **115,** 782.
VAN DER KLEIJN E. (1969) *Arch. int. Pharmacodyn.* **179,** 225.
VAN HARREVELD A., CROWELL J. and MALHOTRA S.K. (1965) *J. Cell Biol.* **25,** 117.
VAN ORDEN L.S., BURKE J.P., GEYER M. and LODOEN F.V. (1970) *J. Pharmacol. exp. Ther.* **174,** 56.
VANE J.R. (1971) *Nature (Lond.)* **231,** 232.
VERENDAKIS A. and WOODBURY D.M. (1960) In *Inhibition in the nervous system and gamma aminobutyric acid.* Ed. Roberts E. Macmillan, New York.
VICTOR M. (1974) In *Peripheral Neuropathy.* Ed. Dyck P.J., Thomas P.K. and Lambert E.H. Saunders, Philadelphia.
VICTOR M., ADAMS R.D. and COLLINS G.H. (1971) *The Wernicke-Korsakoff syndrome.* Davis, Philadelphia.
VILLENEUVE A. and BÖSZÖRMÉNYI Z. (1970) *Lancet* **1,** 353.
VOGT M. (1972) In *Agonist and antagonist actions of narcotic analgesic drugs.* Ed. Kosterlitz H.W., Collier H.O.J. and Villareal J.E. Macmillan, London.
VOLZKE E., DOOSE H. and STEPHAN E. (1967) *Epilepsia (Amst.)* **8,** 64.
VON REIS G., LILJESTRAND Å. and MATELL G. (1966) *Ann. N.Y. Acad. Sci.* **135,** 409.

WADA J.A., BALZANO E., MELDRUM B.S. and NAQUET R. (1972) *Electroenceph clin. Neurophysiol.* **33,** 520.
WADDELL W.J. and BUTLER T.C. (1957) *J. clin. Invest.* **36,** 1217.
WADE O.L. (1970) *Adverse Reactions to Drugs.* Heinemann, London.

WALKER M.B. (1934) *Lancet* **1,** 1200.

WALL P.D. (1967) *Anesthesiology* **28,** 46.

WALL P.D. and SWEET W.H. (1967) *Science* **155,** 108.

WALSHE J.M. (1969) *Lancet* **2,** 1401.

WALSHE J.M. (1970) *Brit. J. Hosp. Med.* **4,** 91.

WALSHE J.M. (1973) *Quart. J. Med.* **42,** 441.

WALTON J.N. (1969) *Disorders of voluntary muscle.* Churchill, London.

WALTON J.N. and ADAMS R.D. (1958) *Polymyositis.* Livingstone, Edinburgh.

WANG J.J. and PRATT C.B. (1970) *Cancer* **25,** 531.

WARD A.A. (1970) In *L-dopa and Parkinsonism.* Ed. Barbeau A. and McDowell F.H. Davis, Philadelphia.

WARMOLTS J.R. and ENGEL W.K. (1972) *New Engl. J. Med.* **286,** 17.

WATERS W.E. (1974) *The Epidemiology of Migraine.* Boehringer Ingelheim, Bracknell.

WEBB H.E. (1969) *Brit. med. J.* **4,** 603.

WEBER R.B. and REINMUTH O.M. (1972) *Neurology (Minneap.)* **22,** 366.

WEIL-MALHERBE H. and BONE A.D. (1959) *J. Neurochem.* **4,** 251.

WEINER N. (1970) *Ann. Rev. Pharmacol.* **10,** 273.

WEINSTEIN J.D., TOY F.J., JAFFE M.E. and GOLDBERG H.I. (1973) *Neurology (Minneap.)* **23,** 121.

WEISBERG H. (1966) *Gastroenterologica* **105,** 321.

WEISS H.D., WALKER M.D. and WIERNIK P.H. (1974) *New Eng. J. Med.* **291,** 75.

WEISS J.L., NG L.K.Y., CHASE T.N. (1971) *Lancet* **1,** 1016.

WEISS P. and HISCOE H.B. (1948) *J. exp. Zool.* **107,** 315.

WELCH K. and FRIEDMAN V. (1960) *Brain.* **83,** 454.

WHISNANT J.P., MATSUMOTO N. and ELVEBACK L.R. (1973) *Mayo Clin. Proc.* **48,** 194.

WHISNANT J.P., MATSUMOTO N. and ELVEBACK L.R. (1973) *Mayo Clin. Proc.* **48,** 844.

WHITTAKER V.P. (1973) In *The scientific basis of medicine annual reviews 1973.* Ed. Gilliland I. and Peden M. Athlone, London.

WHITTY C.W.M., LISHMAN W.A. and FITZGIBBON J.P. (1964) *Lancet* **1,** 1403.

WILDER B.J., STREIFF R.R. and HAMMER R.H. (1972) In *Antiepileptic Drugs,* Ed. Woodbury D.M., Penry J.K. and Schmidt R.P. Raven Press, New York.

WILLIAMS T.F., WINTERS R.W. and BURNETT C.H. (1966) In *The metabolic basis of inherited disease.* Ed. Stanbury J.B., Wyngaarden J.B. and Fredrickson D.S. McGraw-Hill, New York.

WILLIS W.D. and GROSSMAN R.G. (1973) *Medical Neurobiology.* Mosby, St. Louis.

WILSON L.A. and McKECHNIE A.A. (1966) *Scot. med. J.* **11,** 46.

WILSON S.A.K. (1955) *Neurology.* Butterworths, London.

WINK C.A.S. (1972) *Tegretol in Epilepsy.* Nicholls, Manchester.

WINKLER G.F. and YOUNG R.R. (1971) *Trans. Amer. neurol. Ass.* **96,** 66.

WITHROW C.D. and WOODBURY D.M. (1972) In *Antiepileptic drugs.* Ed. Woodbury D.M., Penry J.K. and Schmidt R.P. Raven Press, New York.

WOLF A. (1936) *Arch. Neurol. Psychiat.* **36,** 382.

WOLF S.M. and DAVIS R.L. (1973) *Arch. Neurol. (Chic.)* **29,** 276.

WOLFF H.G. (1963) *Headache and other head pain.* Oxford University Press, New York.

WOOD L. (1972) *Lancet* **2,** 532.

WOODBURNE R.T. (1961) *Anat. Rec.* **141,** 11.

WOODBURY D.M. (1969) *Epilepsia (Amst.)* **10,** 121.

WOODBURY D.M. and KEMP J.W. (1971) *Psychiat. Neurol. Neurochir.* **74,** 91.

WOODBURY D.M., PENRY J.K. and SCHMIDT R.P. (1972) *Antiepileptic drugs.* Raven Press, New York.

WOODBURY D.M. and SWINYARD E.A. (1972) In *Antiepileptic Drugs.* Ed. Woodbury D.M., Penry J.K. and Schmidt R.P. Raven Press, New York.

WOODRUFF A.W. and DICKINSON C.J. (1968) *Brit. med. J.* **3,** 31.

WURTMAN R.J. (1974) In *Frontiers in catecholamine research.* Ed. Usdin E. and Snyder F. Pergamon, New York.

WURTMAN R.J., CHOW C. and ROSE C.M. (1970) *J. Pharmacol. exp. Ther.* **174,** 351.

YAHR M.D. (1973) *Treatment of Parkinsonism: the role of dopa decarboxylase inhibitors.* Raven Press, New York.

YAHR M.D. (1974). In *Second Canadian–American Conference on Parkinson's Disease.* Ed. McDowell F.H. and Barbeau A. Raven Press, New York.

YAHR M.D. and DUVOISIN R.C. (1968) In *Handbook of Clinical Neurology,* Vol. 6. Ed. Vinken P.J. and Bruyn G.W. North Holland Publishing Co, Amsterdam.

YAHR M.D. and DUVOISIN R.C. (1972) *New Engl. J. Med.* **287,** 20.

YAHR M.D., DUVOISIN R.C., HOEHN M.M., SCHEAR M.J. and BARRETT R.E. (1968) *Trans. Amer. neurol. Ass.* **93,** 56.

YEATES W.K. (1973) In *Bladder control and enuresis.* Ed. Kolvin I., MacKeith R.C. and Meadow S.R. Heinemann, London.

YOSHIDA A. and MOTULSKY A.G. (1969) *Amer. J. hum. Genet.* **21,** 486.

YOUNG D.S., FORRESTER T.M. and MORGAN T.N. (1959) *Lancet* **2,** 765.

YOUNT W.J., UTSINGER P.D., PURITZ E.M. and ORTBALS D.W. (1973) *Med. Clin. N. Amer.* **57,** 1343.

ZACKS S.I. and SHEFF M.F. (1966) *J. Neuropath. exp. Neurol.* **25,** 422.

ZAIMIS E. (1973) *Lancet* **1,** 403.

ZBINDEN G. and RANDALL L.O. (1967) *Advanc. Pharmacol.* **5,** 213.

ZIEGLER D.K. (1972) In *Handbook of Clinical Neurology,* Vol. 11. Ed. Vinken P.J. and Bruyn G.W. North Holland Publishing Co, Amsterdam.

ZUCKER M.B. (1973) In *Cerebral Vascular Diseases.* Ed. McDowell F.H. and Brennan R.W. Grune and Stratton, New York.

INDEX